Calcium Antagonism in Heart and Smooth Muscle

CALCIUM ANTAGONISM IN HEART AND SMOOTH MUSCLE

Experimental Facts and Therapeutic Prospects

ALBRECHT FLECKENSTEIN, M.D.
Professor of Physiology
University of Freiburg
Federal Republic of Germany

A Wiley-Interscience Publication

JOHN WILEY & SONS,
New York   Chichester   Brisbane   Toronto   Singapore

Copyright © 1983 by John Wiley & Sons, Inc.

Library of Congress Cataloging in Publication Data

Fleckenstein, Albrecht.
  Calcium antagonism in heart and smooth muscle.

  "A Wiley-Interscience publication."
  Bibliography: p.
  Includes index.
  1. Calcium—Antagonists—Testing. 2. Cardiovascular
system—Diseases—Chemotherapy. 3. Calcium—Metabolism.
I. Title.

RC684.C34F56   1983   616.1'2061   82-15990
ISBN 0-471-05435-6

Printed in the United States of America

10 9 8 7 6 5 4

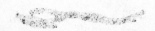

To my wife and research associate,
Professor Gisa Fleckenstein-Grün, M.D.

Preface

"Ions were the powerful tools which life found in the ocean where it originated." This keen statement was made by Albert Szent-Györgyi more than 30 years ago with particular respect to the basic functions of ions in skeletal and heart muscle. The intention was to focus the interest of biologists on the principal involvement of marine ions such as Na, K, Ca, and Mg in a wide variety of vital reactions that are, directly or indirectly, connected with muscular excitation and the production of contractile energy.

Nowadays, it seems remarkable that, within three decades following Dr. Szent-Györgyi's statement, there probably has been more progress in this particular field of research than ever before. Thus the downhill movements of monovalent Na and K ions through the stimulated sarcolemma membrane were proved to be the underlying molecular process of electric membrane excitation, whereas the influx of divalent Ca ions was shown to activate the contractile machinery. Thus the drugs that influence Na conductance alter myocardial excitability. On the other hand, substances acting on the transmembrane Ca channels produce changes in contractile force.

Our studies on sarcolemma membrane biophysics of intact myocardial fibers and smooth muscle cells led 15 years ago to the discovery of a new family of powerful drugs, the Ca antagonists, which can selectively inhibit transmembrane Ca supply so that in the ventricular myocardium, exaggerated tension development and oxygen demand is lowered. Similarly, even minute amounts of Ca antagonists reduce contractile tone of vascular smooth muscle and prevent spastic vasoconstriction, particularly in the extramural section of the coronary bed and on the cerebral arteries.

This monograph offers first of all a systematic treatise about Ca antagonism as a new pharmacodynamic principle with particular reference to its multifaceted manifestations in myocardium, cardiac pacemakers, and vascular smooth muscle. Second, it gives a survey of the powerful organic Ca antagonists that embody this principle as a common basis of their cardiovascular actions. The book deals with both basic research and practical implications. Using the Ca antagonists as tools for physiological investigations, new light has been shed on the fundamental role of Ca ions in myocardial tension development, sinus-node automaticity, atrioventricular impulse conduction, and regulation of coronary and systemic vascular tone. Needless to say, these results have decisively contributed to the rapid progress in current cardiovascular therapy. Thus the Ca antagonists have become the drugs of choice against all types of vasospasm, especially those occurring in the great extramural coronary stem arteries (Prinzmetal's variant angina, angina at rest, and "crescendo angina" with imminent infarction) and against acute hypertensive crises due to an excessive rise in systemic vascular resistance. Moreover, our pathophysiological studies have revealed that most Ca antagonists also exert strong cardioprotective actions in preventing deleterious myocardial Ca overload, which has to be considered the primary etiological factor in the production of cardiac necroses following sympathetic overstimulation, hypercalcemia, and K or Mg deficiency. An abundant uptake of Ca ions has also been found to occur in the myocardium of cardiomyopathic hamsters as early as in the prenecrotic phase of this hereditary disease. Accordingly, a suitable long-term treatment with Ca antagonists provided cardioprotection, not only in cardiomyopathic hamsters, but also in humans suffering from obstructive hypertrophic cardiomyopathy. As recently shown by several authors, intracellular Ca overload seems to be involved even in the course of myocardial-fiber disintegration following anoxia or ischemia. Here again, under certain conditions, functional and structural damage could be minimized with the help of Ca antagonists, even in hypoxic human myocardium during open-heart surgery. A similar prophylactic effect of Ca antagonists has been demonstrated by us in the case of vascular calcinosis of rats due to high doses of vitamin D or dihydrotachysterol, or developing in alloxan-diabetic animals. Interestingly enough, the destruction of vascular smooth muscle produced by these experimental procedures in the arterial media resembles the special form of calcific human arteriosclerosis described by Mönckeberg. With this well-elaborated experimental background and many promising clinical trials, the wide spectrum of beneficial effects of Ca antagonists in coronary heart disease, hyperkinetic disorders, cardiac dysrhythmias, cardiomyopathy, acute myocardial ischemia and anoxia, vascular spasm, hypertension, and, possibly, in certain types of human arterial calcinosis, deserves attentive interest. It is the aim of this book to meet the scientific and the clinical requirements.

The book provides a synopsis of the relevant data on the interactions of Ca with subcellular cardiac fiber constituents. It stresses the crucial role of Ca in the complex system of contractile and regulatory proteins and depicts the control of the cytoplasmic Ca concentration by the sarcoplasmic reticulum and the mitochondria. However, the main accent is on the fascinating recent advances concerning the specific regulatory mechanisms that quantitatively control the transmembrane Ca and Mg supply to the active myocardium and the smooth muscle cells. Thus the book not only aims at cardiologists, but also addresses physiologists, pharmacologists, pathologists, and biochemists interested in the basic biological problems of Ca metabolism in contractile tissues.

ALBRECHT FLECKENSTEIN

Freiburg, West Germany
October 1982

Acknowledgments

The author wishes to thank all those, mostly post-doctoral research fellows, who shared with him the investigatory efforts. The participation of these colleagues in the entire research work on Ca antagonism was of utmost importance as documented best by the host of references in the book. In fact, the individual merits of these associates appear more clearly from the cited publications connected with their names than from any laudatory remarks.

As noted in the figure legends, many of the 202 illustrations in this book originate from previously published work of our laboratory. The author gratefully acknowledges the permission of other publishing companies to reproduce this copyrighted material here. By their courtesy, the following institutions have contributed to this book (the individual numbers of the figures released for reproduction from the different sources are given in parentheses):

1. American Physiological Society, Bethesda, Maryland (13,51,52).
2. Academic Press, London (34,44,46,48,55,56,63,150,169,182A).
3. Editio Cantor, Aulendorf, Germany (Federal Republic) (28,142,152,159, 161,173,174,175).
4. Boehringer, Mannheim, Germany (Federal Republic) (109).
5. Elsevier/North Holland Biomedical Press, Amsterdam (143,144,145, 146,155,156A,157,158,160,164).
6. Excerpta Medica, Amsterdam (27,106,114,116,121,131,196).
7. Pergamon Press, Oxford, England (45,46,47,49).
8. Perimed Verlag, Erlangen, Germany (Federal Republic) (194).
9. Laboratoire de Pharmacologie, Faculté de Médecine, (Prof. R.I. Royer), Nancy, France (88,89).
10. Springer-Verlag, Heidelberg, Germany (Federal Republic) (1–10,14–18, 20–25, 28–33, 35–40, 50, 62–64, 66–69, 72–76, 79, 86, 96, 98, 101, 113, 115,117–120,123–125,137–141,151,170–172,184,186,199–202).
11. Schattauer Verlag, Stuttgart, Germany (Federal Republic) (70,71).

ACKNOWLEDGMENTS

12. Dr. Dietrich Steinkopff Verlag, Darmstadt, Germany (Federal Republic) (122).

13. Thieme Verlag, Stuttgart, Germany (Federal Republic) (87,147,153, 156*B*,162,163).

14. Urban and Schwarzenberg, München, Germany (Federal Republic) (77,91,93,94,95,97,105,109*A*,109*B*,154).

A.F.

Contents

CONTENTS

Introduction

When a muscle responds to a stimulus, a chain reaction of electric, mechanical, and chemical processes is initiated in each excited fiber. Whatever the nature of the stimulus may be, the first event usually consists of a change in the transmembrane electric field at the surface, while, as subsequent phenomena, a rapid rise of tension and many biochemical reactions preceding or following the mechanical activity are observed. The electric responses may be local, in the form of graded depolarizations leading to contractures, or propagated, in the form of action potentials followed by ordinary contractions. But in any case, an inward wave of activation has to be postulated that connects the primary excitation events of the membrane to the mechanical processes in the contractile elements and to the metabolic reactions occurring in the interior of the fibers. Thirty years ago, in a very detailed study, Alexander Sandow (1952) called attention to the possibility that Ca ions might play a key role in this mysterious mechanism of excitation–contraction coupling. He proposed, as a working hypothesis, that an action potential or membrane depolarization of the muscle-fiber surface promotes the entrance of Ca into the myoplasm, and this in turn initiates further reactions leading to the appearance of mechanical activity. Since that time evidence has accumulated rapidly in favor of Sandow's concept. Thus, in a wide variety of excitable cells, the transmembrane exchange of the monovalent cations Na^+ and K^+ can be considered the substantial basis of bioelectric membrane activity, whereas Ca ions are required as mediators when, by this superficial process, intracellular reactions such as muscular contractions are initiated. In fact, Ca is the only physiological ion that when injected at a low concentration into muscle fibers causes shortening (Heilbrunn and Wiercinski, 1947; Niedergerke, 1955; Caldwell and Walster, 1963).

Naturally, Ca ions can exert this messenger function either in a primitive way, by penetrating into the intracellular space across the depolarized cell membrane or, at a more advanced stage of evolution, by being released from intracellularly located endoplasmic stores. Hence certain differences between skeletal, cardiac, and smooth muscle arise because the development of large endoplasmic Ca pools is most prominent in skeletal muscle, whereas myocardial fibers and particularly smooth muscle cells are less specialized in this respect. Because of these peculiarities, excita-

1

tion–contraction coupling of mammalian skeletal muscle does not promptly respond to extracellular Ca withdrawal; intracellular stores still provide sufficient quantities of Ca to guarantee contractile activation even if the Ca supply from outside is reduced. Nevertheless, contractile tension development of skeletal muscle is not totally insensitive to changes in extracellular Ca concentration. Thus, using the frog rectus abdominis muscle, we found that in the absence of free Ca ions, depolarization with high concentrations of K or acetylcholine can no longer produce a sustained contracture. This loss of contractility became particularly obvious after addition of small amounts of Na oxalate or EDTA that chelate Ca. Conversely, supernormal Ca concentrations increase height and duration of the contractile responses. Furthermore, in 1959, Bianchi and Shanes showed that repetitive contractions of frog skeletal muscle were accompanied by a progressive uptake of labeled extracellular Ca.

But in general, myocardial and smooth muscle contractility is much more susceptible to variations in environmental Ca than is tension development of skeletal muscle because the intracellular Ca stores of cardiac tissue and particularly smooth muscle fibers are of rather limited capacity. Thus the degree of contractile activation of these cells is most clearly linked with the availability of Ca from extracellular sources or even appears as a direct function of the quantity of Ca that enters the cell during excitation. Hence contractile energy expenditure of heart muscle can be controlled quantitatively by means of physiological or pharmacological agents that influence transmembrane Ca conductivity. For instance β-receptor-stimulating catecholamines such as epinephrine, norepinephrine, or isoproterenol selectively increase the inward Ca current across the excited myocardial sarcolemma membrane, thus augmenting contractile force. Opposite effects are exerted by the Ca antagonists, to which this book is devoted. These drugs restrict myocardial contractility in parallel with a dose-related reduction of transmembrane Ca influx.

In fact, the new pharmacological family of Ca antagonists comprises the most powerful and specific inhibitors of Ca-dependent excitation–contraction coupling yet discovered. By this basic mechanism, the Ca antagonists damp hyperkinetic hearts and simultaneously act as "musculotropic" relaxants, particularly on vascular smooth muscle, thus exerting vasodilator and spasmolytic effects in coronary and systemic circulation. Moreover, they exhibit broncholytic and tocolytic activities. Nevertheless, myocardium and vascular smooth muscle are certainly the preferential targets of these new drugs. Here the Ca antagonists interfere with excitation–contraction coupling as specifically as curare, for instance, interrupts neuromuscular transmission. Furthermore they affect Ca-dependent automatic impulse discharge from nomotopic and ectopic cardiac pacemaker cells. It is particularly for these reasons that the present monograph concentrates nearly exclusively on the prominent cardiovascular actions of these drugs.

As to the use of Ca antagonists for purely scientific purposes, these drugs are also capable of blocking the Ca influx through excited glandular cell membranes. Although Ca-dependent excitation–secretion coupling is beyond the scope of this book, it is noteworthy that in experiments on isolated tissue samples or perfused glands, suitably high concentrations of certain Ca antagonists (verapamil, D 600) inhibit the release of oxytocin and vasopressin from the depolarized neurohypophysis (Dreifuss, Grau, and Nordmann, 1975; Russell and Thorn, 1974) or the release of insulin from excited B cells in the islets of Langerhans (Devis, Somers, Van Obberghen, and Malaisse, 1975; Matthews and Sakamoto, 1975). Extra calcium easily restores the secretory function even in the presence of the inhibitors. Vera-pamil also interferes with pituitary Ca uptake following *in vitro* depolarizations and thereby suppresses secretion of ACTH and of gonadotropic and thyroid stimulating hormones (Eto, Wood, Hutchins, and Fleischer, 1974). Nevertheless, the drug concentrations required to block excitation–secretion coupling of endocrine glands or to suppress Ca-dependent transmitter release from sympathetic fibers *in vitro* (Haeusler, 1972) are much higher than those that exert cardiovascular actions *in vivo*. Therefore, the influence of Ca antagonists on glandular secretion is more of academic than practical interest.

The Ca antagonists are not uniform in every respect because they exhibit some differences (1) in their relative potencies on myocardium, cardiac pacemakers, or vessels and (2) in the degree of Ca-antagonistic specificity in relation to additional influences on transmembrane Na and Mg conductivity. Nevertheless, the organic Ca antagonists represent a distinct pharmacological family that according to our present knowledge should be subdivided into only two groups:

1. *Group A.* Substances of outstanding Ca-antagonistic potency and speci-ficity such as nifedipine (together with its derivatives niludipine and ni-modipine), verapamil, D 600, and diltiazem.
2. *Group B.* Substances such as prenylamine, fendiline, terodiline, perhex-iline, and caroverine that also possess prominent Ca-antagonistic properties but do not reach the outstanding degree of specificity of group A.

Thus for the sake of a clear-cut terminology, the name *Ca antagonist* is reserved in this book for the substances of group A and group B that are not only of remarkable strength but also qualified for therapeutic purposes in human medicine. However, in addition to the subdivision of the "true" Ca antagonists into class A and class B, it seems feasible to constitute a further group C that comprises substances with *unspecific* Ca-antagonistic side effects. There is indeed a considerable number of agents such as certain β-blockers (as for instance propranolol), barbituric acid, or hydantoine derivatives, as well as local anesthetic, antiarrhythmic, or antifibrillatory drugs that exert Ca antagonism in a secondary way. In most of these cases, Ca antagonism only manifests itself in the form of cardiodepression or arterial hypo-tension if excessive doses are administered. Such Ca-antagonistic side effects may be particularly interesting for pharmacological or toxicological reasons. However, the designation of a substance as a Ca antagonist is justified only if this quality distinctly prevails. The same reservation must also be made with respect to a number of inorganic agents such as La, Co, Ni, and Mn salts that are frequently used on isolated myocardium, pacemaker tissues, or vascular smooth muscle to interfere with transmembrane Ca movements. These agents have to be considered useful tools for basic research on a cellular level. However, if administered to the whole animal, they exhibit a host of accessory toxic effects, so any therapeutic use is precluded. Obviously these metal salts too do not exert Ca antagonism in a sufficiently specific and innocuous form. In consequence, they should not be called by the name *Ca antagonists*.

There has also been some other terminological confusion in recent years in that besides the original term *Ca antagonist* introduced by us in the years 1967 to 1969, certain synonyms were proposed such as "slow-channel blocker," "calcium-channel blocker," "calcium-entry blocker," "calcium blocker," and so forth. All these alternative terms refer to the fact, established in our laboratory in the years 1970 to 1972, that the fundamental action of these drugs consists of a dose-related selective inhibition of the transsarcolemmal inward Ca current through the so-called "slow channels." In a strictly scientific sense, these synonyms may be acceptable, but from a medical point of view, they are misleading, since a real blockade of the Ca channels is incompatible with life. One can certainly abolish the cardiac actions of β-adrenergic catecholamines, histamine, or acetylcholine by an adequate receptor blockade without lethal consequences. However, a blockade of the Ca channels would suppress vital functions such as sinoatrial or atrioventricular node automaticity, atrioventricular conduction, and generation of systolic force, as well as active tension in the vascular walls. Hence a true Ca-channel blockade would lead to cardiac pacemaker arrest, myocardial contractile failure, and vascular paralysis. In our opinion, it would be irrational to designate a new family of therapeutically useful drugs by names that allude to the extreme case of a Ca-channel blockade that is only producible *in vitro* with huge overdoses but can never occur in a living animal. In reality, the medical use of Ca antagonists aims at *normalization* of transmembrane Ca influx in case the latter has reached, under pathological conditions, an excessive intensity. This applies to hyperkinetic heart dysfunction, ectopic pacemaker activity, myocardial Ca overload (leading to necrotization), vascular spasms, hypertension, arterial smooth muscle calcinosis, and so forth. Needless to say, in the treatment of these Ca-dependent cardiovascular disorders, Ca-channel blockade has to be strictly *avoided*. Thus there is no reason for abandoning the term *Ca antagonist*, which undoubtedly covers the therapeutic actions of these drugs more accurately than any of the alternative terms.

CHAPTER ONE

The Fundamental Role of Calcium in Myocardial High-Energy-Phosphate Metabolism and Contraction

It is generally assumed that the mechanical activity of heart muscle, like that of other contractile tissues, is closely linked to the metabolism of high-energy phosphates, especially adenosine triphosphate (ATP) and creatine phosphate (CP). The splitting of ATP by the Ca-activated myofibrillar ATPase is believed to be the primary source of contraction energy, ATP being instantaneously restored at the expense of CP. Subsequently, ATP and CP are resynthesized by a long chain of rapid recovery reactions that conserve, in the form of high-energy phosphate bonds, the free energy available from the aerobic and anaerobic substrate breakdown. Even if this principle of contractile energy production is formulated, as above, in the simplest possible way, two fundamental prerequisites are apparent:

1. An adequate supply of ATP, in heart muscle particularly by means of oxidative phosphorylation.
2. Enough free Ca ions so that ATP can be readily utilized by the contractile system.

Hence two alternative types of contractile cardiac failure exist that result either from high-energy-phosphate exhaustion or Ca deficiency (Fleckenstein, 1964a, 1967, 1968a,b,c; Fleckenstein, Döring, and Kammermeier, 1966/1967).

1.1. CONTRACTILE DISORDERS DUE TO CARDIAC HIGH-ENERGY-PHOSPHATE PENURY

Many authors have shown that the characteristic loss of cardiac contractility during anoxia or ischemia is intimately correlated with a steep fall in the myocardial CP and ATP contents (Fawaz, Hawa, and Tutunji, 1957; Fleckenstein, Janke, and

Gerlach, 1959; Thorn, Heimann, Müldener, Isselhard, and Gercken, 1959; Szekeres and Schein, 1959, Isselhard, 1960; Lamprecht, Michal, and Nägle, 1961; Döring and Kammermeier, 1961; Benson, Evans, Hallaway, Phibbs, and Freier, 1961; Feinstein, 1962; Nägle, Hockerts, and Bögelmann, 1964). For instance, in our experiments on thoracotomized guinea pigs, rats, and cats, the CP concentration was reduced in the myocardium of the left ventricle by about 80 to 90% after artificial respiration had been stopped for 1 min under normothermic conditions. The ATP concentration decreases more slowly, so that only about $1/3$ of the normal ATP of the myocardium was lost within 3 min. The inorganic phosphate concentration changes in the opposite direction. Practically identical results were obtained in the ischemic myocardial tissue of cats after coronary occlusion or if pure nitrogen was administered by a respiration pump. The acute CP and ATP breakdown in the apical region of two cat hearts within 1 and 2 min, respectively, after ligature of both coronary arteries is shown in Figure 1. Although the myocardial CP is always more rapidly exhausted than the ATP fraction, the degradation of the ATP fraction also becomes nearly complete when the duration of asphyxia or ischemia is extended to 10 or 15 min (Figure 2). But if, on the other hand, air respiration is resumed with a delay of no longer than 3 to 4 min, the recovery of CP is nearly as quick as its breakdown. The restoration of the ATP concentration is usually somewhat retarded.

The concomitant alterations of cardiac contractility consist not only of a reduction in systolic force but also of an acute increase in the diastolic volume of both ventricles. This dilation is partly due to the reduction of systolic output. But apart

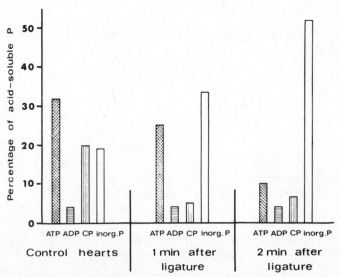

FIGURE 1. Breakdown of myocardial creatine phosphate (CP) and ATP within 1 and 2 min, respectively, following the ligature of both coronary arteries. Analytical data obtained from the apical region of the left ventricular myocardium of two cats. From Fleckenstein, Janke, and Gerlach (1959).

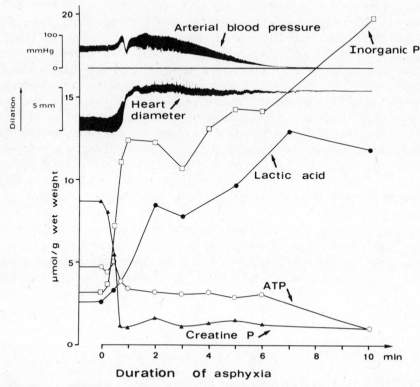

FIGURE 2. Concentration changes of the most prominent acid-soluble-phosphate fractions of the guinea pig myocardium during the course of prolonged asphyxia. The rise in lactic acid concentration roughly parallels that of inorganic phosphate. Acute ventricular dilation occurs within 60 sec simultaneously with CP breakdown. Complete loss of systolic contractility and drop of arterial blood pressure to zero takes place within 6 min. From Fleckenstein, Döring, Janke, and Byon (1975).

from this, the deficiency of high-energy phosphates clearly affects the diastolic tonus. The acute dilation of anoxic or asphyctic hearts has been described by many authors (Mathison, 1910; Fühner and Starling, 1913; Zondek, 1919; Gremels and Starling, 1926; Jarisch and Wastl, 1926; Barcroft, 1927; Takeuchi, 1925; Loewy and Mayer, 1926; Strughold, 1930; Rushmer, 1961; Büchner and Iijima, 1961). According to Takeuchi's results and our own observations, the maximum ventricular expansion is reached when the oxygen saturation of the blood falls to almost zero. Opitz and Schneider (1950) reported dilation at a venous pO_2 of 12 mm Hg. As to the critical oxygen saturation of the arterial blood at which contractile failure develops, the figures differ more widely: 50% according to Jarisch and Wastl (1926) and Allela (1958); 40% according to Gremels and Starling (1926); 30% according to Bretschneider (1958); and 10 to 20% according to Gorlin and Lewis (1954) and Mercker (1943). Probably with regard to these widely scattered data, no serious attempt has been made by these authors to correlate the development of cardiac incompetence with definite alterations in myocardial metabolism. However, in focusing on the high-energy phosphates, it clearly turned out that there is a surprisingly close interrelationship between the myocardial CP content and diastolic ventricular volume (Fleckenstein, 1960; Döring and Kammermeier, 1963; Fleckenstein, 1964a). Figure 3 shows the striking correlation between the mechanical behavior of a beating guinea pig heart *in situ* and the changes in the high-energy-phosphate content of the myocardium both in the state of asphyxia and thereafter during postasphyctic recovery. As indicated by the steep upward deflection of the upper curve, the acute dilation of the ventricles reaches its maximum within 60 sec together with the breakdown of the CP fraction. This rapid loss of diastolic tone clearly precedes the loss of systolic contractility, because in the case of prolonged anoxia or asphyxia, the asystolic arrest of the hearts occurs only after a delay of at least 6 min (Figure 2). If, on the other hand, anoxia or asphyxia is limited to 3 to 4 min, both contractility and heart diameter return to normal as soon as the CP supply is restored after resuming respiration.

Anoxic ventricular dilation is most obvious in hearts with the pericardium removed. Such ventricles are often so greatly expanded that within 1 min of anoxia, the tricuspid valve becomes insufficient. If, however, in our experiments on guinea pigs the degree of dilation was restricted by the surrounding intact pericardium,

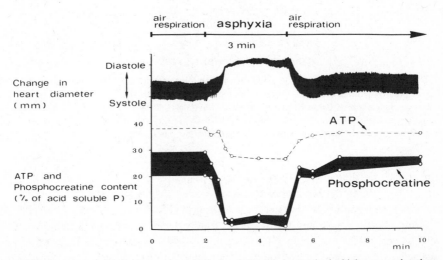

FIGURE 3.　Time correlation between mechanical activity and changes in the high-energy-phosphate content of the guinea pig myocardium in a state of asphyxia and thereafter during postasphyctic recovery. Obviously the acute ventricular dilation and the reduction in contraction amplitude during the first minute of asphyxia coincide completely with the drop in CP. Accordingly, contractility and heart diameter return to normal as soon as the CP supply is restored after resuming respiration. The concentrations of CP, ATP, and inorganic phosphate were analyzed in 32 asphyctic or postasphyctic left ventricles (open-chest preparations). The values are expressed as percentage of the total acid-soluble phosphorous of the blood-free cardiac tissue. The absolute control values obtained on 32 nonasphyxiated hearts were as follows: ATP, 4.6 ($\pm$ 0.1); CP, 8.3 ($\pm$ 0.25); inorganic phosphate, 3.2 ($\pm$ 0.1) μmol/g. All values shown are means $\pm$ SE of the mean. From Fleckenstein, (1960) and Fleckenstein, Döring, and Kammermeier (1966/1967).

not more than about 60% of the maximum heart diameter could be measured in full anoxia. Under these circumstances anoxic valvular dysfunction was less frequent. Additional observations were also made on a considerable number of heart–lung preparations with constant heart rates and stabilized arterial and venous blood pressures. The principal result was essentially the same as with hearts *in situ:* Anoxic ventricular dilation depends neither on a reduction of cardiac frequency nor on changes in blood pressure but merely on a decrease in contractile diastolic tone caused by high-energy-phosphate deficiency. In the case of local anoxia, the loss of tone may even be confined to only part of the ventricular wall. This results in local ventricular bulging, a well-known phenomenon that can be experimentally produced by ligature of a coronary branch (see Kerber and Abboud, 1975) or clinically observed in infarcted hearts. The recent introduction of two-dimensional echocardiography has made the recognition of this special type of regional cardiac dilation easier (Eaton, Weiss, Bulkley, Garrison, and Weisfeldt, 1979). Obviously the myocardium is dilated as long as the CP concentration is at an insufficient level. Further observations have shown that an acute ventricular dilation can also be brought about by other factors that exhaust the CP store, for example, carbon monoxide inhalation or metabolic inhibitors (NaCN, fluoroacetate, 2,4-dinitrophenol). Figure 4 represents experiments in which after treatment with these poisons, the hearts were frozen for chemical analysis just at the peak of ventricular dilation (Döring, Kammermeier, and Byon, 1962). The data demonstrate that again in all these cases the breakdown of CP was most closely related to the increase in heart diameter.

In contrast to CP concentration, the ATP concentration seems to be less critical. Thus during postasphyctic recovery of animal hearts after prolonged periods of

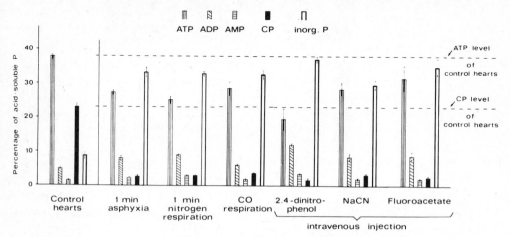

FIGURE 4. Exhaustion of CP and decrease in ATP at the peak of ventricular dilation produced by asphyxia, respiration of pure nitrogen, respiration of air with 4% (vol) CO, or IV injection of 30 mg/kg 2,4-dinitrophenol, 9 mg/kg NaCN, 25 mg/kg fluoroacetate. Values shown are means ± SE of the mean. From Döring, Kammermeier, and Byon (1962).

standstill, we were able to show that complete restoration of the strength of contraction requires a full CP supply, whereas ATP concentration may remain considerably below normal. Nevertheless, this ATP reduction can become a limiting factor in reviving the anoxic hearts if more than 50 to 60% of the original ATP has definitely disappeared (Kammermeier, 1964). The adenosine nucleotides of the normal and asphyctic myocardium can easily be visualized in 260-nm light after separation on paper. As can be seen from Figure 5, a large amount of ATP is broken down during prolonged asphyxia, since the large spot that represents ATP in the chromatogram of the control heart is reduced to $^1/_5$ of the normal size after an oxygen lack of 15 min at 37°C. This breakdown goes beyond adenosine diphosphate (ADP) and adenosine monophosphate (AMP). As shown in our laboratory by Gerlach, Deuticke, and Dreisbach (1963), the progressive degradation of ATP in anoxic hearts rapidly leads to the formation of adenosine, inosine, hypoxanthine,

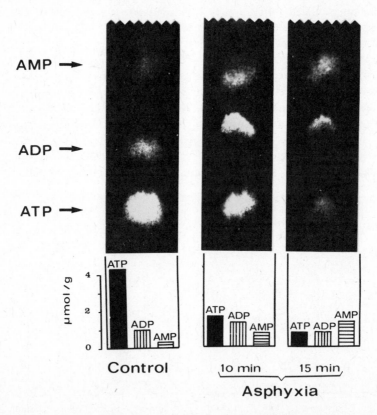

FIGURE 5. Progressive breakdown of myocardial ATP produced by asphyxia of a duration of 15 min. After separation on paper, the UV-absorbing nucleotides ATP, ADP, and AMP were visualized by the photoprint technique of Markham and Smith (Biochem. J. *45*, 294, 1949) at a wavelength of 260 nm. Obviously, the big UV-absorbing spot, which represents ATP, in the control chromatogram decreases more and more in the chromatograms of asphyctic hearts. In addition, the total amount of adenosine nucleotides diminishes because of further degradation. From Fleckenstein (1963b).

and xanthine (Table 1). But apart from ADP and AMP, only adenosine is suitable for rapid ATP resynthesis in the postasphyctic recovery period, whereas the formation of inosine, hypoxanthine, or xanthine signifies a practically irreversible ATP loss. The minimum amount of ATP that has to be resynthesized from residual ADP, AMP, and adenosine when myocardial contractility should reappear is approximately 40% of the original ATP content. Therefore, the possibility of reanimation of an anoxic or ischemic heart becomes progressively worse as the degradation of the nucleotides proceeds. A similar anoxic breakdown has also been found for the guanine nucleotides, again leading to the appearance of xanthine, and for the uridine nucleotides, which are eventually degraded to uracil (Gerlach, Deuticke, and Dreisbach, 1963).

In summarizing our observations, we stress that the contractile failure in cases of asphyxia, anoxia, or ischemia after ligature of the coronary arteries, or under the influence of inhibitors of glycolysis, respiration, or phosphorylation clearly has a biochemical basis. In fact any interruption of the high-energy-phosphate supply, as indicated by an exhaustion of CP, leads to almost immediate disorders of cardiac contractility. Interestingly enough, phosphate-bond energy is utilized by the contractile system not only to cover the expenses of systolic work but also to maintain cardiac diastolic tone. The correlation between changes in diastolic tone and myocardial CP content is particularly evident. The changes in ATP content, on the other hand, do not exhibit such an obvious connection with the mechanical events. But this can be explained by:

1. The fact that ATP, being the immediate energy source for contraction, is instantaneously restored at the expense of CP.
2. The assumption that only a minor fraction of ATP, probably amounting to about $1/5$ to $1/4$ of the total ATP content of the myocardium, is directly concerned with contraction and consequently equilibrates with CP.

TABLE 1.   Pathways of Myocardial Nucleotide Degradation in Asphyxia[a]

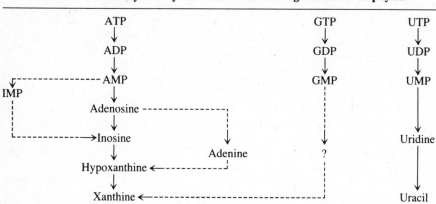

[a]Gerlach, Deuticke, and Dreisbach (1963).

Apart from the contractile function, structural integrity cannot be maintained when the high-energy-phosphate pools are empty. Therefore, all factors that interfere with the high-energy-phosphate supply finally produce cellular destruction and rigor that manifest in isolated myocardium as a progressive irreversible rise in basal tone. The involvement of high-energy phosphates in myocardial cell regeneration and in the maintenance of structural integrity is discussed in Chapter 3.

1.2. CALCIUM DEPENDENCY OF HIGH-ENERGY-PHOSPHATE UTILIZATION AND OXYGEN DEMAND OF THE BEATING HEART

The important role of Ca in sustaining myocardial contractility was first appreciated in 1882 by Sidney Ringer. He found that Ca-free saline leads to cardiac arrest of isolated frog hearts. As reported by Locke and Rosenheim (1907) and later by Mines (1913), Ca withdrawal impairs primarily mechanical performance, whereas the bioelectric process of ventricular excitation may persist. Figure 6 shows one of our own experiments in which an electrically stimulated rabbit papillary muscle was put into a Ca-free Tyrode solution. Single-fiber action potentials and isometric mechanograms were continuously recorded. As expected, isometric peak tension fell to almost zero within 14 min in a Ca-free environment, whereas the action potentials did not change appreciably. However, the mechanical function of the cardiac fibers was rapidly restored on return to a normal Ca-containing medium.

Overwhelming evidence has accumulated in the last two decades that Ca ions are required during excitation to activate the biochemical processes that utilize ATP for contraction. The rapid rise in free intracellular Ca resulting from the increased transmembrane Ca influx and a simultaneous liberation of Ca from endoplasmic stores initiates the splitting of ATP by the Ca-dependent ATPase of the myofibrils

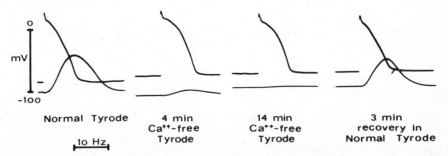

FIGURE 6. Complete loss of contractility of an isolated rabbit papillary muscle in a Ca-free Tyrode solution at 37°C. Rapid recovery in ordinary Tyrode solution containing 2mM Ca. Rate of stimulation: 3 shocks/min. Potentials were measured with intracellular microelectrodes of conventional type. Isometric tensions were recorded with a transducer valve (RCA 5734). The solutions were vigorously gassed with 95% O_2 and 5% CO_2. Thereby a rise in basal tone ("calcium-paradox" according to Zimmerman and Hülsmann, 1966) that may occur upon return of Ca-deprived myocardium into a Ca-containing medium could be avoided. Besides previous Ca withdrawal, a certain degree of hypoxia seems to be another prerequisite that must be fulfilled before the "calcium-paradox" develops. From Fleckenstein (1963a).

so that phosphate-bond energy is transformed into mechanical work. As shown directly on isolated frog muscles and beating rabbit auricles, the Ca-deficient fibers exhibit a striking insufficiency to split their high-energy-phosphate compounds in the excited state (Fleckenstein, Schwoerer, and Janke, 1961; Fleckenstein and Schwoerer, 1961; Fleckenstein, 1963a, 1968a,b,c; Schildberg and Fleckenstein, 1965). But after addition of Ca, the high-energy-phosphate utilization is normalized. If, on the other hand, the extracellular Ca concentration is increased above normal, more Ca is taken up, so that both splitting of high-energy phosphates and contractility are potentiated. Figure 7 demonstrates, for instance, the stepwise decline in CP content and augmentation of orthophosphate content due to an increase in the extracellular Ca concentration. The experiments were carried out on isolated rabbit auricles at a constant stimulation rate of 200/min. Isometric tension was also increased by the rise in Ca concentration up to a maximum of about 10 mM, a value fivefold above normal. Ca concentrations that were still higher than that value activated the splitting of high-energy phosphates even more, but failed to produce a proportional augmentation of tension. This drop in efficiency signifies the beginning of exhaustion and seems to be a natural consequence of the progressive breakdown of CP. Nevertheless, there is no doubt that the Ca ions not only trigger the contractile process but also control quantitatively the output of mechanical tension by regulating the amount of ATP that is metabolized during activity.

It is a well-known fact that the increased consumption of high-energy phosphates in the cell also gives rise to intensified glycolytic and oxidative reactions that thereafter have to refill the high-energy-phosphate stores. This explains why the

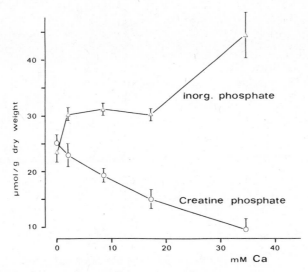

FIGURE 7. Influence of increasing extracellular Ca on the CP and inorganic-phosphate content of the atrial myocardium (32 isolated rabbit auricles) at a constant rate of stimulation of 200 shocks/min. Simultaneously with the loss of CP, the ATP concentration was also reduced from a maximum of 15.3 ($\pm$ 0.7) μmol/g dry weight at zero Ca to 9.0 ($\pm$ 0.9) μmol/g in the Ca-rich Tyrode solution with 34.6 mM Ca. Temperature, 30°C. From Schildberg and Fleckenstein (1965).

whole chain of metabolic recovery processes and particularly the rate of respiration of active heart muscle is also highly "Ca-sensitive." Figure 8 demonstrates the rates of oxygen consumption of isolated frog ventricular strips and of cat papillary muscles at rest and during stimulation, both in ordinary Ringer solution and in a Ca-free medium. Obviously, oxygen uptake at rest does not differ appreciably whether or not the surrounding fluid contains Ca. However, if stimulation begins, the oxygen consumption rises sharply, but only in presence of Ca, whereas it remains more or less at resting level in the Ca-deprived myocardium, which responds electrically but not mechanically to stimulation. If, on the other hand, the Ca concentration is

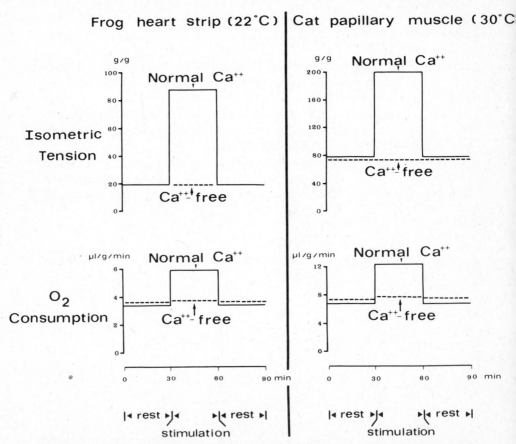

FIGURE 8. Mean O_2 consumption of 14 isolated frog ventricular strips and 11 cat papillary muscles at rest and during activity both in ordinary Ringer solution with 1.8 mM Ca and in a Ca-free medium. The rates of O_2 consumption were calculated from O_2-tension measurements in the surrounding fluid using a platinum electrode. Simultaneously, the mechanical activity was registered by recording the isometric tension with an inductive force transducer. The contractility of the Ca-deprived preparations was negligible during the stimulation period, whereas electric excitability persisted. The stimulation rate was 24/min (frog ventricular strips) and 60/min (cat papillary muscles). From Byon and Fleckenstein (1965), Fleckenstein (1963a), and Fleckenstein, Döring and Kammermeier (1966/1967).

Isometric peak tensions

(attained in 180 single contractions at different Ca concentrations)

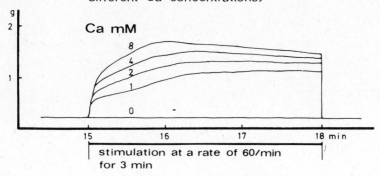

stimulation at a rate of 60/min for 3 min

Oxygen consumption

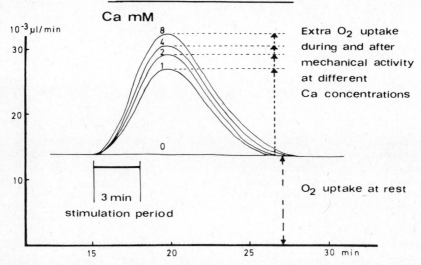

FIGURE 9. Variation in extracellular Ca content. Parallel changes in isometric peak tension and additional consumption of oxygen due to mechanical activity (exceeding the oxygen uptake at rest) of a rabbit papillary muscle in Tyrode solutions of different Ca concentrations (0, 1, 2, 4, and 8 mM). The muscle (1.6 mg wet weight) was incubated at rest in the different media each time for 20 min and then stimulated for 3 min at a frequency of 60/min. Measurements of the rates of oxygen consumption (with a platinum electrode) and of mechanical tension (with a mechanoelectronic displacement transducer) were made in a flow respirometer at 30°C throughout the experiment. There is a time lag between the mechanogram and the registration of oxygen consumption because it takes several minutes before the interstitial fluid of lowered oxygen content is completely washed out of the muscle and reaches the downstream-placed oxygen electrode. The solutions were not changed before the respiration rates had returned to resting level after each stimulation period. From Byon and Fleckenstein (1969).

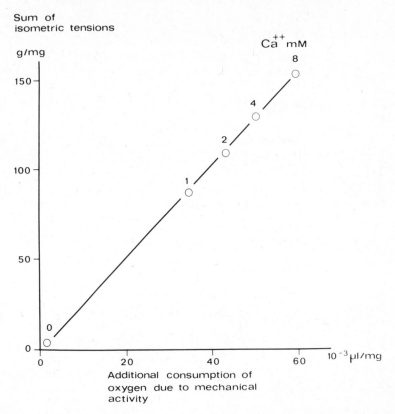

FIGURE 10.   Variation in extracellular Ca content. Linear correlation between isometric tension and the additional consumption of oxygen (due to mechanical activity) of a rabbit papillary muscle in Tyrode solutions of different Ca concentrations (0, 1, 2, 4, and 8 mM). The graph shows the sum of the isometric peak tensions produced during each stimulation period (3 min) plotted against the corresponding additional consumptions of oxygen during and after stimulation. Figure 10 represents an evaluation of the experiment shown in Figure 9. From Byon and Fleckenstein (1969).

increased above normal, the energy output of the excited myocardium will be further intensified. Thus alterations in the extracellular Ca concentration generally lead to parallel changes in the following three parameters:

1. The amount of ATP consumed in the contractile system.
2. The magnitude of mechanical tension developed.
3. The extra uptake of oxygen related to the contractile force generated.

For instance, in the Ca-concentration range between 0 and 8 mM, there is a strictly linear relationship between isometric tension development of rabbit papillary muscles and the concomitant increase in oxygen uptake above resting level (see Figures 9 and 10). At a Ca concentration of about 10 mM, the maximum tension development was reached. In quiescent heart muscle, on the other hand, resting tension, high-energy-phosphate turnover, and basal oxygen consumption proved to be rather insensitive to changes in extracellular Ca. This is easily understood because at rest (1) transmembrane Ca conductivity is rather small and (2) ATP serves purposes other than contraction and therefore is metabolized along Ca-independent pathways.

1.3.   INTERACTIONS OF CALCIUM WITH ISOLATED CONTRACTILE AND REGULATORY PROTEINS

The findings obtained using intact myocardial tissue agree with the results obtained using subcellular muscle constituents such as isolated myofibrils or contractile proteins, which were also found to require the addition of Ca for shortening (syneresis, superprecipitation) and maximum ATPase activity. However, very extensive studies showed that the involvement of Ca in these reactions is highly complex. As generally accepted, the fundamental macromolecular process that underlies contraction consists of an interaction of myosin and polymerized actin (F actin). Myosin is a fibrous protein (H.H. Weber, 1934). F Actin is built from monomeric G actin, a small globular protein.

The rapid development of basic research on muscle contraction during the last three decades was initiated in 1942 by A. Szent-Györgyi. He discovered that myosin and F actin combine *in vitro* to form a colloidal actomyosin gel that exerts ATPase activity and, in analogy with muscle contraction, shrinks (syneresis) when ATP is split (Szent-Györgyi, 1947). Using this model as well as isolated myofibrils, a number of further successful steps toward the elucidation of the contractile machinery were taken. It was found and confirmed by several authors that the ATPase activity of "native" actomyosin preparations could be inhibited by Ca removal with EDTA or EGTA, whereas "synthetic" actomyosin, made by combining myosin with vigorously purified actin, was insensitive in this respect (see Perry and Grey, 1956; A. Weber and Winicur, 1961; A. Weber and Herz, 1963; Seidel and Gergely, 1963). Hence the conclusion was justified that a "regulatory" protein that is responsible for the susceptibility to Ca had probably been removed or destroyed during the actin purification.

These observations recalled earlier investigations of Bailey. In 1948 he had discovered a new helical protein, named tropomyosin, that was able to combine with actin and possibly to regulate the interaction between myosin and actin. The problem was finally solved by Ebashi and his group in the years 1964 to 1967. Starting from Bailey's crude tropomyosin preparation, they succeeded in isolating "troponin" a new protein with specific Ca-binding properties (Ebashi and Ebashi, 1964; Ebashi and Kodama, 1965; Ebashi, Ebashi, and Kodama, 1967). Troponin operates as the determinant Ca-receptive protein within the troponin–tropomyosin complex. There is, however, a mutual influence of the two regulatory proteins on each other because in the presence of Ca ions, troponin produces maximum activation of the actomyosin ATPase only in a 1 : 1 combination with tropomyosin. Interestingly enough, troponin is composed of three polypeptide chains (TNC, TNT, and TNI) with specific subfunctions (Greaser and Gergely, 1971; see Table 2).

TABLE 2. Contractile and Regulatory Proteins[a]

Protein	Isolation and First Description	Molecular Weight	Molecular Properties	Intracellular Distribution
Myosin	H.H. Weber (1934)	500,000	Interaction to form the actomyosin complex of a molecular weight greater than 20,000,000	Constituent material of the thick myofibrillar filaments of the A bands of the sarcomere
Actin (F actin)	A. Szent-Györgyi (1947)	1,500,000		Constituent material of the thin myofibrillar filaments connected with the Z-line structure of the sarcomere
Tropomyosin	K. Bailey (1948)	70,000	Integral constituent of the Ca-binding troponin-tropomyosin complex.	
Troponin	S. Ebashi, F. Ebashi, and A. Kodama (1967)		Ca-free troponin blocks myosin–actin interaction and myofibrillar ATPase activity. If troponin as specific Ca-receptor protein binds Ca, the blockage is relieved and contraction occurs.	Close attachment to the F-actin molecules in the thin myofibrillar filaments
Composed of 3 polypeptide chains of different subfunctions[b]	TNC: Ca-binding polypeptide	18,000		
	TNT: Tropomyosin-combining polypeptide	37,000		
	TNI: Polypeptide that inhibits actin–myosin interaction	23,000		

[a]For more details see the review articles of W. Hasselbach and H.H. Weber (1965); S. Ebashi and M. Endo (1968); A.M. Katz (1970); and A. Weber and J.M. Murray (1973).
[b]M.L. Greaser and J. Gergely (1971).

In summary, there are four distinct proteins that take part in the contraction cycle of the myofibrils: (1) myosin, (2) actin, (3) troponin, and (4) tropomyosin. When Ca is absent, Ca-free troponin blocks both myosin–actin interaction and myofibrillar ATPase activity so that the myofibrils are kept in the relaxed state. But if, on the other hand, Ca ions come into contact with the myofibrils, Ca troponin is formed, and the blockage of myosin–actin interaction and ATPase activity is relieved. Hence contraction occurs.

Further cogent evidence concerning the key role of Ca in the function of muscle was obtained, quite unexpectedly, from studies that had originally been undertaken to elucidate the mechanism of relaxation. The investigations were initiated by Marsh in 1951 when he discovered during the preparation of isolated myofibrils that a "relaxing factor" was present in the supernatant fraction. This relaxing factor was able to reverse syneresis of actomyosin, that is, to redisperse the actomyosin gel into the original components and to suppress actomyosin ATPase activity. The relaxing factor seemed to be a soluble protein, possibly of enzymatic nature (myokinase, creatine phosphokinase), but subsequent studies by Kumagai, Ebashi, and Takeda (1955) disproved this. They demonstrated that in reality the relaxing effect is exerted by granules in the supernatant fraction that possess a membrane-bound ATPase activity of their own, quite distinct from that of myofibrils or mitochondria. In fact, the ATPase of the relaxing granules was shown to be part of an ATP-driven Ca pump, which concentrates Ca in the interior of these corpuscles (Hasselbach and Makinose, 1961; Ebashi and Lipmann 1962). With this discovery, the time was ripe to integrate the different pieces of evidence into a functional concept: Obviously the relaxing granules remove Ca ions from the cytoplasm. In the presence of oxalate, which sequesters Ca in the granules, the concentration difference between the extragranular and intragranular Ca concentrations can reach a ratio of 1 : 6000 (Hasselbach and Makinose, 1961). Hence the relaxing granules are able to lower the Ca concentration of the surrounding fluid to such a critical extent ($\sim 10^{-7}\ M$) that the myosin–actin interaction is blocked as it occurs under the influence of Ca-chelating agents (EDTA, EGTA). The Ca-pumping granules originate from fractionized sarcoplasmic reticulum (Ebashi and Lipmann, 1962). Therefore the conclusion was justified that the sarcoplasmic reticulum (SR) serves as an intracellular Ca pool from which Ca ions can be released to cause contraction or are reabsorbed to produce relaxation.

However, in living muscle, myosin and actin do not interact as randomly distributed molecules, because natural contraction is a highly oriented process in which myosin and actin participate in the form of orderly arranged subcellular structures. In fact, as independently shown by A.F. Huxley and Niedergerke and by H.E. Huxley and Hanson in 1954, the myofibrils as the proper contractile elements contain two kinds of filaments of different diameter that slide along each other during contraction. The thick filaments (110 Å) are composed of an orderly array of myosin molecules and form the so-called A bands in the light microscope. The thin filaments (50 Å), on the other hand, are composed of a double helix of actin molecules and in addition contain the troponin–tropomyosin complex. Each thick filament is encircled by six thin ones and bears a large number of regularly spaced short lateral

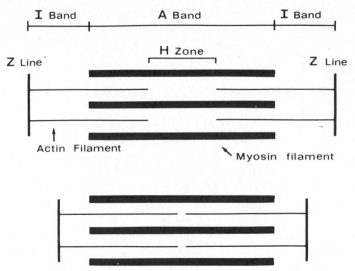

FIGURE 11.   Scheme of muscle contraction according to the sliding-filament mechanism proposed by A.F. Huxley and Niedergerke (1954) and H.E. Huxley and Hanson (1954).

projections that extend toward the thin filaments. The lateral projections consist of the heads of myosin molecules and serve to build cross bridges with the actin filaments when ATP and Ca ions are present. The sliding-filament mechanism of contraction is now generally accepted (Figure 11). The theory assumes that the formation of cross bridges is a repetitive process by which the thin actin filaments, which are attached to the Z-line structure, are drawn along the thick myosin filaments in the direction of the center of the sarcomere so that the total sarcomere length diminishes (H.E. Huxley, 1969). Calcium ions obviously initiate the crucial act of cross-bridge formation from which contraction results.

The conclusion is justified that in the intact heart muscle fiber, a fundamental correlation exists between the number of cross bridges produced, the quantity of ATP split, the magnitude of isometric peak tension developed, and the extra amount of oxygen consumed in connection with consecutive ATP resynthesis. By this molecular interaction, Ca-dependent contractile performance and metabolic activity are firmly linked together.

1.4.   CONTROL OF CALCIUM SUPPLY TO THE CONTRACTILE SYSTEM BY THE MYOCARDIAL SARCOLEMMA MEMBRANE AND INTRACELLULAR ORGANELLES (SARCOPLASMIC RETICULUM, MITOCHONDRIA)

From the foregoing discussion it is clear that cardiac contraction and relaxation has to be considered a functional consequence of rigidly regulated cyclic changes in the cytoplasmic concentration of free Ca ions. According to the current concept, contraction occurs when the cytoplasmic Ca concentration rises from about 10^{-7} to 10^{-6} or 10^{-5} M, so that more Ca is bound by the myofilaments. Conversely, relaxation is produced when the cytoplasmic Ca concentration returns to 10^{-7} M, whereby myofibrillar Ca binding is reversed. Sarcolemma membrane, mitochondria, and sarcoplasmic reticulum (SR) seem to be the most important subcellular organelles that control the Ca supply to the contractile system.

1.4.1. Transsarcolemmal Calcium Influx

There is no doubt that the initial event in excitation–contraction coupling of heart muscle consists of an increase in the transmembrane permeability of the excited sarcolemma membrane to external Ca. Electrophysiological studies have provided evidence that under normal conditions, two transmembrane inward currents operate during excitation of the mammalian myocardial fibers: (1) a fast influx of Na ions, which produces the rapid upstroke of the action potential and (2) a subsequent slow influx of Ca ions, which first contributes to the electrogenesis of the plateau phase of the action potential and second acts as the decisive link in excitation–contraction coupling. Obviously both currents use separate transmembrane carrier systems, a so-called "fast channel" for Na, and a "slow channel" preferably for Ca (Mascher and Peper, 1969; Mascher, 1970; Beeler and Reuter, 1970a,b). As depicted in later chapters, the principle of action of the new pharmacological family of Ca antagonists is to reduce the transmembrane Ca influx through the slow channel selectively. This effect is directly opposite to that of β-adrenergic catecholamines because one of the most significant results of myocardial β-receptor stimulation consists of a promotion of the slow inward Ca current.

Many observations indicate that the sarcolemma membrane not only regulates the inward diffusion of Ca into the myoplasm but also plays an important role as a Ca-accumulating system. Thus the existence of a superficially located store of rapidly exchangeable Ca has been taken into consideration by many authors (Niedergerke, 1957; Langer and Brady, 1963; Fleckenstein, 1963a; Nayler and Merrillees, 1970/1971; Nayler and Szeto, 1972; Langer, 1973; Langer, Serena, and Nudd, 1975; Dhalla, Ziegelhoffer, and Harrow, 1977; Philipson and Langer, 1979; Philipson, Bers, Nishimoto, and Langer, 1980). However, a further clear distinction still has to be made between two possibilities. The first alternative is that this Ca depot is located in the outer layers of the sarcolemma membrane, that is, at the visible cell surface or, perhaps preferentially, at those parts of the sarcolemma membrane that are invaginated in the form of the T tubules (Figure 12). In this case the superficially located Ca stores would be more confined to the extracellular space than to the interior of the cardiac fibers. The second alternative is that the rapidly exchangeable Ca fraction also comprises Ca that is stored immediately below the sarcolemma, that is, in the subsarcolemmal cisternae that are in close contact with the transverse tubular system. In this case the superficially located Ca stores would also belong, at least in part, to the intracellular space. In other words, a problem that remains to be solved is whether the superficial Ca depots are essentially located outside or inside the sarcolemmal structure that operates, as "slow channel," at the border line between the extracellular and intracellular space.

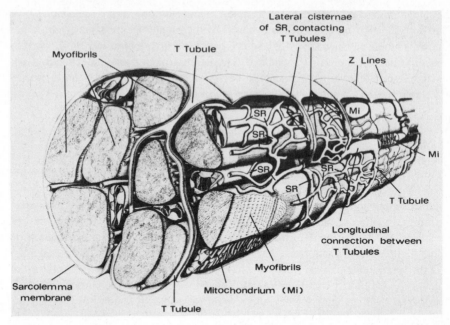

FIGURE 12.   The ultrastructure of a myocardial fiber, modification of a scheme of Nelson and Benson (*J. Cell. Biol.* **16,** 297, 1963).

The more recent observations of Langer and his group (Langer, 1973; Langer, Serena, and Nudd, 1975; Shine, Serena, and Langer, 1971) as well as our own investigations presented in Sections 2.6 to 2.8 have accumulated clear evidence in favor of the first alternative. In fact, as schematically illustrated in Figure 13, a functionally important Ca pool is probably situated in a superficial sheath of the sarcolemma membrane and particularly in the T tubules. Here extracellular Ca is taken up from the interstitial fluid by specific binding sites and deposited in a readily detachable form so that it can be instantaneously made available to the slow channels as soon as depolarization occurs. The ultrastructural analysis has revealed that the myocardial sarcolemma membrane consists of two distinct layers, namely an approximately 500-Å thick, superficially located "basement membrane" and a thin, electron-dense "plasma membrane" underneath (Fawcett and McNutt, 1969). The basement membrane contains plenty of negatively charged free or protein-bound mucopolysaccharide material (Howse, Ferrans, and Hibbs, 1970) with specific affinity for Ca. In this layer, called the *glycocalyx,* a considerably higher Ca concentration in comparison with the extracellular space can be maintained. As pointed out by Langer, Frank, Nudd, and Seraydarian, 1976, the ionization of the carboxyl groups of sialic acid may be a major source of negativity. According to these authors, sialic acid, an amino sugar, probably occupies peripheral terminal positions in the oligosaccharide portions of the glycoproteins that make up a large component of the coat material of the cell surface. This applies even more to the invaginated parts of the cardiac sarcolemma membrane (T tubules). In fact, the T system of

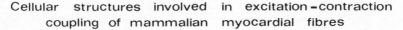

Cellular structures involved in excitation – contraction coupling of mammalian myocardial fibres

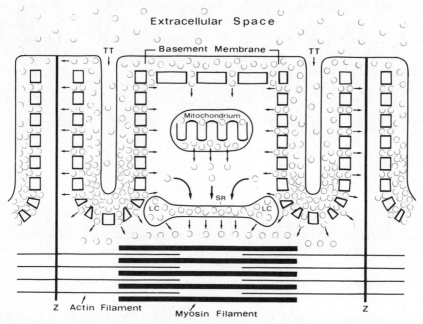

FIGURE 13. Cellular structures involved in excitation–contraction coupling of mammalian myocardial fibers. The balls represent Ca ions. They are taken up from the extracellular space and accumulated in the outer layers of the sarcolemma membrane ("basement membrane"). The highest Ca concentration is probably attained in those parts of the sarcolemma membrane that are invaginated in the form of the T tubules (*TT*). From here the Ca ions enter the interior of the myocardial fibers through the "slow channels" (marked by arrows) as soon as an excitation wave depolarizes the sarcolemma membrane. Simultaneously there is an additional Ca-triggered release of free Ca ions from the SR, particularly at the place of closest contact with the transverse tubular system, that is, at the lateral cisternae. Contraction of the myofibrils sets in when the Ca concentration in the surrounding myoplasm rises from about 10^{-7} to 10^{-6} or 10^{-5} M. The mitochondria seem to participate in the long-term regulation of the intracellular Ca concentration in that they act as a Ca buffer (From Fleckenstein, 1981).

the heart is five times the diameter of that of skeletal muscle, and is filled with Ca-binding mucopolysaccharides, whereas the T tubules of skeletal muscle are virtually empty (Fawcett and McNutt, 1969). However, a further possibility is that the negative charges of *phosphorylated proteins* in the sarcolemma membrane also act as superficially located binding sites for Ca. According to this concept outlined by Wollenberger (1975), β-adrenergic catecholamines, through formation of cyclic AMP, activate a membrane-bound protein kinase, which, in turn, induces phosphorylation of sarcolemma membrane proteins. By this reaction, the number of fixed negative phosphate groups that recruit Ca ions from the extracellular space is increased. Thus β-adrenergic catecholamines augment superficial Ca binding on membrane structures outside the slow channels or even in the slow channels. In any case, β-adrenergic catecholamines fill the superficial Ca pools with more loosely bound Ca ions that can instantaneously be mobilized upon depolarization in order to intensify the slow inward current and to potentiate contractile force. Observations from our laboratory indicate that, in fact, epinephrine and isoproterenol increase the capacity of the superficial Ca store so that the Ca uptake from the environment and the subsequent transsarcolemmal influx are facilitated. By this action, the β-adrenergic catecholamines

1. Neutralize the symptoms of Ca deficiency as long as traces of Ca are available from the interstitial fluid (for more details, see Section 2.8 and Figures 14, 51, and 52.

2. Guarantee a sufficient Ca supply to the slow channels even at rather high stimulation rates.

3. Accelerate the recovery of the transmembrane Ca current considerably when Ca is readmitted to previously Ca deprived myocardium.

During the last decade the question whether or not the slow transmembrane inward current provides sufficient amounts of Ca to make the myofibrils contract has aroused much interest. On the basis of biochemical studies on Ca binding, ATPase activity, and tension development of isolated contractile systems, several research groups have calculated that a myoplasmic Ca concentration of about 50 to 100 μmol/kg heart weight is necessary for full tension development by the myocardium (Weber and Herz, 1963; Katz and Repke, 1967; Katz, 1970; Solaro, Wise, Shiner, and Briggs, 1974). However, these high values clearly contrasted with the much lower figures that were derived from measurements of the transmembrane Ca influx into intact myocardial fibers using ^{45}Ca or electrophysiological methods as, for instance, the voltage-clamp technique. In fact, the gain in Ca, as calculated by Grossman and Furchgott (1964), Langer (1964), Nayler (1967), and others from the influx of labeled Ca in mammalian hearts, only ranged between 0.5 and 2.7 μmol/kg per beat (see Nayler and Merrillees, 1970/1971). Similarly, the Ca uptake, as indicated by the net transfer of positive charges through the slow membrane channels, generally did not amount to more than 5 to 10 μmol/kg heart weight per impulse (Reuter, 1973; Trautwein, 1973). However, these low figures may not reflect the true situation, because there are several difficulties in quantitation. The currently used techniques for measuring Ca influx may deliver erroneously low results if the uptake of labeled Ca during depolarization is partially compensated by Ca extrusion during repolarization. Moreover, it is unlikely that the slow inward current, as determined by voltage-clamp measurements, really represents the total amount of Ca entering the myocardial cell upon depolarization, because the inflow of Ca may be partially masked by an outflow of K ions.

Nevertheless, in spite of this uncertainty, one is generally inclined to believe that the transmembrane Ca influx, although it operates as the decisive regulator of myocardial contraction, does not by itself provide enough Ca to fully activate the contractile machinery. Hence it was argued that the Ca ions that are supplied to the myofibrils for the activation of contraction not only originate from the superficially located membrane pool but also from intracellular storage sites, particularly

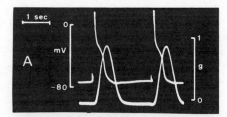

Ringer's solution
(2.5 mM Ca)

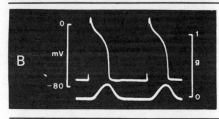

Ca-deficient
(0.5 mM Ca)
Ringer's solution
for 22 min

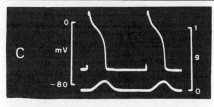

Ca-deficient
(0.5 mM Ca)
Ringer's solution
for 43 min

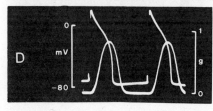

Recovery of contractility
within 2 min after
addition of adrenaline (5μg/ml)
to Ca-deficient (0.5 mM Ca)
Ringer's solution

FIGURE 14.   Restoration of contractile force of partially Ca deprived frog ventricular myocardium by addition of adrenaline to the Ca-deficient medium. From Antoni, Engstfeld, and Fleckenstein (1960).

SR and possibly also from mitochondria. Most Ca that is stored in these intermediate depots probably enters the cell through the slow channel and therefore is discernible with the voltage-clamp technique. However, further passage of Ca from these intracellular pools to the myofilaments cannot be followed in intact cells by means of electrophysiological methods. Thus research on intracellular Ca movements is preferably carried out on disintegrated systems (skinned fibers, fractionated cardiac tissue, isolated subcellular organelles), although the evidence thereby obtainable is indirect and sometimes controversial.

1.4.2. Sarcoplasmic Reticulum (SR)

The most important depot of intracellularly mobilizable Ca seems to be located in the SR, which surrounds every myofibril from Z line to Z line, and particularly in the lateral cisternae that contact the T tubules (see Figure 12). Because the action potential depolarizes the sarcolemma membrane even at the depth of the T tubules, the lateral cisternae represent that part of the SR that is most closely exposed to the influence of the excitatory process and the simultaneous transmembrane currents of ions. The close proximity of the transverse tubular system to the lateral cisternae of the SR has prompted the idea that a Ca release from the SR might be directly induced by a spread of the electric excitatory process beyond the limits of the T tubules. Accordingly, Lee, Ladinsky, Choi, and Kasuya (1966) have shown that isolated SR when electrically stimulated *in vitro* loses Ca. Although in this case the experimental conditions were rather unphysiological, the possibility of a Ca release from the SR produced by alterations of the electric charge of the sarcotubular membranes cannot be disregarded.

However, several investigators have suggested as an alternative that the small quantity of Ca entering the cell through the slow channel could trigger the release of a larger amount of Ca from the SR, and this then would permit full myofilament activation (Endo, Tanaka, and Ogawa, 1970; Ford and Podolsky, 1970). This concept of a "Ca-triggered" Ca release from the SR was further substantiated by Fabiato and Fabiato in recent years (1975, 1977, 1978). They demonstrated on skinned cardiac cells from adult human, dog, cat, rabbit, and rat hearts and from fetal and newborn rat ventricles that a constant correlation exists between the parameters measuring the Ca accumulation by the SR and Ca-induced release of Ca from the SR. The minimum free Ca concentration that triggered a transient contractile response via Ca-induced Ca release from the SR was found to be around or below $10^{-7} M$, a concentration of Ca considerably lower than that required for activating contraction of the myofibrils directly, that is, 10^{-6} to $10^{-5} M$. In agreement with this, selective destruction of the SR with the non-ionic detergent Brij[58] (Orentlicher, Reuben, Grundfest, and Brandt, 1974) rendered the skinned cardiac fibers insensitive to the trigger effect of $10^{-7} M$ Ca, but still allowed a regular direct activation of the myofibrils by $10^{-6} M$ Ca. The Ca-induced release of Ca from the SR seems to be a gradated response that is quantitatively correlated to the amount of "trigger Ca" that comes into contact with the SR, rather than an all-or-none process. The meaning of these observations on skinned myocardial fibers is that the SR probably not only operates as a "relaxing system" by Ca accumulation (Hasselbach and Makinose, 1961; Ebashi and Lipmann, 1962), but also participates in the activation of contraction by a Ca-induced Ca release. The major unsolved problem is whether the behavior of the SR of these skinned cardiac cells is representative of that of intact myocardial fibers (for more details, see the recent review by Endo, 1977).

Admittedly, the role of the SR in inducing contraction is not as well documented by *in vitro* studies as its involvement in relaxation. So no precise information is available about the specific mode of action by which an electric excitation wave or the transmembrane Ca current may displace Ca from the SR. Nevertheless, the conclusion is inevitable that the delivery of Ca by the SR for contraction is in some way the retroversion of those processes that induce relaxation. The reactions leading to the release of Ca may even be a reversal of some biochemical steps that are involved in the mechanisms of Ca uptake or Ca binding. It should be noted in this connection that the terms *Ca uptake* and *Ca binding* by the SR were used primarily to indicate different experimental procedures but, in addition, may also signify differences in the biochemical mechanisms. So the Ca accumulation by the SR in the presence of precipitating anions such as oxalate or phosphate is usually referred to as *uptake,* whereas accumulation in the absence of such anions is referred to as *binding.* However, apart from this technical point of view, studies on ATP dependence and drug susceptibility have revealed that "uptake" and "binding" of Ca may also differ by the nature of the processes involved. Whereas Hasselbach and Makinose (1961) were putting more weight on "Ca uptake," Ebashi and Endo (1968) have argued that "Ca binding" in the absence of oxalate or phosphate might be of greater physiological significance. Thus there is still some uncertainty about whether "Ca uptake" or "Ca binding" reflects the natural situation more precisely.

Special attention should be paid to the work of A. Schwartz (1970/1971), who studied the rate of Ca binding on highly active fractions of SR that had been isolated from canine heart muscle. This author showed by dual-beam spectrophotometry using murexide as an indicator of the free-Ca-ion concentration (Ohnishi and Ebashi, 1963) that after addition of ATP, approximately 100 μmol Ca/kg of ventricular myocardium can be bound at body temperature within 200 msec (average relaxation time of mammalian ventricle). This would mean that, in fact, the rate of Ca binding by the SR of dog hearts is sufficiently high to completely remove, within one contraction cycle, an amount of Ca from the contractile system that is equivalent to that needed for full tension development (i.e., 50 to 100 μmol Ca/kg cardiac tissue weight, as mentioned above). It has for a long time been accepted that the reabsorption of free Ca into the SR is the crucial event in relaxation of skeletal muscle. In cardiac muscle, however, the SR is scarcely developed, and active Ca accumulation is less intense than that in skeletal muscle, both in the presence of oxalate (Fanburg, Finkel, and Martonosi, 1964; Inesi, Ebashi, and Watanabe, 1964) and in the absence of a precipitating anion (Katz and Repke, 1967; Pretorius, Pohl, Smithen, and Inesi, 1969; Weber, Herz, and Reiss, 1967). This discrepancy has occasionally led to some scepticism with respect to the functional significance of the SR in the myocardial fibers. After all, the relevant data of Schwartz seem to indicate that in cardiac muscle too, Ca binding by the SR fulfills the quantitative requirements for being considered to represent the real relaxing mechanism.

Interestingly enough, β-adrenergic catecholamines not only increase cardiac tension development by enhancing transsarcolemmal Ca influx, but also accelerate cardiac relaxation, probably by intensifying intracellular Ca reuptake. Extensive studies have shown that the catecholamines produce an earlier onset and a more rapid course of relaxation and are even able to suppress K-induced contractures in frog and mammalian myocardium (Kavaler and Morad, 1966; Tritthart, Fleckenstein, Kaufmann, and Bayer, 1968; Morad, 1969; Morad and Rolett, 1972). The relaxing system can even be selectively stimulated by β-adrenergic catecholamines in the intact myocardium of frogs, guinea pigs, cats, and monkeys. If, for instance, isolated papillary muscles from cats (Kavaler and Morad, 1966) or rhesus monkeys (Tritthart, Fleckenstein, Kaufmann, and Bayer, 1968) had been caused by previous incubation in a medium of high Ca and reduced Na concentration to develop maximum isometric peak tension, β-adrenergic catecholamines were virtually unable to induce a further increase in contractile force. But in this situation they were still capable of enhancing the rate of relaxation: Isometric tension then decayed so precipitously under the influence of β-mimetic drugs that relaxation preceded rather than followed membrane repolarization. The catecholamines, while speeding up relaxation, tend even to retard repolarization in that they prolong the partially Ca-dependent plateau phase of action potential (see Figures 15 and 16). All these effects were quickly reversed by adrenergic β-receptor blockade (Figures 17 and 18). In contrast with catecholamines, no other agents that increase cardiac contractile force (excessive concentration of external Ca, cardiac glycosides, caffeine, theophylline) were able to induce a similar acceleration of relaxation in our experiments.

These observations suggested that the β-adrenergic catecholamines are really involved in the physiological control of cardiac relaxation. Their promoter effect on the relaxing system can be clearly dissociated from the particular actions of catecholamines on systolic tension development and the plateau phase of action potential, that is to say, from those catecholamine actions that are nowadays under-

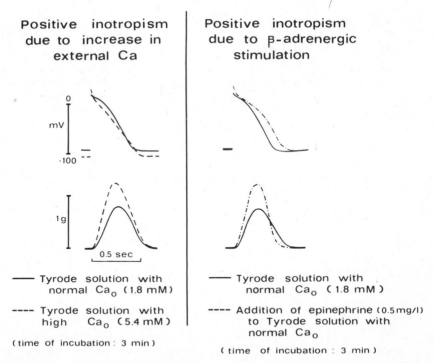

FIGURE 15. Dissociation of relaxation from repolarization upon β-receptor stimulation in isolated rhesus monkey papillary muscles. Paradoxical speeding up of relaxation with simultaneous retardation of repolarization, a typical feature of the positive inotropism produced by β-adrenergic catecholamines. Contrarily, the normal time correlation between action potential and mechanogram is not altered when an equivalent positive inotropic response is evoked by increasing the external Ca concentration. From Tritthart, Fleckenstein, Kaufmann, and Bayer (1968).

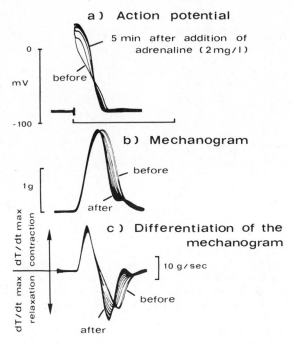

FIGURE 16.   Isolated rhesus monkey papillary muscle pretreated for 40 min with a modified (11 mM Ca, 102 mM Na) Tyrode solution to guarantee maximal tension development without β-adrenergic stimulation. Thus addition of adrenaline to this special solution does not further increase contractile force but produces the following phenomena within 5 min: (*a*) prolongation of the plateau of action potential, (*b*) paradoxical abbreviation of the relaxation phase of the mechanogram, (*c*) selective increase in the rate of relaxation (dT/dt_{max}). The stimulation rate was 2/min at 35°C. From Tritthart, Fleckenstein, Kaufmann, and Bayer (1968).

stood to result from the catecholamine-induced increase in the slow transsarcolemmal inward Ca current. Hence we concluded in 1968 that (1) the enhancement of relaxation is due to a sarcolemma-independent catecholamine effect that is exerted on intracellular structures, and (2) this effect might consist of an intensification of the ATP-dependent Ca reuptake into the SR by way of a "cocatalytic" action of catecholamines on the "granular transport ATPase." A similar hypothesis was later put forward by Morad and Rolett (1972). In fact, many subsequent papers from different laboratories have substantiated the essence of these suggestions (see Kirchberger, Tada, Repke, and Katz, 1972; Kirchberger, Tada, and Katz, 1974; Katz, Repke, Tada, and Corkedale, 1974; Tada, Kirchberger, Repke, Katz, 1974; Tada, Kirchberger, and Katz, 1975; Nayler and Berry, 1975; Fedelesova and Ziegelhöffer, 1975; Dhalla, Anand, and Harrow, 1976). From these excellent investigations it is now clear that β-adrenergic catecholamines facilitate Ca accumulation by the cardiac SR. As to the mechanism of action, catecholamines probably activate a cyclic-adenosine-3′,5′-monophosphate-dependent protein kinase of the SR so that following an increased formation of phosphoproteins, more Ca can be bound, presumably

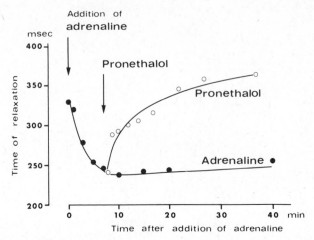

FIGURE 17. Specific abbreviation of the relaxation time of isolated rhesus monkey papillary muscles (N = 12) from 330 to 240 msec, on the average, within 7 min following addition of adrenaline (2 mg/l) to a modified (11 mM Ca, 102 mM Na) Tyrode solution. Subsequent adrenergic β-receptor blockade on 6 muscles with pronethalol (15 mg/l) rapidly neutralized the promoter effect of adrenaline on relaxation without lowering contractile force. From Tritthart, Fleckenstein, Kaufmann, and Bayer (1968).

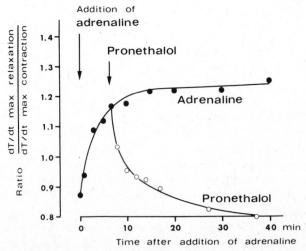

FIGURE 18. Specific increase in the ratio ($dT/dt_{\text{max relaxation}}$)/($dT/dt_{\text{max contraction}}$) produced by adrenaline (2 mg/l) on 12 isolated rhesus monkey papillary muscles in a modified (11 mM Ca, 102 mM Na) Tyrode solution. Subsequent adrenergic β-receptor blockade on 6 muscles with pronethalol (15 mg/l) abolished the adrenaline affect. From Tritthart, Fleckenstein, Kaufmann, and Bayer (1968).

at the surface of the SR structures. This in turn seems to stimulate the (granular) Ca-transport ATPase that eventually transfers and accumulates Ca in the SR in order to induce relaxation. The abundant research work on the molecular mechanism of active Ca transport by SR of skeletal and heart muscle has been reviewed by Tada, Yamamoto, and Tonomura (1978) with particular respect to the recent developments.

1.4.3. Mitochondria

In contrast with skeletal muscle, the myocardium contains many mitochondria, which are greater in mass than the less-developed cardiac SR. Moreover the highest specific activity following intraperitoneal injection of ^{45}Ca was measured in the cardiac mitochondria rather than in the SR (Patriarca and Carafoli, 1968). To investigate the mechanism of Ca accumulation in heart mitochondria, studies were carried out by many authors on the isolated organelles or on intact myocardial tissue (Slater and Cleland, 1953; Lehninger, 1970; Brierley, Murer, and Bachmann, 1964; Sanadi, 1965; Chance, 1965; Patriarca and Carafoli, 1968; Dhalla, McNamara, and Sulakhe, 1970; Horn, Fyhn, and Haugaard, 1971). In fact, Ca can be accumulated by the mitochondria by two principal distinct processes: (1) passive, energy-independent binding of Ca to the surface of the mitochondrial membrane and (2) active, energy-dependent Ca accumulation followed by an anion-dependent transfer of Ca into the intramitochondrial space. The energy-dependent mitochondrial Ca accumulation is respiration supported and/or requires an ATP-driven Ca pump. In this way the mitochondria are capable of lowering the cytoplasmic free-Ca concentration in case it rises above the normal level. As shown in *in vitro* studies, cardiac mitochondria are even able to remove bound Ca from troponin, thereby producing relaxation—an action that is comparable to that of the SR (Carafoli, Dabrowska, Crovetti, Tiozzo, and Drabikowski, 1975; Affolter, Chiesi, Dabrowska, and Carafoli, 1976).

Most authors are, however, still reluctant to accept the hypothesis that the mitochondria might be directly involved in the acute beat-to-beat regulation of the myoplasmic Ca concentration (see Kitazawa, 1976). Nevertheless, the great mass of cardiac mitochondria provides a large capacity for Ca binding and accumulation. Thus the mitochondria probably operate as a slow, but rather efficient, Ca buffer that tends to prevent the myoplasmic Ca concentration from a disproportionate rise. But even with respect to this action there are certain limitations. For instance, the mitochondrial respiratory and phosphorylation activities are highly sensitive to an excessive intramitochondrial Ca uptake (Chance, 1965). In fact, the mitochondria are badly damaged both morphologically and functionally as soon as the accumulated Ca reaches a critical level. Then the mitochondria exhibit cristolysis, swelling, and vacuolization simultaneously with a loss of respiratory control and an inhibition of ATP synthesis. In other words, excessive Ca binding by the cardiac mitochondria produces permanent alterations of these organelles and even a persistent calcification that is incompatible with the reversible character of a Ca buffer system, at least at an advanced stage of mitochondrial Ca accumulation (see Section 3.2 and Figures

92 and 93). Hence the statement is justified that the significance of the cardiac mitochondria as a physiological control mechanism of the cytoplasmic Ca concentration is accepted in principle, however still controversial in its details.

1.4.4.   Transsarcolemmal Calcium Extrusion

Obviously the myocardial fibers not only need intracellular uptake mechanisms (SR, mitochondria) for the control of the myoplasmic free-Ca concentration but also a system of Ca extrusion from the cell that counterbalances the transsarcolemmal Ca influx through the slow channel. Otherwise a steady gain in myoplasmic Ca during cardiac activity would kill the mitochondria and thereby the cell (for details see Chapter 3). This system of Ca extrusion is necessary to keep the oscillations of the myoplasmic Ca concentration during the contraction–relaxation cycle within the relatively low physiological range. Thereby a hyperactivation of the contractile machinery, a luxury consumption of ATP (and oxygen), and mitochondrial damage can be avoided. Calcium extrusion from the cardiac cell has to be considered an active process of variable intensity depending on the level of the myoplasmic free-Ca concentration. The aim of this process is to reduce the myoplasmic Ca concentration to such an extent that the intracellular binding sites for Ca in the SR, mitochondria, and myofibrils are kept in a state of rather incomplete saturation. This is even true of the activated contractile elements in normally beating hearts. As a matter of fact, incomplete saturation with Ca is the decisive prerequisite of the positive inotropic action that is exerted by all interventions that produce an increase in the myoplasmic free-Ca concentration above normal. This mechanism of action applies to the augmentation of contractile force that occurs under the following circumstances:

1.   Increase in stimulation rate that intensifies transsarcolemmal Ca supply (positive "staircase" phenomenon).

2.   Increase in transsarcolemmal Ca uptake by raising the external Ca concentration.

3.   Increase in transsarcolemmal Ca influx by facilitating the passage through the slow channel following application of β-adrenergic catecholamines.

4.   Increase in the myoplasmic free-Ca concentration by an intracellular release of Ca from the SR under the influence of caffeine or theophylline.

Under all these circumstances, a higher level of myoplasmic free Ca leads to a higher degree of saturation of the contractile elements, thus producing positive inotropic effects. But probably in every case, the processes of Ca extrusion tend to establish a new equilibrium in that the increment in Ca supply to the myoplasm is balanced by a greater amount of Ca pumped out. Then with only a short delay, a new steady state may be attained in the cardiac cell that is characterized by a somewhat elevated myoplasmic free-Ca concentration, a higher level of contractile and metabolic activity, and an equal intensification of both delivery of Ca to and Ca extrusion from the myoplasm.

The nature of the processes leading to extrusion of Ca is still poorly understood. As proposed by Reuter and Seitz (1968) and Reuter (1974), the efflux of Ca from the myocardium possibly occurs through a carrier mechanism involving a Na–Ca exchange. Several observations seem to indicate that the mechanism of action of cardiac glycosides might consist of an interference with the processes of Ca extrusion or, more precisely, with this Na–Ca exchange (Wilbrandt, 1955; Repke, 1964; Baker, 1972). According to this theory, cardiac glycosides, by inhibiting the Na,K-transport ATPase, increase the Na concentration at the inside of the sarcolemma membrane so that the Na–Ca exchange system that is responsible for Ca extrusion is occupied by Na. Without discussing here the hypothetical details (see Schwartz, Lindenmayer, and Allen, 1975; Biedert, Barry, and Smith (1979), we note that the cardiac glycosides, by inhibiting Ca elimination, would eventually shift the equilibrium between transsarcolemmal Ca influx and extrusion in the same direction as the β-adrenergic catecholamines do in straightforward manner by enhancing the slow inward Ca current. An alternative suggestion is that the cardiac glycosides, by inhibiting the Na,K-transport ATPase, might possibly induce a coupled K-efflux–Ca-influx exchange reaction. Whatever the final answer is, both explanations are consistent with the following facts:

1. Cardiac glycosides, as first proposed by O. Loewi in 1917, exert their positive inotropic effect via an interaction with Ca (see Lee and Klaus, 1971).

2. Cardiac glycosides augment the cytoplasmic free-Ca concentration by acting on an electroneutral exchange mechanism, undetectible by voltage-clamp measurements (see Greenspan and Morad, 1975; McDonald, Nawrath, and Trautwein, 1975), whereas the catecholamine-induced promotion of the slow Ca current is clearly electrogenic.

Hence the promoter actions of β-adrenergic catecholamines and cardiac glycosides on myocardial contractility represent two different ways of increasing the availability of free Ca ions to the myofibrils. Nevertheless, both catecholamines and cardiac glycosides ultimately correspond in that they facilitate the Ca-dependent transformation of phosphate-bond energy into mechanical work (for more details see Section 2.8.5).

CHAPTER TWO

Discovery and Mechanism of Action of Specific Calcium-Antagonistic Inhibitors of Excitation–Contraction Coupling in the Mammalian Myocardium

2.1. HISTORY

Obviously many substances with a positive or negative inotropic action operate by enhancing or inhibiting the function of Ca in the contractile machinery. Whereas β-adrenergic catecholamines and cardiac glycosides intensify the Ca-dependent utilization of high-energy phosphates for contraction, the Ca-antagonistic inhibitors of excitation–contraction coupling act in the opposite direction, thus producing negative inotropic effects.

Electrophysiological and biochemical evidence that a number of drugs can mimic the effects of simple Ca withdrawal on isolated mammalian myocardium and intact hearts *in situ* was presented by Fleckenstein (1964a). This report was based on observations obtained with two new compounds, namely Isoptin® (= iproveratril, later given the generic name verapamil) and Segontin® (prenylamine), as well as studies with high concentrations of certain adrenergic β-receptor blocking agents (propranolol, pronethalol, dichloroisoproterenol) or of barbituric acid derivatives. Under appropriate experimental conditions all these substances did the following:

1. Diminished contractile force without a major change in action potential.
2. Reduced high-energy-phosphate utilization of the contractile system.
3. Lowered extra oxygen consumption during activity.
4. Were easily neutralized by administration of additional Ca, β-adrenergic catecholamines, or cardiac glycosides, that is to say, by measures that were suitable to restore the Ca supply to the contractile system.

The observations led us to suppose that the negative inotropic action of these drugs might consist of an interference with the mediator function of Ca in excitation–contraction coupling of heart muscle. Henceforth the concept of Ca antagonism as a new pharmacodynamic principle arose.

2.1.1. Nonspecific Calcium Antagonism

To further clarify the pertinent problems, our investigations were primarily advanced in two directions (Fleckenstein, Döring, and Kammermeier, 1966/1967, 1968; Fleckenstein, Kammermeier, Döring, and Freund, 1967; Fleckenstein, 1968b,c; Grün, Byon, Kaufmann, and Fleckenstein, 1972). First it appeared necessary to distinguish the negative inotropic drug actions that are due to Ca antagonism from those produced by β-receptor blockade. Secondly it seemed reasonable to search for more drugs that exert Ca antagonism not only as a side effect but in a specific form. As to the differentiation between Ca antagonism and β-blockade, it was in fact not difficult to show that the effective doses of propranolol, pronethalol, or dichloroisoproterenol that directly inhibited Ca-dependent excitation–contraction coupling of guinea pig hearts were roughly 10 times greater than those needed for β-receptor blockade (see Table 3). Accordingly, contractile function returned rapidly to normal upon administration of an extra dose of $CaCl_2$, whereas the β-blockade persisted. On the other hand, some highly potent β-receptor blocking agents such as pindolol, oxprenolol, and sotalol proved to be unable to produce cardiac contractile failure because they did not exert an appreciable Ca-antagonistic

TABLE 3. Substances with Ca-Antagonistic Side Effects on Excitation–Contraction Coupling[a]

Substances	Effective Doses for Causing Contractile Failure of Guinea Pig Hearts (mg/kg)	Effective[b] Doses for Blocking β-Receptors in Guinea Pig Hearts (mg/kg)
Propranolol (Inderal, Dociton)	1.5–6	0.3
Pronethalol (Alderlin, Nethalide)	3–5	0.5
Dichloroisoproterenol	6–25	1.5
Pernocton® (= butylbromallylbarbituric acid)	75	no effect
Luminal® (= phenylethylbarbituric acid)	180	no effect
Nembutal® (= ethylmethylbutylbarbituric acid)	200	no effect
Somnifen® (= diethylbarbituric allylisopropylbarbituric acid)	190	no effect

[a]Fleckenstein, Döring, and Kammermeier (1966/1967).
[b]The "effective" doses for blocking β-receptors indicate, arbitrarily, the amount of substance which completely inhibits the chronotropic action of 0.1 μg isoproterenol on guinea pig hearts (i.v. administration on open chest preparations).

action. Thus the ability of directly interrupting Ca-dependent excitation–contraction coupling of heart muscle certainly had nothing to do with β-receptor blockade.

Ca antagonism as a genuine pharmacodynamic principle was also established in further experiments with high doses of barbiturates. Here too excitation–contraction uncoupling of heart muscle turned out to be a side effect that merely occurs under the influence of supernormal concentrations that are much greater than those required for general anesthesia. In earlier studies on cardiac incompetence produced by barbiturates, some of the criteria of Ca antagonism listed above had already been observed, but remained unexplained. This applies particularly to (1) the selective depression of cardiac contractility by barbiturates without a loss of excitability (Krayer and Schütz, 1932), (2) the high myocardial ATP and CP contents at the climax of barbiturate-induced contractile failure (Wollenberger, 1947; Fawaz and Hawa, 1953; Döring and Kammermeier, 1961), and (3) the easy restitution of contractile force by cardiac glycosides (Krayer, 1931; Schwiegk, 1931) or adrenaline (Krayer and Schütz, 1932) even in the presence of high barbiturate concentrations. Now the concept of Ca antagonism is able to provide a reasonable basis for the understanding of these scattered experimental findings.

Lastly, Ca antagonism is also exerted as a side effect by a number of local anesthetic, antiarrhythmic, or antifibrillatory drugs if they are applied in large negative inotropic doses. With respect to the accessory cardiodepression (and analogous smooth muscle relaxation) that such drugs may produce in a high dosage range, these nonspecific forms of Ca antagonism certainly deserve pharmacological and toxicological interest. As we have suggested, such drugs should pass for "Ca antagonists of group C" (see the introduction).

2.1.2. Specific Calcium Antagonism

The decisive insight, however, into Ca antagonism as a new pharmacodynamic principle resulted from the analysis of the mechanism of action of such compounds that according to our observations are capable of blocking excitation–contraction coupling specifically (see Table 4). "Specifically" means that the Ca-antagonistic inhibitory effects of these compounds on excitation–contraction coupling of heart (and vascular smooth muscle) are so predominant that other pharmacodynamic properties, at least in the therapeutic dosage range, are more or less negligible. Prenylamine (Segontin®) and verapamil (Isoptin®) were the first drugs of this type that attracted our interest beginning in 1964. Prenylamine was still relatively weak and of modest specificity. Nevertheless, increasing doses of prenylamine inhibited Ca-dependent excitation–contraction coupling of isolated papillary muscles from the hearts of rabbits, cats, guinea pigs, and rhesus monkeys by 50 to 70% before the Na-dependent excitatory process was also considerably affected (Fleckenstein, 1964a; Fleckenstein, Kammermeier, Döring, and Freund, 1967; Fleckenstein, Döring, Kammermeier, and Grün, 1968). However the Ca-antagonistic action of verapamil, in comparison with that of prenylamine, proved to be of higher potency and selectivity. In fact, verapamil could completely suppress the contractile function of the isolated myocardium without a major alteration of action potential (Fleckenstein, 1968b,c, see Figure 23). In 1968 we also found that D 600, a methoxy derivative of verapamil, is even more potent than the original compound with respect to its Ca-antagonistic effects on high-energy-phosphate consumption, contractile tension development, and extra oxygen uptake in electrically stimulated papillary muscles or intact hearts. As to the mechanism of action, it was proposed that prenylamine and verapamil exert their negative inotropic influence *"by blocking the movements of Ca from the excited fibre membrane to the contractile system or by competing with Ca for active sites where ATP is split"* (Fleckenstein, Kammermeier, Döring, and Freund, 1967). In 1969, on the basis of these findings with verapamil, D600 and prenylamine, we felt sufficiently entitled to emphasize the existence of a distinct pharmacological group of highly potent inhibitors of excitation–contraction coupling and to designate the members of this new family, with respect to their common mechanism of action, competitive *calcium-antagonists* (A. Fleckenstein, Tritthart, B. Fleckenstein, Herbst, and Grün, 1969). At a low extracellular Ca concentration, the Ca-antagonistic drug effects were greatly increased, whereas they promptly disappeared when the Ca content of the interstitial fluid was supernormal. Moreover, it was demonstrated in further studies since 1969 that:

1. The specific Ca antagonists can also block excitation–contraction coupling of uterine and vascular smooth muscle (Fleckenstein and Grün, 1969; Fleckenstein, 1970/1971b; Fleckenstein, Grün, Tritthart, and Byon, 1971; Grün, Fleckenstein, and Byon, 1971a,b, 1971/1972; Grün and Fleckenstein, 1971, 1972; Haeusler, 1972).

2. The Ca antagonists interfere with the uptake of ^{45}Ca into the myocardium (Janke, Fleckenstein, and Jaedicke, 1970; Fleckenstein, 1970/1971a,b).

3. According to voltage-clamp studies with verapamil, D 600, and nifedipine, the Ca antagonists act as specific inhibitors of the slow transsarcolemmal Ca influx, whereas the fast Na current is not affected (Fleckenstein, 1970/1971a,b); Kohlhardt, Bauer, Krause, and Fleckenstein, 1971, 1972; Kohlhardt and Fleckenstein, 1977).

4. The inhibition of cardiac pacemaker activity and atrioventricular conduction, which is another typical effect of Ca antagonists, is also produced by interference with the electrogenic transmembrane Ca influx into the nodal cells.

Table 4 is a compilation of the specific Ca antagonists that were (with the exception of diltiazem) originally identified in our institute. Some of these substances are chemically related as, for instance, the following:

1. Verapamil and its powerful methoxy derivative D 600, which represent the classical Ca antagonists.

2. Nifedipine (Bay a 1040) and other 1,4-dihydropyridines such as niludipine and nimodipine.

3. Prenylamine and two other diphenylamines, namely fendiline (Sensit®) and terodiline (Bicor®) with a nearly equal Ca-antagonistic efficacy.

Of the 1,4-dihydropyridines, compound Bay a 1040 (generic name, nifedipine; trade name, Adalat®) was the first substance of outstanding Ca-antagonistic potency that even surpassed in our experiments the potency of verapamil and D 600 (Fleckenstein, 1970/1971a,b,; Fleckenstein, Tritthart, Döring, and Byon, 1972; Grün and Fleckenstein, 1972; Fleckenstein, Grün, Byon, Döring, and Tritthart, 1975; Fleckenstein, 1975; Fleckenstein-Grün and Fleckenstein, 1975). Later on niludipine (Bay a 7168) and nimodipine (Bay e 9736) proved to be other 1,4-dihydropyridine derivatives that also possess strong Ca-antagonistic properties on heart and particularly vascular smooth muscle (Fleckenstein, Fleckenstein-Grün, Byon, Haastert, and Späh, 1979; Hashimoto, Takeda, Katano, Nakagawa, Tsukada, Hashimoto, Shimamoto, Sakai, Otorii, and Imai, 1979; Kazda, Hoffmeister, Garthoff, and Towart, 1979; Kodama, Hirata, Toyama, and Yamada, 1980). Ryosidine, a fluorinated compound of this series was nearly indistinguishable from nifedipine in a recent unpublished study of our laboratory.

In addition, diltiazem, perhexiline maleate, and caroverine, although they are

TABLE 4. Specific Ca-Antagonistic Inhibitors of Excitation–Contraction Coupling in Myocardium and Vascular Smooth Muscle Identified (with the Exception of Diltiazem)[a] in the Physiological Institute Freiburg[b]

Group A : Calcium Antagonists of Outstanding Specificity

Criteria : Inhibition by 90 to 100% of Slow Inward Ca²⁺-Current without Concomitant Influence on Transmembrane Na⁺ Conductivity

TABLE 4. *(Continued)*

Group B: Calcium Antagonists of Satisfactory Specificity

Criteria : Inhibition by 50 to 70 % of Slow Inward Ca Current <u>before</u> fast Na Influx is also affected.

Prenylamine (Mol. wt. 329.46)	**Terodiline** (Mol. wt. 281.0)
Fendiline (Mol. wt. 315.46)	**Perhexiline** (Mol. wt. 277.50)

Caroverine (Mol. wt. 366.49)

[a]The Ca-antagonistic faculties of diltiazem were found by Japanese researchers (Nakajima, Hoshiyama, Yamashita, and Kiyomoto, 1975).
[b]The substances listed in this table were generously supplied by the following pharmaceutical companies under the respective trade names: *Knoll AG, Ludwigshafen, Germany (Federal Republic)*—Verapamil hydrochloride = Isoptin, Methoxyverapamil hydrochloride (D 600) = Gallopamil; *Bayer AG, Leverkusen, Germany (Federal Republic)*—Nifedipine (Bay a 1040, Adalat), Niludipine (Bay a 7168), Nimodipine (Bay e 9736); *Sanol Schwarz GmbH, Monheim, Germany (Federal Republic)*—Ryosidine; *Tanabe Seiyaku Ltd, Osaka, Japan*—Diltiazem hydrochloride = Herbesser; *Farbwerke Hoechst AG, Frankfurt am Main, Germany (Federal Republic)*—Prenylamine = Segontin; *Dr. Thiemann AG, Lünen, Germany (Federal Republic)*—Fendiline hydrochloride = Sensit; *Kabi AB, Stockholm, Sweden*—Terodiline hydrochloride = Bicor; *Richardson Merrell, Inc., Cincinnati (Ohio, USA)*—Perhexiline maleate = Pexid; *Medichemie AG, Serumwerk AG, Basel-Ettingen, Switzerland*—Caroverine fumarate.

not related structurally to any of the foregoing drugs, had to be classified as Ca antagonists. Diltiazem was introduced by Japanese researchers (Sato, Nagao, Yamagushi, Nakajima, and Kiyomoto, 1971) and identified as a Ca antagonist by Nakajima, Hoshiyama, Yamashita, and Kiyomoto (1975). The cardiovascular pharmacology of perhexiline maleate had been studied by Hudak, Lewis, and Kuhn (1970) before the mechanism of action was clarified by Fleckenstein-Grün, Fleckenstein, Byon, and Kim (1976). Similarly, the Ca-antagonistic properties of caroverine were recognized by us several years after its introduction as a smooth muscle relaxant (Hornykiewicz, Hitzenberger, and Zellner, 1963).

Regarding the considerable differences in chemical structure, any attempt to attribute the Ca-antagonistic activity to a distinct molecular configuration is probably in vain. However, as discussed in the introduction, the Ca antagonists listed in Table 4 should be subdivided into groups A and B, according to criteria unrelated to their chemical constitution but corresponding to the strength and specificity of their Ca-antagonistic activities.

According to this classification, *group A* comprises the most potent and specific Ca antagonists such as nifedipine, niludipine, nimodipine, ryosidine, verapamil, D 600, and diltiazem. These substances are capable of inhibiting Ca-dependent excitation–contraction coupling of the mammalian ventricular myocardium by 90% and more before the fast Na influx during the rising phase of the action potential is also affected. Moreover, they do not interfere with the transsarcolemmal Mg conductivity (see Section 2.7).

Group B, on the other hand, includes prenylamine, fendiline, terodiline, perhexiline, and caroverine. These drugs are somewhat less potent and specific. Thus under their influence a concomitant inhibition of the Na-dependent excitatory process sets in when Ca-dependent contractile tension development of isolated papillary muscles has been reduced by 50 to 70%. However, such serious degrees of contractile depression can never be observed *in vivo* as long as the drug concentrations remain in the therapeutic dosage range. Thus the inhibitory influence of the Ca antagonists of group B on the fast transmembrane Na influx is therapeutically rather irrelevant. Whether the same is also true of the inhibitory effect of the Ca antagonists of group B on the transmembrane Mg influx needs further examination (See Section 2.7).

The classification of the Ca antagonists into two groups takes account of the fact that there are certain differences with respect to specificity and scope of their actions on the myocardial fiber membrane. Nevertheless, from a more general point of view, it is clear that, irrespective of such peculiarities, all Ca antagonists listed in Table 4 represent functionally related prototypes of a well-defined new category of drugs. There are some indications that cinnarizine and flunarizine also belong to group B. However, the poor water solubility of the latter agents did not allow us a satisfactory electrophysiological analysis on isolated myocardial tissue.

The young family of Ca antagonists is steadily growing. But unfortunately, among true Ca antagonists, drugs were also recently launched under this name that in reality lack Ca-antagonistic specificity. For instance, tiapamil (Ro 11.1781) reduces both the Na-dependent action-potential parameters and the Ca-dependent contractile responses of mammalian papillary muscles with almost equal strength. Moreover lidoflazine (which was also claimed by its producers to be a Ca antagonist) turned out in our studies to represent a predominantly Na-antagonistic rather than a Ca-antagonistic agent. Thus there is an urgent need for proper verification by a series of crucial tests on myocardium and vascular smooth muscle with electrophysiological, biochemical, and isotope techniques before a new compound can be accepted as a "specific Ca antagonist." To meet these requirements, solid criteria are worked out in the following chapters on which a reliable judgment of the specificity of a presumptive Ca antagonist should be based.

2.2. PRELIMINARY CHARACTERIZATION OF CALCIUM ANTAGONISTS BY THEIR INFLUENCE ON THE CARDIAC MECHANOGRAM

The original reports on marked cardiodepressant influences of prenylamine (Lindner, 1960), verapamil (Haas and Härtfelder, 1962), compound D 600 (Haas and Busch, 1967), and nifedipine (Vater, Kroneberg, Hoffmeister, Kaller, Meng, Oberdorf, Puls, Schlossmann, and Stoepel, 1972) did not offer an explanation of the specific mode of action. The same was true of the introductory papers on fendiline, terodiline, and perhexiline maleate, which also did not contribute to the understanding of the fundamental mechanism, and even worse: Verapamil and D 600 were erroneously launched as adrenergic β-receptor blocking agents. Thus the first indication that these substances might directly interfere with Ca-dependent excita-

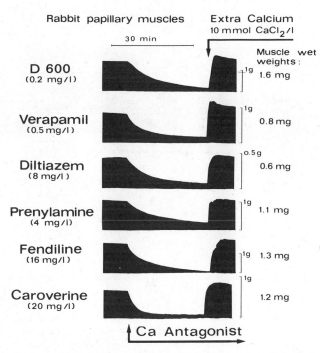

FIGURE 19.   Decrease in isometric-contraction amplitude of isolated, electrically stimulated rabbit papillary muscles during 30 min under the influence of various Ca antagonists in Tyrode solution with 2 mM Ca. Rapid restitution of contractile force to the original strength in the presence of the Ca antagonists by means of increasing the extracellular Ca concentration up to 12 mM. Stimulation frequency, 30/min; temperature, 30°C. Collection of mechanograms by Byon and Fleckenstein.

tion–contraction coupling came from our observations on isolated atria and papillary muscles that promptly recovered from drug-induced contractile incompetence upon addition of extra Ca. Figure 19 shows a series of typical tests with various Ca antagonists on electrically stimulated rabbit papillary muscles. As is a common feature of all Ca antagonists, contractile tension development was reduced by suitable drug concentrations to a very low level within 30 min and then restored to normal or even supernormal values as soon as the extracellular Ca concentration was increased from 2 to 12 mM in the presence of the inhibitors. Another experiment with different concentrations of nifedipine on a rabbit papillary muscle is shown in Figure 20. Here a drug concentration as low as 0.1 mg/l (3×10^{-7} M) was capable of reversibly lowering contractile force by approximately 95%.

Nevertheless, we stress that such simple mechanograms can provide only a preliminary orientation rather than definite evidence of a true Ca-antagonistic drug action because there are two distinct types of negative inotropism that both can be

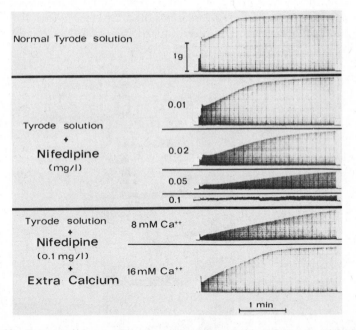

FIGURE 20. Depression of contractility of a rabbit papillary muscle (1.7 mg wet weight) in Tyrode solution containing 2 mM CaCl$_2$ by increasing concentrations of nifedipine (0.01–0.1 mg/l). Isometric tension measurements were made at a stimulation frequency of 60/min each time for 3 min after previous exposure of the muscle to the different media for 20 min. After the onset of stimulation, the normal isometric tensions in the absence of nifedipine, as well as the reduced tensions in the presence of nifedipine, continuously increased from beat to beat toward their individual maxima. This augmentation of developed tension reflects a cumulative progression in the saturation of the contractile system with Ca. Thus the more the transmembrane Ca influx is reduced by higher nifedipine concentrations, the longer the attainment of the individual tension maxima is retarded. Conversely, extra Ca in the presence of nifedipine not only restores contractility, but also shortens the time lag between onset of stimulation and the attainment of maximum tension. From Fleckenstein, Tritthart, Döring, and Byon (1972).

neutralized with extra calcium. *The first type* results from an abbreviation of membrane excitation, that is to say of the plateau phase of the action potential. This leads to a decrease in Ca supply to the contractile system due to restriction of the length of time of transmembrane Ca entry (and intracellular Ca release). For instance, low concentrations of acetylcholine can exert their negative inotropic actions on frog hearts and mammalian atria merely by an abbreviation of the action potential. In this case Ca conductivity of the depolarized membrane and all other steps of excitation–contraction coupling may remain completely intact (Fleckenstein, 1963a; Antoni and Rotmann, 1968; see Figures 21 and 22). Contractile force recovers promptly upon addition of extra calcium in the presence of acetylcholine, whereas the short action potentials persist (Figure 22). Here the steeper gradient of Ca influx apparently compensates for the abbreviation of the time of Ca entry.

The second type of negative inotropism, which is characteristic of the Ca antagonists, results from direct inhibition of Ca-dependent excitation–contraction coupling. In this case, contractile force declines selectively, whereas the original height and the duration of the action potentials are not decisively altered. When excess Ca is administered, contractile tension development is also restored. Thus both the fibers with abbreviated action potentials and those with deficient excitation–contraction coupling behave similarly, in that contractile force recovers, at least in part, if the extracellular Ca concentration rises above normal. From this it becomes obvious that a suitable differentiation of the mechanisms of action of negative inotropic agents requires the use of modern electrophysiological techniques such as recording of single-fiber action potentials with intracellular microelectrodes, registration of isometric tension development with mechanoelectronic transducers, and in addition direct measurements of the transmembrane cation conductivities with suitable voltage-clamp techniques and other methods. Moreover, studies on negative-inotropic drugs must also include observations on the most important metabolic parameters such as cardiac oxygen consumption and high-energy-phos-

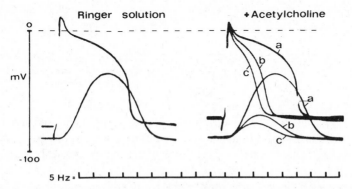

FIGURE 21. Depression of contractile force of isolated frog ventricular myocardium by abbreviation of the action potential in an acetylcholine-containing Ringer solution. Registration of single-fiber action potentials and isometric mechanograms as in Figure 6. From Fleckenstein (1963a); Antoni and Rotmann (1968).

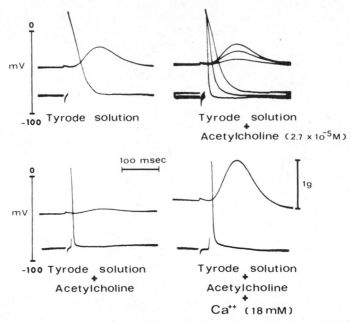

Figure 22. Depression of the contractile force of isolated atrial tissue of a guinea pig by abbreviation of the action potential in an acetylcholine-containing Tyrode solution. Restitution of the strength of contraction by addition of excess Ca without an appreciable reprolongation of action potential. From Antoni and Fleckenstein; see Fleckenstein, (1963a).

phate contents during the development of contractile depression. Otherwise no reliable information is obtainable about whether the diminution in mechanical-energy output is caused by direct respiratory inhibition, leading to high-energy-phosphate exhaustion, or results from a blockade of Ca-dependent high-energy-phosphate utilization, leading to supernormal cardiac ATP and CP concentrations.

2.3. SPECIFIC EXCITATION–CONTRACTION UNCOUPLING OF HEART MUSCLE BY CALCIUM ANTAGONISTS

Specific Ca-antagonistic inhibitors of excitation–contraction coupling reduce the contractile response of the myocardium without considerable alterations of the bioelectric excitation process as long as excessive concentrations are avoided. To illustrate this effect, a number of typical experiments on isolated cat and guinea pig papillary muscles are shown in Figures 23 to 28. For instance, Figure 23 represents a typical experiment with verapamil on an isolated guinea pig papillary muscle, published by Fleckenstein in 1968. As shown from top to bottom, contractility was selectively suppressed by increasing concentrations of verapamil. With $1 \times 10^{-5}\ M$ verapamil, the contractile responses completely disappeared, whereas

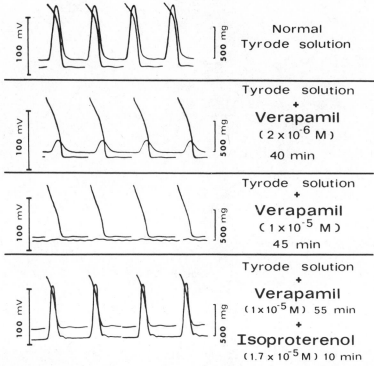

FIGURE 23. Selective loss of cardiac contractility under the influence of a high overdose of verapamil, and the reversal of this effect by isoproterenol. Experiments on an electrically driven (2 shocks/sec) isolated papillary muscle of a guinea pig in Tyrode solution with 2 mM Ca. Methods as in Figure 6. From Fleckenstein 1968b,c).

the single-fiber action potentials persisted. However, with isoproterenol, in the lowest part of Figure 23, the height of the mechanical responses was restored to normal. Isoproterenol promotes the Ca influx so that the effect of verapamil is overcome. All Ca antagonists of group A are similarly selective in blocking myo-cardial tension development. As another example, Figures 24A and B represent two experiments on cat papillary muscles in which an 80% loss of contractility was obtained by 400 μg nifedipine/l, whereas the height and the shape of the single-fiber action potentials practically did not change. As shown on the right side of these figures, contractility was restored by extra Ca (upper curve) or by isoproterenol (lower record). With a higher dose of nifedipine (1 mg/l ≈ 3 × $10^{-6}M$), contractility was totally abolished (Figure 24C). But resting potential and the action-potential parameters such as upstroke velocity and height of the overshoot, indicating the transmembrane Na influx, remained completely unaffected. Only the plateau of the action potential appeared to be abbreviated by nifedipine, because the Ca ions cannot continue to contribute to the maintenance of depolarization during the late phase of the plateau when the transmembrane Ca conductivity has been blocked

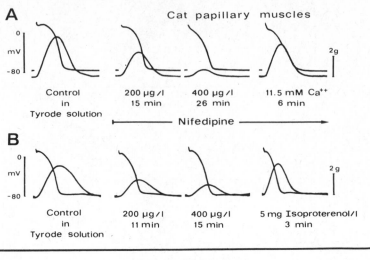

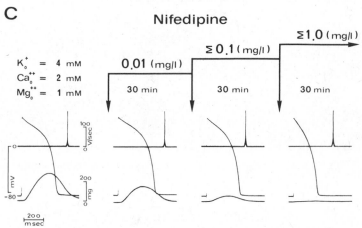

FIGURE 24. (*A*) and (*B*) Selective inhibition of contractile force of 2 isolated cat papillary muscles in normal Tyrode solution with 2 mM Ca under the influence of nifedipine (200 μg/l initially, and then 400 μg/l for further depression). Restoration of contractility by additional Ca (experiment A) within 6 min or by isoproterenol (experiment B) within 3 min. (*C*) Complete excitation–contraction uncoupling of a guinea pig papillary muscle by a stepwise increase of the nifedipine concentration from 0.01 to 0.1 and finally 1 mg/l. The upstroke velocity of the action potentials (dV/dt_{max} = 175 V/sec), indicating the fast Na influx, did not change at all [see upper curve in (*C*)]. Single-fiber action potentials and isometric contractions were measured using the same techniques as in Figure 6. Records A and B from Fleckenstein, Tritthart, Döring, and Byon (1972).

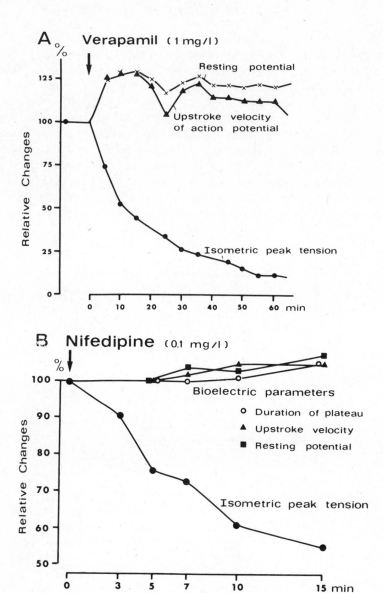

FIGURE 25. (A) Selective reduction of the Ca-dependent contractile force of a guinea pig papillary muscle to 1/10 of normal by 1 mg/l verapamil within 60 min, while the upstroke velocity (dV/dt_{max}) and the height of the overshoot of the cardiac action potential, which indicate the transmembrane Na influx, do not decrease. Continuous microelectrode recordings were taken from the same cardiac fiber for 90 min in Tyrode solution containing 2 mM Ca. The absolute values (100%) at the beginning of the experiment were as follows: resting potential (-75 mV), dV/dt_{max} (130 V/sec), isometric peak tension (700 mg). Temperature 36°C. Frequency of stimulation 2/sec. From Fleckenstein (1970/1971a). (B) Selective inhibition by 0.1 mg/l nifedipine of the contractile force of a cat papillary muscle without reduction of resting potential and without influence on velocity of rise (dV/dt_{max}) and duration of the plateau of action potential (at a height of 50%). Experimental procedure as in (A). From Fleckenstein, Tritthart, Döring, and Byon (1972).

(as depicted in following chapters). In the latter experiment with nifedipine, each molecule of the Ca antagonist neutralized approximately 700 Ca ions so that the papillary muscle finally behaved as in a Ca-free medium. The graphs in Figure 25 represent quantitative evaluations of typical experiments with verapamil and nifedipine on guinea pig and cat papillary muscles respectively. Again, resting potential and upstroke velocity of the action potential persisted, whereas contractility declined. Another experiment, shown in Figure 26, is equally impressive. Here the contractility of an isolated guinea pig papillary muscle was totally suppressed by a relatively large dose of diltiazem (30 mg/l). However, with additional Ca at the end of the experiment, the height of the mechanical responses returned to normal. The Ca antagonists of group B also spare the Na-dependent excitatory processes in a low dosage range as long as Ca-dependent contractile tension development is

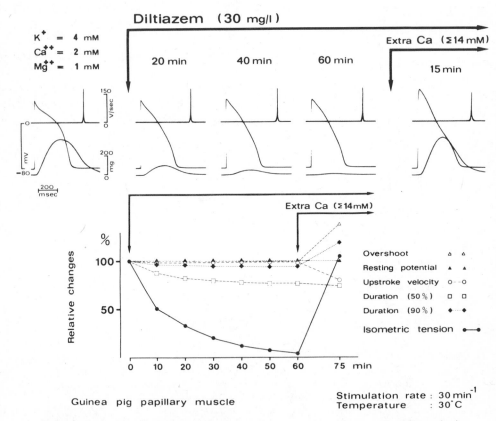

FIGURE 26. Selective suppression of contractility of a guinea pig papillary muscle without reduction of resting potential and by diltiazem on velocity of rise (dV/dt_{max}) of action potential. At the end of experiment, restitution of contractility is attained by elevation of Ca concentration of the diltiazem-containing Tyrode solution from 2 to 14 mM. Evaluation of the experiment in the lower part of the figure. General experimental procedure as in Figure 24C. From Fleckenstein and Späh (1981/1982).

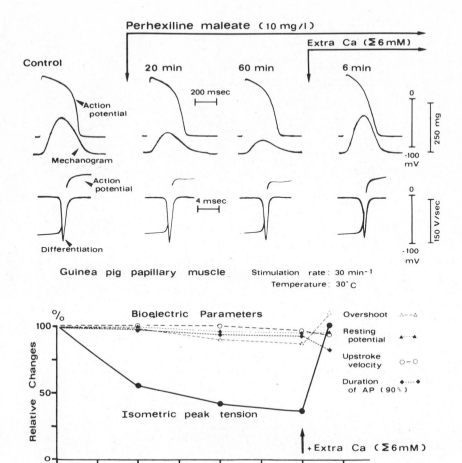

Figure 27. Selective inhibition of the contractility of an electrically stimulated guinea pig papillary muscle under the influence of perhexiline maleate (10 mg/l) in Tyrode solution containing 2 mM Ca. Whereas within 60 min the isometric-contraction amplitude is reduced to approximately 40% of its initial value, the action-potential parameters [upstroke velocity, overshoot, duration of action potential (measured at 90% repolarization)] and the resting potential are only slightly affected. The differentiation curve (downward deflection) directly indicates that the Na-dependent maximal rate of rise of the action potentials (approx. 140 V/sec) remains nearly constant. Subsequently, rapid restitution of contractility under the influence of additional Ca (increase of the extracellular Ca concentration to 6 mM). An evaluation of the experiment is shown in the lower graph. Obviously, the bioelectrical parameters are much less influenced than isometric tension development (initial values prior to administration of perhexiline maleate always 100%). Intracellular microelectrode insertion in one single myocardial fiber for a period of 90 min. From Fleckenstein-Grün, Fleckenstein, Byon, and Kim (1976).

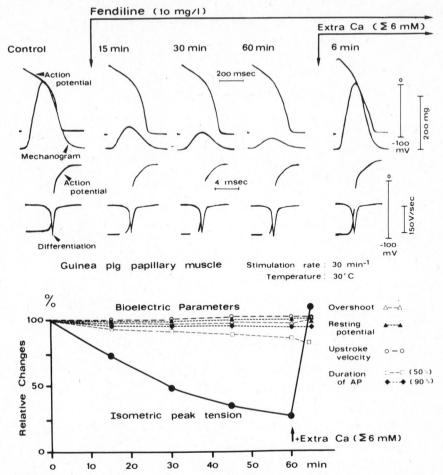

FIGURE 28. Selective inhibition of the contractility of an electrically stimulated guinea pig papillary muscle under the influence of fendiline (10 mg/l) in Tyrode solution with 2 mM Ca. The isometric contraction amplitude falls within 60 min to about 25% of the initial value, but the action-potential parameters (upstroke velocity, overshoot, and duration of action potential, the latter being measured at 90% repolarization) as well as the resting potential remain nearly unchanged. Only the plateau of the action potential (measured at 50% repolarization) seems slightly abbreviated. Subsequently a rapid restitution of contractility is attained by addition of extra Ca (increase in Ca content to 6 mM). A graphic evaluation of the experiment is given in the lower part of the figure. Intracellular microelectrode insertion in one single myocardial fiber for a period of 90 min. From Fleckenstein, Fleckenstein-Grün, and Byon (1977).

not depressed by more than 50 to 70%. Pertinent examples are shown in Figures 27 and 28 with the use of perhexiline maleate and fendiline. If, however, higher degrees of contractile inhibition are produced by stronger concentrations of Ca antagonists of group B, the Na-dependent action-potential parameters (maximal rate of upstroke $= dV/dt_{max}$; height of overshoot) are also significantly lowered.

2.4. SELECTIVE SUPPRESSION OF THE TRANSSARCOLEMMAL INWARD CALCIUM CURRENT BY CALCIUM ANTAGONISTS

Although it was clear from the foregoing studies that the Ca antagonists restrict the Ca supply to the contractile system, for some years the exact site of action remained a matter of speculation. When, however, in 1970 methods became available to measure the transsarcolemmal Na and Ca currents independently of each other, the first problem to be examined was whether the Ca antagonists specifically interfere with the slow transsarcolemmal Ca inward current. The electric device used in our experiments corresponded to Stämpfli's (1954) classical sucrose-gap technique in a modification of Haas, Kern, and Einwächter (1970). The separation of the trans-membrane Na and Ca currents was done according to the conditioning-clamping technique described by Reuter and Beeler (1969). In these experiments the membrane was depolarized in a first clamping step by 30 to 50 mV for about 400 msec to elicit the fast transient Na inward current. Then, in a second clamping step, the membrane potential was further decreased by 20 mV. This causes the appearance of another inward current. Because the Na-carrying system becomes inactivated during the course of the first depolarization step, the second inward current is mainly due to an influx of Ca. Thus, in confirmation of the observations of Reuter and Beeler (1969) and Mascher and Peper (1969), the second inward current disappeared in a Ca-free medium and, conversely, increased when the extracellular Ca concentration was augmented. However, the decisive result of our studies consisted of the observation that verapamil and compound D 600 suppress the transsarcolemmal Ca current in the same dosage range as that at which they inhibit contractile tension development (Kohlhardt, Bauer, Krause, and Fleckenstein, 1971, 1972). For instance, verapamil (2 mg/l) or D 600 (0.5 mg/l) reduced the Ca currents by 60 to 70% within 20 min. In some cases D 600 blocked the Ca currents completely. However, the Ca-antagonistic drug effects could be neutralized or even overcompensated by addition of excess Ca to the bathing fluid. But in contrast to their strong inhibitory effect on the passive transmembrane Ca movements, verapamil and D 600, in corresponding concentrations, did not block the fast Na current.

The graphs in Figures 29 and 30 demonstrate in detail the influence of D 600 and verapamil on the transmembrane Ca and Na currents. The flow intensities are expressed in μAmp. on the abscissa and plotted against the clamped-membrane potentials on the ordinate. As can be seen from the left parts of the figures, the current–voltage-relationship curves of the transmembrane Ca currents were shifted by D 600 and verapamil to very low values. But when the extracellular Ca con-

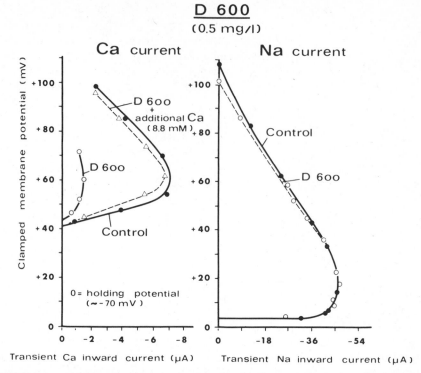

FIGURE 29. Current–voltage-relationship curves of the slow transmembrane Ca current and the fast Na current under the influence of D 600 (0.5 mg/l). Observations on an isolated trabecula from the right ventricle of a cat. By addition of D 600 to normal Tyrode solution containing 2.2 mM CaCl$_2$, the current–voltage-relationship curve of the slow inward Ca current is shifted to very low values, indicating a strong inhibition of the transmembrane Ca influx through the slow channel. By increasing the extracellular Ca concentration up to 8.8 mM, the effect of D 600 on the transmembrane Ca current is nearly neutralized. The influence of D 600 on the fast Na inward current is negligible. Temperature, 32°C; pH, 7.35. From Kohlhardt, Bauer, Krause, and Fleckenstein (1972).

centration was increased in the D 600- or verapamil-containing medium from 2.2 up to 8.8 mM, the Ca currents returned almost completely to their control heights. Quite similar results were obtained in more-recent experiments with nifedipine (Kohlhardt and Fleckenstein, 1977). The fast Na conductivity, on the other hand, was not altered by the drugs, as shown on the right side of the figures. Here the current–voltage-relationship curves of the fast inward Na currents were practically identical regardless of whether the Ca-antagonistic drugs had been added or not. This is particularly true of the physiologically most important range of depolarizations up to 50 mV that are decisive for the initiation of action potentials. Needless to say, the refractoriness of the passive transmembrane Na movements to verapamil, D 600, and nifedipine explains the fact that these drugs lack an appreciable influence

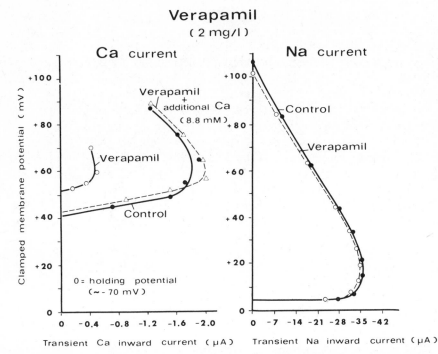

FIGURE 30. Current–voltage-relationship curves of the slow transmembrane Ca current and the fast Na current under the influence of verapamil (2 mg/l). With this dose the transmembrane Ca conductivity is reduced to a similar extent as with 0.5 mg/l D 600. There is again no significant change in the fast Na current. The measurements were carried out on a trabecula from the right ventricle of a cat. Experimental procedures as in Figure 29. From Kohlhardt, Bauer, Krause, and Fleckenstein (1972).

on the Na-dependent bioelectric membrane parameters of the mammalian ventricular myocardium.

In this respect the Ca antagonists differ fundamentally from local anesthetic agents: It is well known that local anesthetics stabilize the resting potential of nerve and muscle-fiber membranes by blocking the Na–K exchange (Fleckenstein and Hardt, 1949; Shanes, 1950; Fleckenstein, 1955). According to Weidmann's observations (1955), cocaine, procaine amide, and quinidine reduce the maximum upstroke velocity of the action potential in Purkinje fibers. This had led to the assumption that local anesthetics and related drugs interfere with the rapid Na influx. In fact, local anesthetics as well as many other substances that inhibit cardiac membrane excitation retard the rising phase of the action potentials in atrial or ventricular fibers (Vaughan Williams, 1965; Fleckenstein, 1969a; Tritthart, B. Fleckenstein, and A. Fleckenstein, 1970/1971). Thus it was not surprising that local anesthetics such as procaine and lidocaine (xylocaine), in contrast with specific Ca antagonists, predominantly interfere with the fast transmembrane inward Na current.

One of our experiments with lidocaine (50 mg/l) is shown in Figure 31. Here only the current–voltage-relationship curve of Na was typically shifted toward lower values (from -30 to -20 μAmp. at 30 mV depolarization), whereas no change in Ca conductivity occurred. Apparently the decrease in Na influx reduces the excitability of the myocardial cell without directly impairing the contractile response. The Na-antagonistic membrane action of procaine and xylocaine resembles to some extent that of tetrodotoxin, which also inhibits, in a still more specific way, the excitatory Na movements in nerve, skeletal muscle, and myocardium.

The differential susceptibilities of the transmembrane Na and Ca currents to specific inhibitors demonstrate that the influxes of these cations during excitation are independent of each other. Therefore, in the mammalian myocardium the existence of separate channels for Na and Ca has to be assumed. As a functional consequence of these independently operating transport systems, it is possible to increase or decrease cardiac contractile force by inotropic substances, which act as

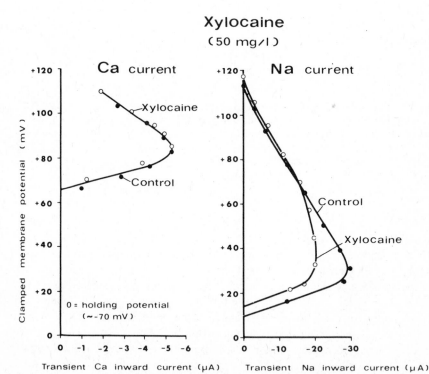

FIGURE 31. Current–voltage-relationship curves of the slow transmembrane Ca current and the fast Na current under the influence of xylocaine (50 mg/l) on a right ventricular trabecula of a cat. In contrast to the Ca antagonists D 600 and verapamil, compounds with a predominantly local anesthetic action such as xylocaine (lidocaine) are able to reduce the Na conductivity of the myocardial fiber membrane without interfering with the slow Ca current. Hence lidocaine inhibits Na-dependent excitation much more than Ca-dependent contractile force. Experimental procedure as in Figures 29 and 30. From Kohlhardt, Bauer, Krause, and Fleckenstein (1972).

promoters (β-adrenergic catecholamines) or inhibitors (Ca antagonists) of the Ca current without concomitant effects on Na-dependent excitation.

The divalent Sr ions that are capable of replacing Ca in excitation–contraction coupling also use the slow channel when they penetrate into the myocardial fibers (Kohlhardt, Haastert, and Krause, 1973). This implies that a blockade of the slow channel produced by Ca-antagonistic agents also abolishes the influx of Sr, provided the sarcolemma membrane is intact. On the other hand, Ni, Co, or Mn ions block the slow channel by themselves because they probably compete with Ca for certain active sites in this particular carrier system. Kaufmann and Fleckenstein had already reported in 1965 that 2 mM NiCl$_2$ or CoCl$_2$ when added to an ordinary Tyrode solution with 1.8 mM Ca produce a nearly complete loss of contractility of electrically stimulated guinea pig papillary muscles, whereas resting and action potentials remain practically unchanged. Excitation–contraction uncoupling took place within 30 min and could be rapidly reversed by increasing the external Ca concentration up to 3.8 mM (see Figure 32). Later observations of Ochi (1970), Mascher (1970), and Vitek and Trautwein (1971) established that divalent Mn ions too are capable of blocking cardiac excitation–contraction coupling by interference with

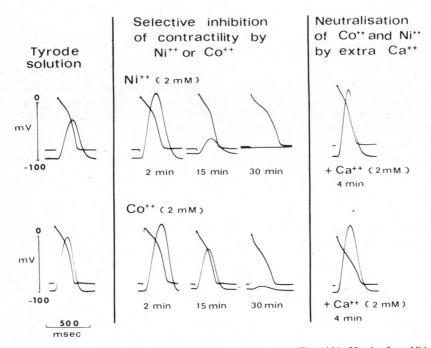

Figure 32. Isolated guinea pig papillary muscles lose their contractility within 30 min after addition of 2 mmols NiCl$_2$ or CoCl$_2$/l normal Tyrode solution containing 1.8 mM Ca, whereas the single-fiber action potentials persist. The effects of Co and Ni can be rapidly neutralized by an extra dose of 2 mmols CaCl$_2$/l, so that contractility recovers within 4 min. Rate of stimulation, 30 shocks/min; temperature, 33°C. Methods as in Figure 6. From Kaufmann and Fleckenstein (1965).

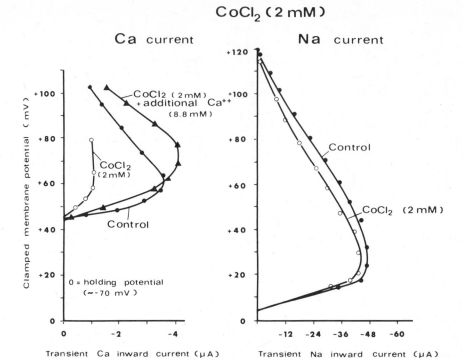

FIGURE 33. Current–voltage relationships of both the slow Ca and the fast Na inward currents obtained on a trabecula from the right ventricle of a cat using the voltage-clamp technique. The ordinate shows the clamped (depolarized) potential; 0 indicates the holding potential (approximately −70 mV). By addition of $CoCl_2$ (2 mmol/l) to a normal Tyrode solution with 2.2 mM $CaCl_2$ the current–voltage-relationship curve of the slow Ca inward current is shifted to lower values, indicating a reduced transmembrane Ca conductivity. By increasing the extracellular Ca concentration up to 8.8 mM the effect of Co on the transmembrane Ca current is more than compensated. The influence of Co on the fast Na inward current is relatively weak. Additional Ca reduced the transmembrane Na conductivity even more. From Kohlhardt, Bauer, Krause, and Fleckenstein (1973).

the slow Ca current. The pertinent voltage-clamp data from our laboratory concerning the Ca-antagonistic action of Co ions are represented in Figure 33 (Kohlhardt, Bauer, Krause, and Fleckenstein, 1973). The trivalent rare-earth element La is also a well-known inhibitor of the slow inward current. Lanthanum was found to selectively eliminate contractility of perfused rabbit ventricular muscle in a concentration as low as 4×10^{-5} M (Sanborn and Langer, 1970). Nevertheless, in comparison with the most efficient organic Ca antagonists, the inhibitory action of La appears rather modest. According to our observations, La (4×10^{-5} M), D 600 (1×10^{-6} M), and nifedipine (3×10^{-7} M) are equipotent. This means that in comparison with La, nifedipine is at least 100 times, and D 600 approximately 40 times, stronger.

2.5. QUANTITATIVE CORRELATION BETWEEN INHIBITION BY CALCIUM ANTAGONISTS OF TRANSMEMBRANE CALCIUM INFLUX AND CONTRACTILE TENSION DEVELOPMENT

The foregoing voltage-clamp studies demonstrated that the organic Ca-antagonists can selectively block the slow inward Ca current and that the effective drug concentrations correspond approximately to those that inhibit cardiac contractility. However, the experimental device was not sufficiently subtle for deciding the following:

1. Whether the measurable decrease of transsarcolemmal Ca influx caused by Ca antagonists really determines the degree of contractile inhibition in a strictly quantitative manner.

2. Whether excitation–contraction uncoupling by Ca antagonists is so predominantly due to this specific action on the slow Ca channel that an additional interference with intracellular Ca movements can practically be disregarded.

Several attempts have been made to solve these pending problems. It was shown in our laboratory (Weder and Grün, 1973) that the possibility of controlling contractile force by Ca antagonists is lost in skinned myocardial fibers that have been prepared by glycerin-water extraction or according to Winegrad's (1971) technique. In such skinned fibers, the Ca-antagonistic compounds produced no inhibition when contraction was directly induced by addition of ATP and Ca. This means that the structural integrity of the cardiac sarcolemma membrane is an indispensable prerequisite of the Ca-antagonistic drug action. Obviously, these agents lose their power if the Ca ions have free access to the myofibrils where ATP is split. Hence there is certainly no direct effect of Ca-antagonistic compounds on the Ca-dependent activation of myofibrillar ATPase and on energy transformation in the myofilaments. Similarly, in fractionated SR, all direct attempts to show an inhibitory effect of negative inotropic doses of verapamil on binding, accumulation, or exchange of Ca have failed (Nayler and Szeto, 1972; Entman, Allen, Bornet, Gillette, Wallick, and Schwartz, 1972; Watanabe and Besch, 1974b). Moreover, in isolated cardiac mitochondria, only an excessive concentration of verapamil, more than 1000 times greater than that required to produce contractile failure, suppressed Ca uptake (Frey and Janke, 1975). In other words, evidence of a significant intracellular action of the Ca antagonists listed in Table 4 is hitherto lacking.

Therefore, it appeared more promising to concentrate upon the cardiac sarcolemma membrane and to analyze, under the influence of Ca antagonists, the quantitative correlation between the inhibition of Ca influx and the decrease in contractile force. For this study isolated cat and guinea pig papillary muscles were used in which the fast Na-transport system had previously been blocked. For instance, if the cardiac fiber membrane potential is reduced to -45 mV, the fast inward Na current becomes inactivated, whereas the slow Ca channel continues to respond to electric stimulation. The simplest method to produce this critical degree of depolarization consists of adding excess K into the bathing solution (Mascher, 1970). Such predepolarized myocardial fibers are still capable of conducting propagated impulses. But now the transmembrane bioelectric activity depends on the slow inward current of Ca ions. Hence the rate of rise of Ca-carried action potentials is typically slow. As an example, Figure 34 shows superimposed traces of the electric and mechanical activities of a guinea pig papillary muscle before as well as 2, 4, and 8 min after the K concentration of the Tyrode solution was increased from 4 to 19 mM. Because of the depolarizing effect of this K-rich Tyrode solution, the resting potential dropped within 8 min from -79.7 ($\pm$ 2.6) mV (mean $\pm$ SE of mean, $N = 38$) to -45.2 ($\pm$ 2.8) mV ($N = 58$). *Pari passu* with this partial depolarization, the transition from normal Na-carried action potentials to those mediated by the slow inward Ca current took place. This caused a drastic drop of dV/dt_{max} from 170.4 ($\pm$ 12.3) to only 6.5 ($\pm$ 0.4) V/sec.

Another peculiarity of the Ca-mediated action potentials of partially depolarized myocardial fibers is that they are highly susceptible to changes in the extracellular Ca concentration. Thus upstroke velocity, height, and duration of such action potentials increase when the environmental Ca concentration rises. Conversely, bioelectric activity rapidly disappears in a Ca-deficient medium together with the contractile function. The fundamental influence of *Ca deficiency* on the partially depolarized myocardium is represented in Figure 35. The original records and the graphic evaluation of the experimental data clearly show that, in fact, the bioelectric and the mechanical changes run closely parallel both during the period of Ca withdrawal and thereafter during the recovery phase when the extracellular Ca concentration has been normalized.

The decisive result, however, was that in partially depolarized myocardium, the *Ca antagonists mimic the effects of simple Ca deficiency.* This turned out first in

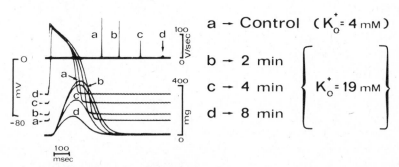

FIGURE 34. Transition within 8 min from fast Na-mediated action potentials to slow Ca-carried action potentials as a consequence of partial depolarization by increasing the external K concentration from 4 to 19 mM. In the upper record the upstroke velocity (dV/dt_{max}) diminishes from 170 to 6 V/sec. Isometric tension is reduced to 1/3 of the original height in the lower record.

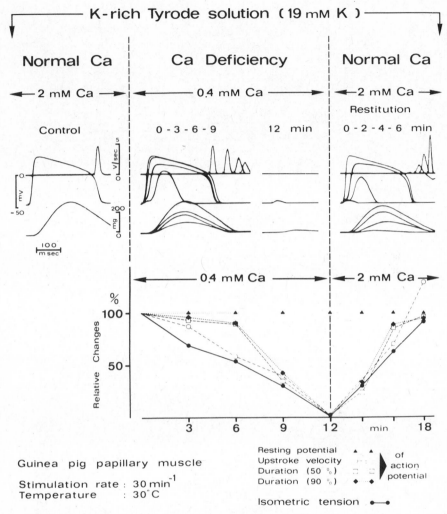

FIGURE 35. Parallel suppression of Ca-dependent electric excitability and contractility of a partially depolarized guinea pig papillary muscle in a K-rich (19 mM) Tyrode solution by lowering the Ca content from 2 to 0.4 mM. The upstroke velocity (= dV/dt_{max}) of the single-fiber action potentials is directly registered in the upper line. Underneath, the superimposed traces of the action potentials and the corresponding mechanograms visualize the progressive decay of the bioelectric and contractile function at time intervals of 3, 6, 9, and 12 min after the muscle has been transferred into the solution with low Ca$_o$ concentration. The graphs in the lower part of the figure represent a quantitative evaluation of the records. The duration of the action potentials was measured at 50 and 90% repolarization. Following readmission of 2 mM Ca at the end of the experiment, there was a full recovery of all bioelectric and mechanical parameters to their original heights (= 100%) within 6 min. The bioelectric activity was recorded during 70 min with an inserted microelectrode on one single myocardial fiber.

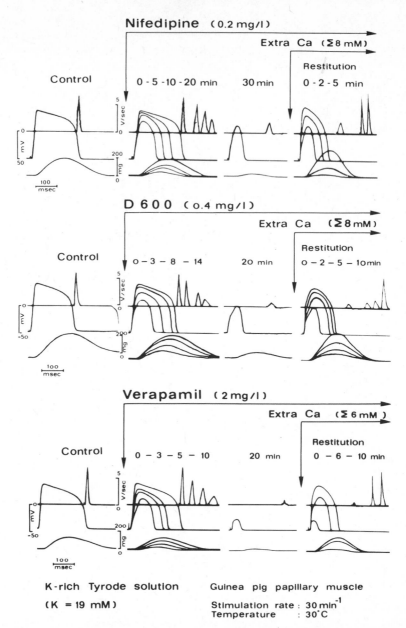

FIGURE 36. Parallel suppression by Ca antagonists of the Ca-dependent bioelectric and mechanical activities of partially depolarized guinea pig papillary muscles in a K-rich (19 mM) Tyrode solution with normal Ca content (2 mM). Three identical experiments with nifedipine (0.2 mg/l), D 600 (0.4 mg/l), and verapamil (2 mg/l). In each experiment the upper registration curve demonstrates the gradual reduction of upstroke velocity (dV/dt_{max}) during an observation period of 20 to 40 min following the addition of the drugs. The superimposed records underneath show the corresponding decrease of height and duration of the Ca-dependent action potentials and of the isometric mechanograms. Finally, the cardiodepressant effects of the Ca antagonists were overcome by raising the Ca content of the K-rich Tyrode solutions from 2 to 6 or 8 mM. The bioelectric records of each experiment were derived from microelectrode insertions on one and the same myocardial fiber lasting for 70 to 120 min. From Späh and Fleckenstein (1978/1980), and Fleckenstein (1981).

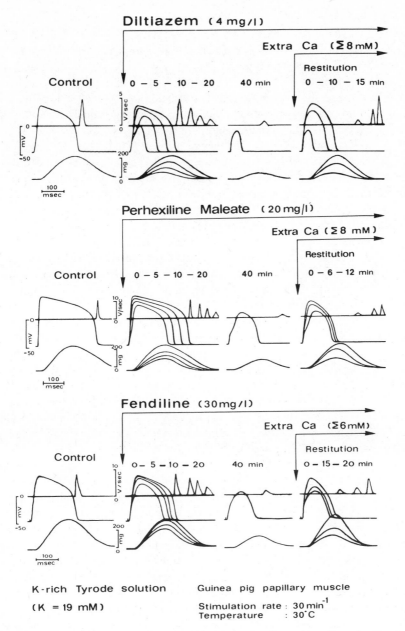

FIGURE 37. Same as Figure 36, however with the use of diltiazem (4 mg/l), perhexiline maleate (20 mg/l), and fendiline (30 mg/l).

experiments with verapamil and D 600 (Tritthart, Volkmann, Weiss, and Fleckenstein, 1973) and later with nifedipine (Kohlhardt and Fleckenstein, 1977). But recent studies of Späh and Fleckenstein (1978/1980) have ascertained that this applies to all Ca antagonists listed in Table 4. Figures 36 and 37 represent observations with nifedipine (0.2 mg/l), D 600 (0.4 mg/l), verapamil (2 mg/l), diltiazem (4 mg/l), perhexiline maleate (20 mg/l), and fendiline (30 mg/l). In all these experiments, the first step consisted of exposing guinea pig papillary muscles, electrically stimulated with 30 impulses/min, to a K-rich (19 mM KCl) Tyrode solution with normal Ca content (2 mM). The time of incubation in the depolarizing solution was 30 min so that the Ca-mediated action potentials and the isometric-contraction amplitudes could reach an absolutely constant steady-state level. Then in a second step, the Ca antagonists were added to the K-rich (19 mM K) Ca-containing (2 mM Ca) Tyrode solution, and the resulting changes in both the Ca-dependent action potentials and the isometric mechanograms monitored. As can easily be seen from the superimposed traces registered with a storage oscilloscope and from a graphic evaluation of the records, Ca antagonists and Ca deficiency produce quite similar effects on the partially depolarized myocardium. Obviously in both cases, the time course of inhibition of the Ca-mediated action potentials coincides with the development of contractile incompetence. On the other hand, when the Ca antagonists are neutralized by increasing the Ca concentration up to 6 or 8 mM, the bioelectric membrane activity of the partially depolarized myocardium again recovers more or less in parallel with the mechanical performance.

Partially depolarized ventricular myocardium offers unique possibilities of testing in this way the quantitative correlation between transmembrane Ca influx, as indicated by the bioelectric parameters of the Ca-mediated action potentials, and the mechanical responses. Thus the upstroke velocity (dV/dt_{max}) of Ca-mediated action potentials indicates the *intensity* of transsarcolemmal Ca influx through the slow channel, whereas the duration of a Ca-mediated action potential marks the *length of time of Ca entry*. The diagrams shown in Figures 38, 39, and 40 prove the existence of a linear relationship between the diminution of isometric tension development (on the ordinate) and the decrease in the bioelectric parameters (on the abscissa) under the influence of various Ca antagonists (verapamil, D 600, nifedipine, prenylamine, fendiline, and diltiazem), irrespective of the nature and the concentration of the individual drug used. In fact, as is evident from the graphs shown in Figures 38 and 39, isometric peak tension always declines to approximately the same extent as the different Ca antagonists inhibit upstroke velocity (dV/dt_{max}) and duration of the Ca-mediated action potentials. Moreover, in Figure 40, the areas of the Ca-mediated action potentials are plotted against the pertinent areas of the Ca-dependent isometric mechanograms. Each area circumscribed by an action-potential trace reflects the approximate amount of transferred Ca, whereas the area of the Ca-dependent isometric mechanograms represents tension time as the most appropriate parameter of contractile performance. As shown in Figure 40, in this case a linear correlation between the reduction of bioelectric and mechanical activity is also established. Hence the conclusion is justified that the various Ca antagonists tested on partially depolarized myocardium inhibit contractile force, as a rule, to

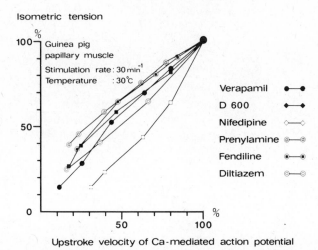

FIGURE 38. Linear relationship between the decrease of isometric peak tension and the reduction of upstroke velocity (dV/dt_{max}) of the Ca-mediated action potentials under the influence of various Ca antagonists. The control data ($= 100\%$) were obtained on partially depolarized guinea pig papillary muscles after incubation in a K-rich (19 mM) Ca-containing (2 mM) Tyrode solution for 30 min. Then each Ca antagonist was applied in different effective concentrations for 20 to 40 min until the definite changes on the Ca-dependent action potentials and mechanograms were measured.

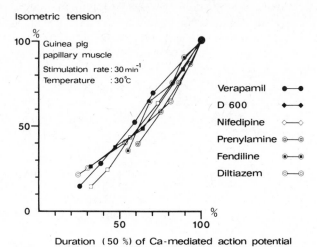

FIGURE 39. Linear relationship between the decrease of isometric peak tension and the reduction of the plateau phase (determined at 50% repolarization) of the Ca-mediated action potentials under the influence of various Ca antagonists. For these measurements the same muscles as in the experiments of Figure 38 were used.

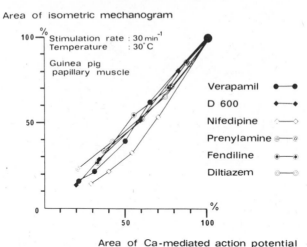

FIGURE 40. Linear relationship between the decrease of the area of the isometric mechanograms and the reduction of the area of the Ca-mediated action potentials under the influence of various Ca antagonists. Experimental procedure as in Figures 38 and 39.

the same extent as they are capable of diminishing the slow transsarcolemmal inward Ca current. In this respect, Ca antagonists and simple Ca withdrawal have identical results. Thus any major influence of Ca antagonists on intracellular Ca movements in addition to their decisive inhibitory effects on transsarcolemmal Ca supply appears very unlikely. Pertinent investigations of other research groups on cat ventricular trabeculae and papillary muscles (Nawrath, Ten Eick, McDonald, and Trautwein, 1977; McDonald and Trautwein, 1978a,b; McDonald, Pelzer, and Trautwein, 1980) as well as on Purkinje fibers (Kass and Tsien, 1975; Siegelbaum, Tsien, and Kass, 1977), have unanimously confirmed that verapamil and D 600 are, in fact, extremely potent inhibitors of the slow Ca-dependent inward current (I_{si}). A concomitant reduction in the delayed outward current (I_k) turned out to be mainly a consequence of a decrease in the intracellular Ca concentration, resulting from the inhibition of I_{si} (Siegelbaum, Tsien, and Kass, 1977).

2.6. INVERSION BY CALCIUM ANTAGONISTS OF THE POSITIVE-STAIRCASE PHENOMENON—ANOTHER MANIFESTATION OF THE BLOCKADE OF TRANSSARCOLEMMAL CALCIUM SUPPLY

The strength of myocardial contraction usually grows with a higher stimulation frequency (positive-staircase phenomenon). This is also true of partially depolarized myocardium. As shown in Figure 41, the isometric-contraction amplitude of an isolated guinea pig papillary muscle in a K-rich (19 mM) Ca-containing (2 mM Ca)

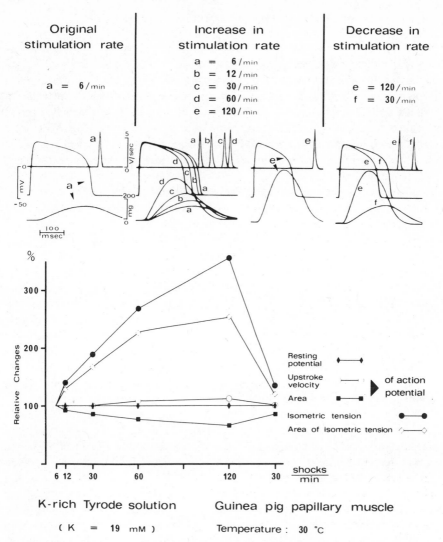

FIGURE 41. Large augmentation of the isometric mechanograms ("positive staircase phenomenon") of a partially depolarized guinea pig papillary muscle by increasing the rate of stimulation from 6 to 12, 30, 60, and finally 120 shocks/min in a Tyrode solution with 19 mM K and 2 mM Ca. At the high stimulation frequency of 120/min, isometric peak tension amounted to almost 360% of the original value measured at 6 shocks/min (= 100%). But regarding the concomitant changes of the Ca-dependent action-potential parameters, there was only a slight increase in upstroke velocity (dV/dt_{max}), whereas the plateau phase and the total circumscribed area of the action potentials were even diminished. When the stimulation rate was then reduced, all changes were rapidly reversed. The observations indicate that the intracellular Ca accumulation that underlies the positive staircase phenomenon is not due to an increase in the quantity of Ca entering the myocardial fibers per single membrane excitation, but only results from the closer succession of the Ca-carrying action potentials at higher stimulation rates.

Tyrode solution rose to almost 350% of the original height (= 100%) when the rate of stimulation was gradually increased from 6 to 120/min. However, in accordance with earlier reports (Beeler and Reuter, 1970b; Ochi and Trautwein, 1971), the slow inward current did not reflect the large intensification of the mechanical responses. In fact, as indicated by the rate of upstroke of the Ca-mediated action potentials, the slow inward Ca current was fully activated in our experiments at a stimulation frequency of 6/min and did not change in magnitude when contractile force was doubled at a stimulation rate of 60/min. Only at a stimulation frequency of 120/min, a slight increase of dV/dt_{max} occurred simultaneously with a more than threefold augmentation of isometric tension, whereas the duration of the Ca-mediated action potentials even diminished. Hence the amount of Ca transported through the slow channel per action potential is relatively independent of heart rate and does not undergo major changes as long as an excessive stimulation frequency is avoided. The positive-staircase phenomenon is certainly caused by a Ca accumulation in the cytoplasm that leads to a higher degree of Ca saturation of the sarcoplasmic, mitochondrial, and myofibrillar binding sites. Then contractile force grows until a new steady state is reached between intensified Ca uptake and extrusion. However, this intracellular Ca accumulation that manifests as the staircase phenomenon is only a consequence of the more rapid succession of the Ca-carrying action potentials rather than the result of an increase in Ca influx per impulse.

But there is a fundamental change as soon as a Ca antagonist is administered. In fact, one of the most obvious actions of a Ca-antagonistic drug is to reverse the positive-staircase phenomenon and to induce a rapid cessation of contractility if partially depolarized myocardium is subjected to an increased rate of stimulation. Two typical experiments are shown in Figure 42. Here, under the influence of nifedipine (0.2 mg/l) and verapamil (1 mg/l), contractile force gradually declined to zero in consequence of a rise in stimulation frequency from 30 to 150 impulses/ min. Contractile failure always develops in such experiments *pari passu* with a progressive inability to produce Ca-mediated action potentials. Accordingly, there was again in all these cases a clear parallelism between the decrease of the bioelectric parameters (upstroke velocity, amplitude, and duration of the Ca-mediated action potentials) and the height of isometric peak tension (see Figure 43). The observations clearly show that under the influence of Ca antagonists, even a partial or latent blockade of the transmembrane Ca supply may become highly evident in the form of a negative-staircase phenomenon when the heart muscle is forced to make more frequent contractions.

Concerning the mechanism of action, it has already been pointed out that the Ca ions that enter the myocardial fiber through the slow channel are probably derived from an intermediate pool of superficially stored Ca ions in the outer layers of the sarcolemma membrane (see the scheme in Figure 13). The assumption is justified that the Ca antagonists, apart from a direct inhibitory action on the slow channel, also interfere with the processes of Ca binding at the myocardial fiber surface. So it was found by Nayler and Szeto (1972) that isolated cardiac sarcolemma membranes could be depleted of bound Ca by verapamil. According to Williamson, Woodrow, and Scarpa (1975), there are two different types of Ca storage in cardiac

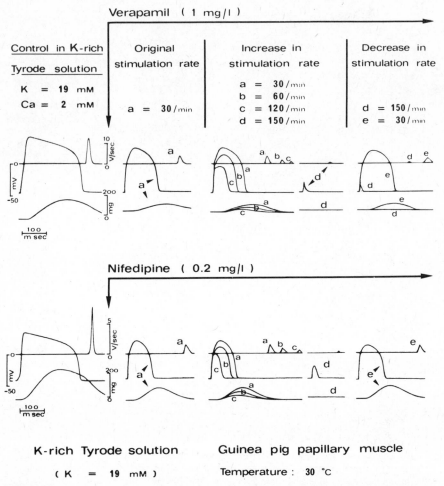

FIGURE 42. Pretreatment of two partially depolarized guinea pig papillary muscles with verapamil or nifedipine leads to a parallel breakdown of the Ca-mediated action potentials and isometric mechanograms as soon as the rate of stimulation is increased from 30 to 60, 120, and finally 150 shocks/min. Obviously small concentrations of verapamil (1 mg/l) or nifedipine (0.2 mg/l) are not only capable of inverting the normal positive staircase phenomenon into a negative one, but also of suppressing the electrogenesis of Ca-mediated action potentials at higher stimulation frequencies. From Späh and Fleckenstein, unpublished.

sarcolemma membranes, one at low- and another at high-affinity binding sites. Verapamil specifically inhibits low-affinity Ca binding (Williamson, Woodrow, and Scarpa, 1975). The effective verapamil concentration proved to be as low as 1,4 μM (Will and Schirpke; see Wollenberger, 1975). On the other hand, high-affinity Ca binding at the isolated myocardial sarcolemma membranes is not affected by verapamil. Thus the reduction in transsarcolemmal Ca transport that is brought about by verapamil and other Ca antagonists may result from the adverse effects

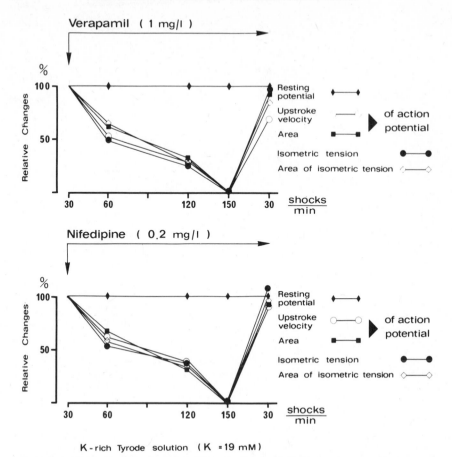

FIGURE 43. Perfect overlap of the progressive breakdown of the bioelectric and mechanical parameters of two partially depolarized guinea pig papillary muscles, pretreated with verapamil or nifedipine, following an increase in stimulation rate from 30 to 60, 120, and 150/min. Apparently the negative staircase phenomenon is closely correlated with a progressive deficiency in transsarcolemmal Ca supply through the slow channel as indicated by the almost complete disappearance of the Ca-mediated action potentials at a stimulation frequency of 150 shocks/min. This seems to be due to exhaustion of certain superficial Ca depots in the outer layers of the sarcolemma membrane. On the other hand, the bioelectric and mechanical functions of the verapamil- or nifedipine-pretreated muscles recover again in parallel upon return to the original stimulation rate of 30/min. The graphs represent evaluations of the experiments of Figure 42.

these drugs exert on the Ca-accumulating activity of these membrane-located storage sites. If this hypothesis is correct, then a principal action of the Ca antagonists would consist of impairing the Ca-binding capacity or the refilling of the superficial Ca depots in the sarcolemma membrane so that the availability of Ca to the slow channels is critically diminished. Under these conditions, high stimulation rates probably produce a precipitous exhaustion of the superficial Ca pool so that both electrogenic Ca influx and contractile force rapidly decline in parallel.

2.7. DISTINCTION BETWEEN CALCIUM ANTAGONISTS OF GROUP A AND GROUP B BY MEANS OF THEIR DIFFERENT INFLUENCES ON MYOCARDIAL TRANSMEMBRANE MAGNESIUM CONDUCTIVITY

During our investigations on partially depolarized guinea pig papillary muscles in a K-rich (19 mM KCl) Tyrode solution, it turned out that after suppression of fast-channel-mediated Na conductivity, action potentials could still be produced not only with Ca, but also with Mg ions as transmembrane electric-charge carriers. The latter effect is illustrated in Figure 44. Here, all electric or mechanical responses to any strength of stimulation disappeared within 6 min after the Ca content of the K-rich Tyrode solution had been lowered from 2 to 0.4 mM. But to our surprise, electric excitability recovered promptly upon addition of suitable amounts of MgCl$_2$ to the Ca-deficient K-rich Tyrode solution. For instance, at a Mg concentration of 14 mM, propagated Mg-carried action potentials with a fairly great overshoot appeared. When the Mg concentration was gradually augmented from 14 to 19 or 24 mM, there was even a further increase of overshoot height and duration of the Mg-mediated action potentials. However, as shown in Figure 45, the Mg-mediated action potentials differed considerably from those carried by Ca ions with respect to the following points:

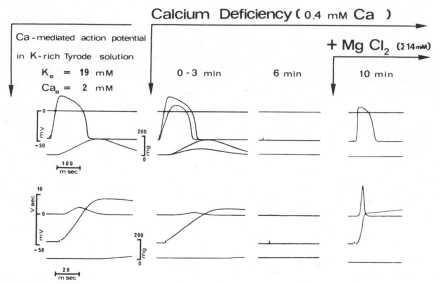

FIGURE 44.   Loss of electric excitability of a partially depolarized guinea pig papillary muscle in a K-rich (19 mM) Tyrode solution with low Ca (0.4 mM) within 6 min. Restitution of conducted action potentials by increasing the Mg concentration of the Ca-deficient solution up to 14 mM. The high-speed records of the rising phase and of the upstroke velocity (dV/dt_{max}) of the action potentials, in the lower part of the figure, show that the onset of the excitatory process is particularly rapid if carried by Mg. From Späh and Fleckenstein (1979).

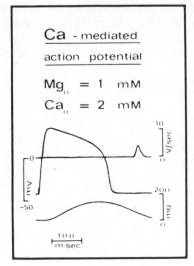

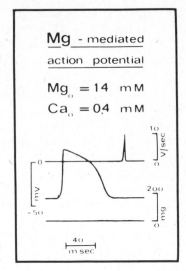

	Ca - mediated action potential	Mg - mediated action potentials		
	2 mM Ca_o	14 mM Mg_o	24 mM Mg_o	34 mM Mg_o
Upstroke velocity (V/sec)	6.5 ± 0.4	21.2 ± 3.5	33.7 ± 4.2	45.5 ± 4.7
Overshoot (mV)	35.3 ± 2.7	11.2 ± 2.6	22.8 ± 3.4	30.4 ± 5.3
Duration of action potential 50% Repolarisation (msec)	196.2 ± 12.6	63.6 ± 3.8	68.2 ± 4.5	75.3 ± 5.1
Duration of action potential 90% Repolarisation (msec)	218.7 ± 15.7	68.5 ± 4.7	77.8 ± 5.3	83.5 ± 5.6
Isometric tension (mg/mg muscle)	188.9 ± 13.2	<u>no</u> mechanical activity		

FIGURE 45. Characteristics of action potentials of partially depolarized guinea pig papillary muscles mediated by Ca or Mg ions. From Späh and Fleckenstein (1979).

1. The Mg-mediated action potentials are characterized by a rather high rate of rise, which is about three to seven times greater than that of Ca-carried action potentials. Obviously Mg ions pass the membrane with a comparably higher speed.

2. The duration of Mg-mediated action potentials is always shorter, that is, only about 40% of the Ca-carried action potentials.

3. The Mg-mediated action potentials never induce any mechanical response.

Taking account of further differences in drug susceptibility and voltage dependence, the conclusion was inevitable that in partially depolarized guinea pig myocardium after inactivation of the fast Na channel, two separate transmembrane carrier systems continue to operate, one for Ca, and another for Mg ions.

Naturally, in this situation, the question arose how specifically Ca antagonists can discriminate between the transmembrane Ca and Mg fluxes. The answer that we have obtained is clear: The highly specific Ca antagonists of group A, such as verapamil, D 600, diltiazem, nifedipine, and its derivatives niludipine, nimodipine, and ryosidine, selectively suppress the slow Ca currents but do not inhibit the Mg conductivity. By contrast, all Ca antagonists of group B tested so far (prenylamine, fendiline, terodiline, perhexiline maleate, caroverine) affect both the electrogenic Ca *and* Mg currents and therefore abolished both Ca- and Mg-carried action potentials.

The particular influences of the Ca antagonists of groups A and B could even be studied simultaneously in single experiments using "mixed" Ca/Mg-mediated action potentials (see Figure 46). This particular type of action potential appears regularly upon stimulation of partially depolarized papillary muscles in a K-rich Tyrode solution with 19 mM K, 2 mM Ca, and 14 mM Mg. Mixed action potentials are characterized by a biphasic upstroke: The first rapid phase is produced by the electrogenic inflow of Mg ions, followed by a second phase that is due to the slow inward current of Ca. Thus there is always a clearly visible notch in the rising phase of the mixed action potentials that signifies the point of transition from the first Mg-dependent to the second Ca-dependent part. The biphasic nature of the action-potential upstroke becomes even more evident if the bioelectric membrane activity is registered with a higher speed and, in addition, differentiated to visualize the individual rates of rise during the two successive upstroke phases. Then two distinct peaks of upstroke velocity will appear in the records, that is, a sharp Mg peak (*1*) at the beginning of the action potential, and a second blunt Ca peak (*2*) behind. In fact, in our experiments the highly specific Ca antagonists of group A only suppressed the Ca peak (*2*) together with contractility, but left the Mg peak (*1*) totally unchanged (Späh and Fleckenstein, 1979; Fleckenstein and Späh, 1981/1982). The selective abolition of the Ca peak (*2*) by nifedipine, D 600, verapamil, and diltiazem is shown in Figures 47 and 48. On the other hand, the Ca antagonists of group B are apparently unable to discriminate sufficiently between the two divalent cations. Thus in all our experiments with prenylamine, fendiline, terodiline, perhexiline maleate, or caroverine, the Mg peaks (*1*) were drastically lowered together with the Ca peaks (*2*). Figure 49 shows pertinent experiments with caroverine and perhexiline maleate.

In conclusion, only the Ca antagonists of group A, represented by verapamil and D 600, nifedipine and other 1,4-dihydropyridines as well as diltiazem fulfill the ultimate expectations on Ca-antagonistic specificity in that they can totally block the transsarcolemmal inward Ca current without any inhibitory influence on the myocardial Na and Mg conductivities. Hence the agents of group A have to be considered the top Ca antagonists. Interestingly enough, this judgment is not only based on our rather sophisticated studies of myocardial transmembrane ion movements, but also corresponds with clinical experiences. As a matter of fact, even on purely empirical grounds, clinical interest centers more and more on the drugs of group A.

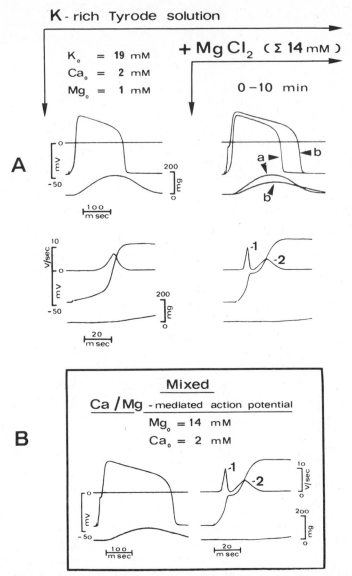

FIGURE 46. (A) Transformation within 10 min, of a pure Ca-mediated action potential, *a*, of a partially depolarized guinea pig papillary muscle to a mixed Mg/Ca-carried action potential, *b*, by increasing the Mg content of a K-rich (19 m*M*) Ca-containing (2 m*M*) Tyrode solution from 1 to 14 m*M*. As is obvious from the notch in the upper record of the mixed action potential and from the step in the lower (more rapid) tracing, there is a first quick phase of upstroke produced by the transmembrane influx of Mg and a second slow phase due to the entry of Ca. Accordingly, the differentiation curve reveals a sharp Mg-dependent peak, *1*, of dV/dt_{max} at the beginning of the mixed action potential and a subsequent blunt peak, *2*, related to the slow inward Ca current. Overshoot and duration of a mixed action potential, *b*, are always considerably greater than those of a pure Ca-mediated action potential, *a*. Nevertheless, the contractile response to a mixed action potential is weaker than that to a pure Ca-carried action potential. (B) Final shape of a mixed Mg/Ca-carried action potential at a steady state after 10 min. Stimulation rate, 30/min; temperature 30°C. From Späh and Fleckenstein (1979).

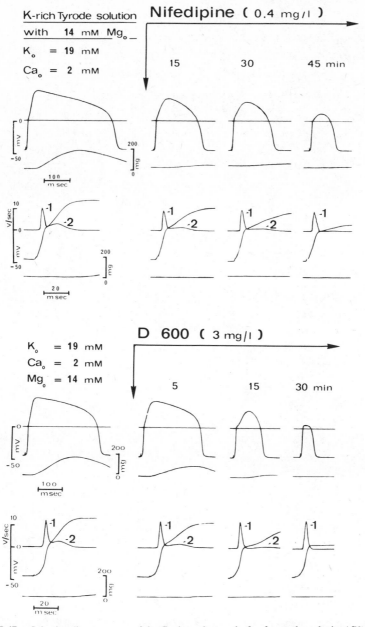

FIGURE 47. Selective disappearance of the Ca-dependent peak, *2*, of upstroke velocity (dV/dt_{max}) of a mixed Mg/Ca-carried action potential under the influence of the powerful Ca antagonists nifedipine and D 600. No effect of nifedipine and D 600 on the Mg-dependent peak, *1*. After 30 to 45 min, the remaining bioelectric activity is exclusively mediated by the Mg influx. Experiments on isolated guinea pig papillary muscles. Stimulation rate, 30/min; temperature 30°C. From Späh and Fleckenstein (1979).

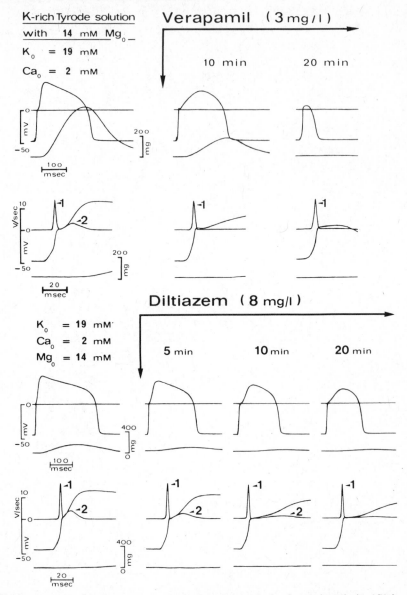

FIGURE 48. Selective suppression of the Ca-dependent peak, *2*, of upstroke velocity (dV/dt_{max}) of mixed Mg/Ca-carried action potentials by verapamil and diltiazem. No influence on the Mg-peak, *1*. Experimental procedure as in Figure 47. From Späh and Fleckenstein (1979) and Fleckenstein and Späh (1981/1982).

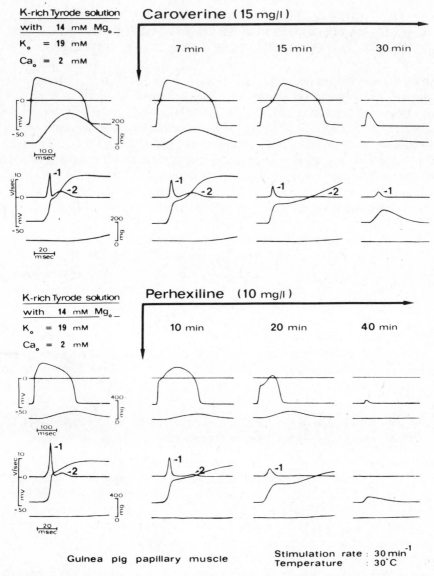

K-rich Tyrode solution
with 14 mM Mg_o
K_o = 19 mM
Ca_o = 2 mM

Caroverine (15 mg/l)

7 min   15 min   30 min

K-rich Tyrode solution
with 14 mM Mg_o
K_o = 19 mM
Ca_o = 2 mM

Perhexiline (10 mg/l)

10 min   20 min   40 min

Guinea pig papillary muscle

Stimulation rate : 30 min^{-1}
Temperature : 30°C

FIGURE 49. The Ca antagonists of group B do not discriminate between divalent Ca and Mg ions. Therefore, caroverine and perhexiline (maleate) inhibit simultaneously both the Mg-dependent peak, *1*, and the Ca-dependent peak, *2*, of the mixed Mg/Ca-carried action potentials. Experimental procedures as in Figure 47. From Fleckenstein and Späh (1981/1982).

2.8.   NEUTRALIZATION OF THE INHIBITORY ACTION OF CALCIUM ANTAGONISTS ON TRANSSARCOLEMMAL CALCIUM INFLUX AND CONTRACTILITY BY CALCIUM PROMOTERS

As already noted in the foregoing chapters, the inhibitory effects of Ca antagonists on myocardial tension development can be readily overcome not only by increasing the extracellular Ca concentration above normal but also by administration of β-adrenergic catecholamines. Moreover in our experiments, some indirectly acting sympathomimetics as well as nicotine, histamine, and dibutyryl cylic AMP proved to be capable of neutralizing the cardiodepression exerted by Ca antagonists. Although the particular mode of action is not identical, all these "Ca promoters" eventually restore the transmembrane Ca supply. There are two principal criteria that are indicative of a potentiation of the myocardial slow inward Ca current:

1.   A positive inotropic effect within a large range of membrane potential, even in a Ca-deficient solution or in the presence of Ca antagonists.

2.   A parallel recovery of both Ca-mediated action potentials and contractile force in partially depolarized myocardium after previous depression with high extracellular K concentrations, low Ca concentrations, or Ca antagonists.

As depicted in the following sections, the Ca antagonists and the Ca promoters counteract each other by their opposite influences on the myocardial fiber membrane in almost every respect.

2.8.1.   Promotion of the Slow Calcium Current by Direct or Indirect β-Receptor Stimulation with Sympathomimetic Amines or Nicotine

The action of β-adrenergic catecholamines is the clearest, because in this case the recovery of contractility apparently results from the resuscitation of the slow inward Ca current. Partially depolarized myocardium is again very suitable for the simultaneous registration of Ca-mediated action potentials (roughly indicating intensity, duration, and magnitude of transsarcolemmal Ca inflow) and the mechanical responses. In fact, even in the absence of Ca-antagonistic agents, administration of β-adrenergic catecholamines largely amplifies the Ca-carried action potentials and the isometric mechanograms. As an example, Figure 50 shows two rather old experiments from our laboratory on partially depolarized papillary muscles excised from a guinea pig and a rhesus monkey heart. Both muscles had eventually become inexcitable in a K-rich Tyrode solution. But as soon as adrenaline was added, they regained the ability to conduct propagated action potentials and contracted vigorously. In publishing these striking observations, Engstfeld, Antoni, and Fleckenstein (1961) stressed that these action potentials exhibited very unusual characteristics and differed from normal Na-carried action potentials by the low level of resting potential (-40 to -45 mV) at which they could be elicited, as well as by an extremely small upstroke velocity and propagation rate. Needless to say, the pe-

Isolated papillary muscles

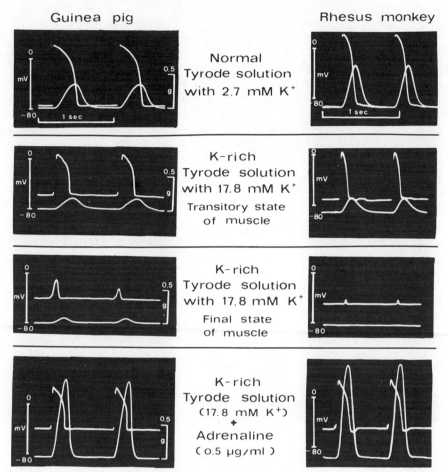

FIGURE 50. Restitution by adrenaline of propagated action potentials and of isometric contractile responses of even supernormal height on partially depolarized guinea pig and rhesus monkey papillary muscles in a K-rich Tyrode solution (17.8 m*M* K, 1.8 m*M* Ca) at 35°C. From Engstfeld, Antoni, and Fleckenstein (1961) and Antoni and Engstfeld (1961).

culiarities of this special type of adrenaline-supported action potentials depicted by us in 1961 and the circumstances of their origin in partially depolarized myocardium were consistent with the nowadays well-known features of Ca-mediated action potentials. In fact, extensive subsequent studies on the specific nature of the adrenaline-supported action potentials have definitely established that in this case the Ca ions act as the decisive electric-charge carriers (see Reuter, 1965; Vassort, Rougier, Garnier, Sauviat, Coraboeuf, and Gargouil, 1969; Carmeliet and Vereecke, 1969; Mascher, 1970; Pappano, 1970; Reuter, 1974; Thyrum, 1974; Schneider and Sperelakis, 1975). Accordingly, the action potentials restored by β-adrenergic stimulation were insensitive to tetrodotoxin, but varied directly with the external Ca concentration.

The same revival of electric excitability, impulse conduction, and contractility as with adrenaline can also be induced, according to our observations on K-polarized papillary muscles and atria, with the help of many other sympathomimetic amines. A list of the effective substances presented by Fleckenstein (1964b) is given in Table 5. Interestingly enough, not only the first group of sympathomimetic amines with a direct β-receptor-stimulating action (adrenaline, noradrenaline, isoproterenol, neosynephrine, epinine, and etilefrine) but also the second group of indirect sympathomimetrics *("Neurosympathomimetics")* that comprises β-phenylethylamine, tyramine, amphetamine, methamphetamine, and pholedrine proved to be highly efficient. The latter substances merely operate as releasers of endogenous sympathetic transmitters, especially noradrenaline from neuronal or other depots (Fleckenstein and Burn, 1953; Fleckenstein, 1953; Fleckenstein and Stöckle, 1955; Muscholl, 1966). Therefore, all these indirect catecholamines lost their restorative power in catecholamine-depleted hearts after the animals had been pretreated for some days with reserpine. Nicotine is another positive inotropic agent that behaved in our experiments on partially depolarized myocardium like an indirect "neurosympathomimetic" agent, that is to say, was neutralized by adrenergic β-receptor blockade or previous catecholamine depletion, thus confirming earlier reports of Bassett and Gelband, (1974). On the other hand, K-depolarized heart muscle preparations dissected from nonreserpinized control animals still fully responded to the catecholamine releasers even if the isolated tissue had been washed in a K-rich Tyrode solution for many hours.

Obviously the normal heart is able to store considerable amounts of adrenaline and noradrenaline along the interstitial ramifications of sympathetic neurons and, under certain conditions, even in the myocardial fibers. Thus autoradiographic studies of Leder and Fleckenstein (1963/1965) on rats revealed that after intravenous administration of one single acute dose of ^{14}C-labeled noradrenaline, most of the injected radioactivity accumulated within 1 min in the cardiac musculature (besides a somewhat smaller uptake in the renal cortex, suprarenal medulla, and pineal gland). Iversen (1965) designated this rapid myocardial catecholamine accumulation "uptake 2." When, however, only a small dose of ^{14}C-labeled noradrenaline was infused slowly over a period of 20 min, the radioactivity of the ventricular wall was predominantly centered in the interstitial space, corresponding to the location of neuronal or chromaffine tissue structures. The observations are consistent with quantitative data from other laboratories that also pointed to the large capacity of normal hearts for catecholamine storage (Holtz, Kroneberg, and Schümann, 1951; Muscholl, 1959; Titus and Dengler, 1966). After all, it is clear that small, isolated papillary muscles from normal guinea pig, rabbit, cat, or monkey hearts still yield enough catecholamines to maintain or restore the Ca transport through the slow channel, if one of the indirectly acting sympathomimetic agents listed in Table 5 or nicotine is administered.

TABLE 5. List of Direct and Indirect Sympathomimetics that Lead to Recovery of Propagated Action Potentials in Partially K-Depolarized Guinea Pig, Rat, Rabbit, Cat, or Monkey Papillary Muscles and Atria[a]

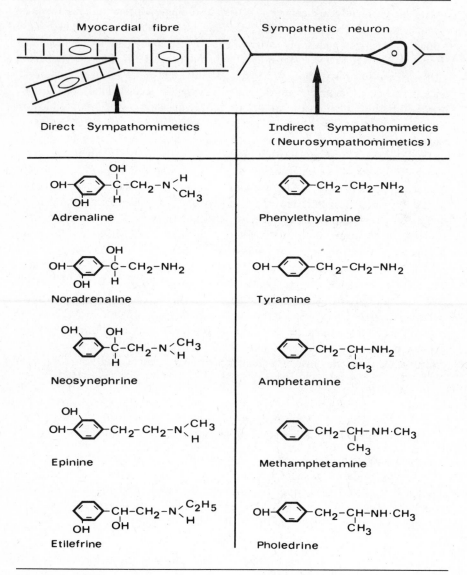

[a]Fleckenstein (1964b).

2.8.2. Promotion of the Slow Calcium Current by H₂-Receptor Stimulation with Histamine

It is well known that histamine too exerts positive inotropic effects in guinea pig and rabbit hearts (Trendelenburg, 1960). Accordingly, histamine was found to stimulate the slow Ca current and to restore the electric and mechanical activity of partially depolarized guinea pig myocardium just like β-adrenergic catecholamines (Houki, 1973; Vornovitskii, Ignat'eva, and Khodorov, 1974; Inui and Imamura, 1976). Hence upstroke velocity, height, and duration of Ca-mediated action potentials as well as contractile force of partially depolarized papillary muscles are increased by histamine in a form that is indistinguishable by electrophysiological techniques from the effects of β-adrenergic catecholamines such as adrenaline or isoproterenol. However, the receptors involved are different, since the positive inotropic action of histamine on the ventricular myocardium is insensitive to adrenergic β-receptor blockade, whereas it can be suppressed specifically by H₂-receptor antagonists such as burimamide, metiamide, or cimetidine. However, the cardiac histamine receptors are not homogenous. For instance, the chronotropic pacemaker effects depend on H₁-receptor activation (Reinhardt, Wagner, and Schümann, 1974; Steinberg and Holland, 1975; Ledda, Fantozzi, Mugelli, Moroni, and Mannaioni, 1974). But as far as tension development in the ventricular myocardium is concerned, clear evidence of a decisive involvement of the histamine H₂-receptors exists. This even applies to embryonic chick ventricular myocardial cells (Josephson, Renaud, Vogel, McLean, and Sperelakis, 1976). Thus stimulation of histaminergic H₂-receptors is a second principal way of increasing the ventricular slow inward Ca current besides the promotion of β-adrenergic mechanisms. Therefore, in our experiments histamine was also capable of neutralizing the negative inotropic effects of Ca deficiency or of Ca antagonists (see Figures 52 and 53).

2.8.3. Key Role of Cyclic AMP as Mediator between β- or H₂-Receptor Stimulation and the Promotion of Transsarcolemmal Calcium Supply

Although sympathomimetic amines and histamine act on different receptors, there is increasing evidence in support of the hypothesis that the decisive biochemical reaction that all these drugs induce is identical, namely the formation of cyclic AMP. The concept that cyclic AMP eventually mediates the increase in transsarcolemmal Ca supply is based on the following observations:

1. All β-adrenergic catecholamines tested so far augment the cyclic AMP content of cardiac tissue (Sutherland, Robison, and Butcher, 1968; Kukovetz and Pöch, 1972; Kukovetz, Pöch, and Wurm, 1973; Tsien, Giles, and Greengard, 1972; Watanabe and Besch, 1974a, b, 1975).

2. Histamine too, but only by stimulation of H₂-receptors, increases the cyclic AMP levels in ventricular myocardium (Klein and Levey, 1971; McNeill

and Muschek, 1972; McNeill and Verma, 1974; Reinhardt, Schmidt, Brodde, and Schümann, 1977).

3. The promoter action of β-adrenergic catecholamines or histamine on Ca-mediated ventricular action potentials and contractility is quantitatively correlated with the elevation of the cyclic AMP concentration. The rise in cyclic AMP levels precedes the restoration of contractility in partially depolarized hearts (Watanabe and Besch 1974a, b, 1975; Reinhardt, Schmidt, Brodde, and Schümann, 1977). On the other hand, blockade of adrenergic β-receptors or H_2-receptors inhibits the positive inotropic actions of β-sympathomimetics and histamine to a similar extent as it reduces the increases in the cyclic AMP concentration.

4. Cyclic AMP directly administered as dibutyryl cyclic AMP or by iontophoresis mimics the effects of both β-adrenergic and H_2-receptor stimulation in ventricular myocardium and Purkinje fibers, in that it enhances transsarcolemmal inward Ca current and contractile force (Skelton, Levey, and Epstein, 1970; Kukovetz and Pöch, 1970; Drummond and Hemmings, 1972; Tsien, 1973; Meinertz, Nawrath, and Scholz, 1973a, b; Entman, 1974; Reuter, 1974). These actions of cyclic AMP are insensitive to β- or H_2-receptor blockade and to previous catecholamine depletion of the hearts with reserpine (see Table 6).

Hence the conclusion is justified that the stimulation of adrenergic β-receptors or histaminergic H_2-receptors leads to activation of adenylate cyclase, which, in turn, produces cyclic AMP as a "second messenger." The further sequence of events is still a matter of speculation. However, as already discussed in Section 1.4.1, cyclic AMP is likely to promote phosphorylation of sarcolemmal proteins by a membrane-bound protein kinase, thus augmenting the number of fixed negative charges suitable for Ca accumulation in the outer layers of the sarcolemma membrane (see Figure 13). Thereby the capacity of these superficial Ca stores would be enlarged so that the uptake of free Ca ions from the interstitial fluid would be increased and the subsequent transsarcolemmal influx through the slow channel potentiated. This new concept necessarily implies that the promoters of the slow Ca current, by accumulating Ca at superficially located binding sites outside the slow channel, strengthen the driving force of the slow inward Ca current rather than simply increasing the passive transmembrane Ca conductivity of the excited sarcolemma membrane. Or in other words, the suggestion seems reasonable that the promoters of the slow Ca influx listed in Tables 5 and 6 not only favor transmembrane Ca movements along a preexisting concentration gradient from outside to inside the myocardial fiber, but steepen this gradient. This hypothesis could explain how the Ca promoters are able to restore the slow inward Ca current not only in the presence of Ca antagonists but also in a Ca-deficient medium after the slope of the normal Ca gradient has been critically lowered. The latter effect was shown in Figure 14, using adrenaline. Our more recent experiments, represented in Figures 51 and 52, illustrate the resuscitation of the Ca-mediated action potentials and of the concomitant contractile

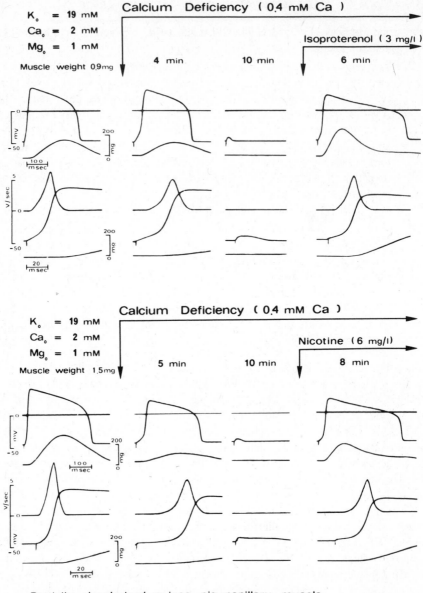

FIGURE 51. Suppresion of Ca-mediated action potentials and contractility of two partially depolarized guinea pig papillary muscles by immersion in a Ca-deficient (0.4 mM Ca) K-rich (19 mM K) Tyrode solution for 10 min. After cessation of the bioelectric and mechanical activities, a more or less complete recovery was obtained by adding isoproterenol or nicotine into the Ca-deficient media.

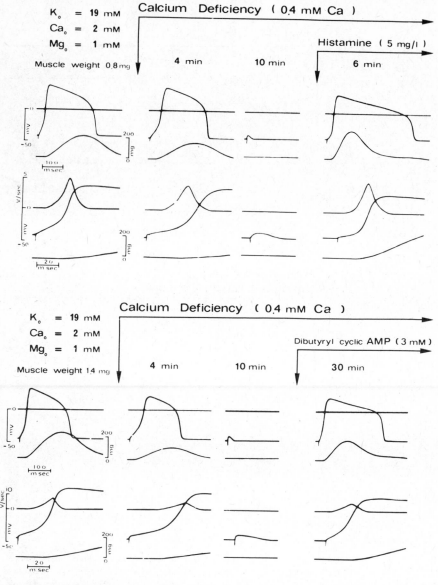

Partially depolarized guinea pig papillary muscle
Stimulation rate : 30 min^{-1} Temperature : 30 °C

FIGURE 52. Same as Figure 51, however with the use of histamine or dibutyryl cyclic AMP. Isoproterenol, nicotine, and histamine (as well as all other Ca-promoters listed in Table 5) are fully effective within 6 to 8 min, whereas the restitution with dibutyryl cyclic AMP always requires 25 to 30 min. This is probably due to the slow rate of transformation of dibutyryl cyclic AMP into cyclic AMP.

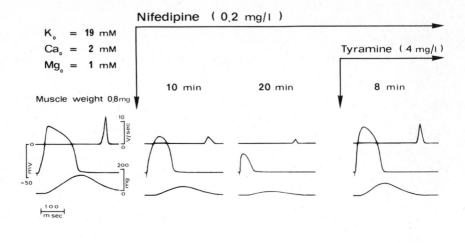

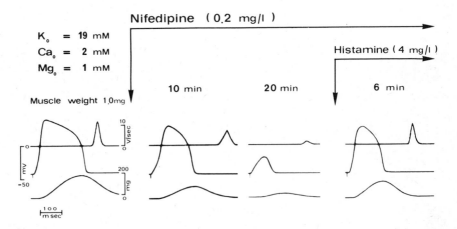

Partially depolarized guinea pig papillary muscle

Stimulation rate : 30 min^{-1} Temperature : 30 °C

FIGURE 53. Suppression by nifedipine (0.2 mg/l) of the Ca-mediated action potentials and mechanical responses of two partially depolarized guinea pig papillary muscles in a K-rich (19 m*M*) Tyrode solution with normal Ca content (2 m*M*). After the muscles had been exposed to the nifedipine-containing media for 20 min, the Ca promoters tyramine or histamine were added in order to restore the bioelectric and mechanical activity. In fact, as in the case of simple Ca deficiency (see Figures 51 and 52), all Ca promoters listed in Tables 5 and 6 proved to be capable of inducing a parallel recovery of the Ca-mediated action potentials and the contractile responses in the presence of the Ca-antagonistic inhibitors.

responses of four partially depolarized guinea pig papillary muscles in a Ca-deficient (0.4 m*M* Ca) Tyrode solution with the help of the Ca promoters isoproterenol, nicotine, histamine, and dibutyryl cyclic AMP. Analogous observations on four partially depolarized guinea pig papillary muscles pretreated with the Ca antagonists nifedipine or verapamil are shown in Figures 53 and 54. Here the Ca promoters tyramine, histamine, nicotine, and dibutyryl cyclic AMP were used for restitution of the Ca-dependent bioelectric and mechanical functions. Some other pertinent experiments on papillary muscles in normal Tyrode solution can be seen from Figures 23 and 24*B*.

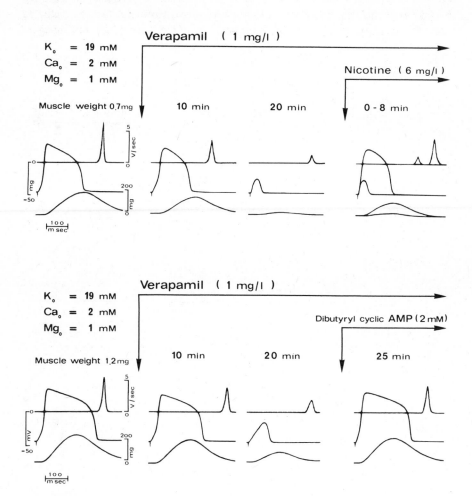

Partially depolarized guinea pig papillary muscle
Stimulation rate : 30 min^{-1} Temperature : 30 °C

FIGURE 54. Same as Figure 53, however with the use of nicotine or dibutyryl cyclic AMP for neutralization of the verapamil effects.

2.8.4. Reciprocal Inhibition of Myocardial Transsarcolemmal Magnesium Conductivity by Calcium Promoters

In the course of our studies on the electrogenic transsarcolemmal Mg movements, an important, hitherto unknown effect of the Ca promoters was discovered. The compounds that potentiate, according to the preceding investigations, the slow inward Ca current in partially depolarized guinea pig papillary muscles are capable of simultaneously blocking all Mg-dependent bioelectric phenomena (Späh and Fleckenstein, 1979). For instance, two experiments are shown in Figure 55 in which Mg-mediated action potentials (see Section 2.7) were totally abolished by adrenaline (1 mg/l) or isoproterenol (0.5 mg/l) within 4 to 5 min. However, the Mg-mediated action potentials were fully restored upon addition of the β-receptor blocking agent

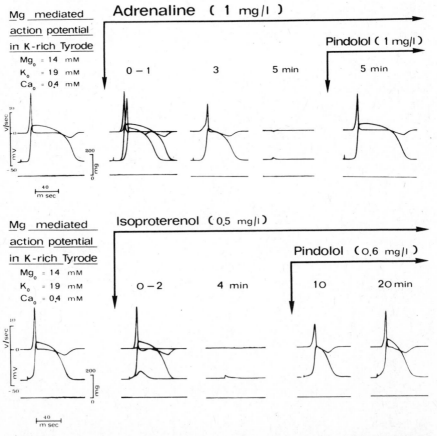

FIGURE 55. Suppression of Mg-mediated action potentials by β-receptor stimulation with adrenaline (upper experiment) or with isoproterenol (lower experiment). Restoration of the Mg-mediated action potentials by β-receptor blockade with pindolol. Parallel changes of upstroke velocity (dV/dt_{max}) in the upper tracing of each experiment. Guinea pig papillary muscles; stimulation rate, 30/min; temperature, 30°C. From Späh and Fleckenstein (1979).

pindolol. An identical suppression of the electrogenic Mg movements was also obtained with all other types of Ca promoters yet tested (further β-adrenergic catecholamines; noradrenaline releasers such as tyramine or nicotine; dibutyryl cyclic AMP; histamine). The histamine-induced inhibition of the Mg-mediated action potentials could be neutralized only by H_2-receptor blockade with burimamide, metiamide, or cimetidine, whereas the inhibitory effect of dibutyryl cyclic AMP was removable merely by washing the agent off. The drug concentrations and the circumstances under which the Mg-dependent bioelectric activity disappeared corresponded exactly to those under which the slow inward Ca current approached its maximum. This indicated that always when the slow Ca current rises above normal following β- or H_2-receptor stimulation or administration of dibutyryl cyclic AMP, there is simultaneously an inhibition of the transsarcolemmal Mg-ion conductivity. Hence activation of the slow inward Ca current seems to be correlated with a reciprocal suppression of the Mg influx. Or in other words, cyclic AMP seems to potentiate the transsarcolemmal influx of Ca at the expense of Mg. Conversely, following blockade of adrenergic β-receptors or histaminergic H_2-receptors, the high catecholamine- or histamine-stimulated Ca fluxes return to normal while the transsarcolemmal Mg conductivity recovers.

Further decisive evidence came from extensive studies on "mixed" Mg/Ca-mediated action potentials that allow a *simultaneous* assessment of the electrogenic Mg and Ca fluxes on partially depolarized guinea pig myocardium (see Section 2.7). In fact, as shown in Figure 56, adrenaline (via β-receptor stimulation) or dibutyryl cyclic AMP (in a more direct way) influence the Mg-dependent peak (*1*) in the differentiation curve (dV/dt_{max}) *reciprocally* to the Ca-dependent peak (*2*). Whereas the sharp Mg peak (*1*) progressively declines, the blunt Ca peak (*2*), mirroring the transmembrane Ca current, largely increases together with the isometric mechanogram. Simultaneously, the Mg-dependent rapid initial upstroke phase and the notch in the mixed Mg/Ca action potentials disappear. Figure 57 represents two analogous experiments with the noradrenaline releasers tyramine and nicotine. There is again a tremendous potentiation of the Ca peak (*2*) and the contractile responses while the Mg peak (*1*) vanishes. If, however, the isolated papillary muscles originate from guinea pigs pretreated during some days with reserpine for catecholamine depletion, tyramine and nicotine lose their power (see Figure 58). Then neither the Mg peak (*1*) nor the Ca peak (*2*) changes. But the reserpine pretreatment does not, of course, interfere with the responsiveness of these peaks to adrenaline. Lastly, the typical reciprocity of the Mg/Ca-conductivity changes also manifests itself under the influence of histamine (see Figure 59). Here, again, the enormous enlargement of the Ca peak (*2*) is conpensated for by a complete disappearance of the Mg peak (*1*). Histamine obviously acts by H_2-receptor stimulation, since H_2-receptor blockade with cimetidine reverses the histamine effects, whereas the H_1-receptor blocking agent bamipine (Soventol®) is ineffective.

Concerning the physiological significance of these observations, one should remember that the Ca and Mg ions are natural competitors: They counteract each other as far as accumulation by the myocardial fibers is concerned (for more details see Section 3.5) and also exert opposite functional effects with respect to their

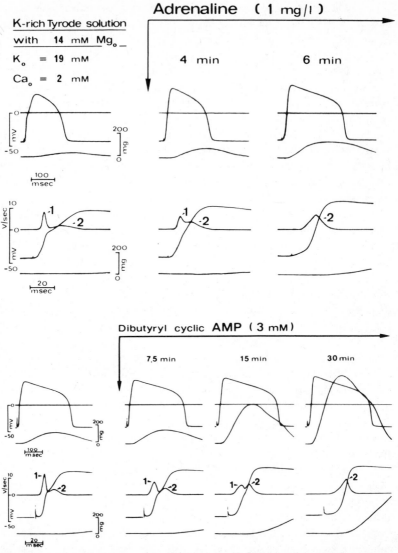

FIGURE 56. Reciprocal effects of adrenergic β-receptor stimulation with adrenaline or of administration of dibutyryl cyclic AMP on the Mg- and Ca-mediated bioelectric membrane activities. Suppression of the Mg-dependent peak, *1*, of upstroke velocity (dV/dt_{max}) of mixed Mg/Ca-carried action potentials simultaneously with a maximum reinforcement of the Ca-dependent peak, *2*. Isometric tension grows with inhibition of transmembrane Mg conductivity and potentiation of Ca inflow. Experiments on partially depolarized guinea pig papillary muscles. Temperature 30°C; stimulation rate, 30/min. From Fleckenstein and Späh (1981/1982).

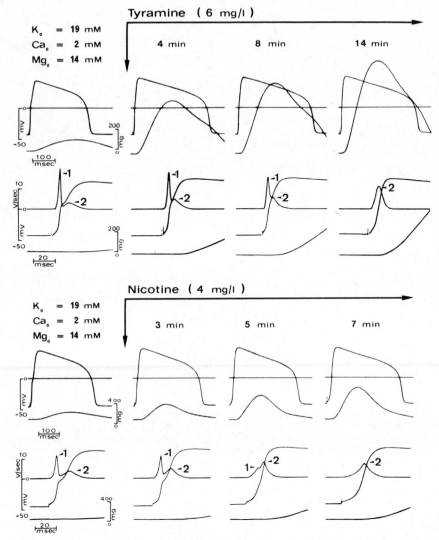

FIGURE 57. Reciprocal influence of the catecholamine releasers tyramine and nicotine on the transmembrane Mg and Ca conductivities of partially depolarized guinea pig papillary muscles. Compensatory suppression of the Mg-dependent peak, *1*, of upstroke velocity (dV/dt_{max}) of mixed Mg/Ca-mediated action potentials, simultaneously with extreme potentiation of the Ca peak, *2*. Experimental conditions as in Figure 56. From Späh and Fleckenstein, unpublished.

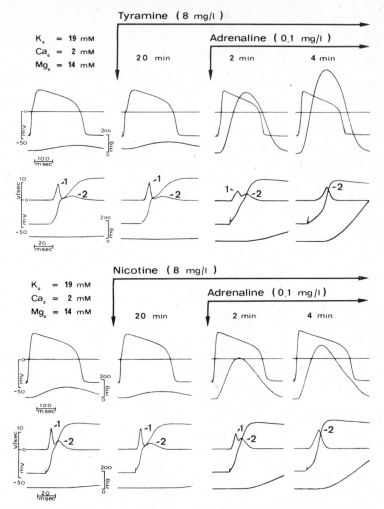

FIGURE 58. Isolated papillary muscles dissected from reserpine-pretreated guinea pigs (daily dose of 0.6 mg reserpine/kg body weight for 3 days). Following catecholamine depletion by reserpine, the catecholamine releasers tyramine and nicotine lose their influence on myocardial Ca and Mg conductivity, whereas the responsiveness to adrenaline not only perists, but even seems to be potentiated. From Späh and Fleckenstein, unpublished.

influence on excitation–contraction coupling. For instance, in skinned ventricular muscle fibers, the Ca-triggered Ca release from the SR is antagonized to a considerable extent when Mg ions are present (Fabiato and Fabiato, 1978). Thus the Ca promoters not only potentiate contractile tension development by enhancing transmembrane Ca supply, but also maximize this effect by restricting the natural Ca-antagonistic influence of Mg.

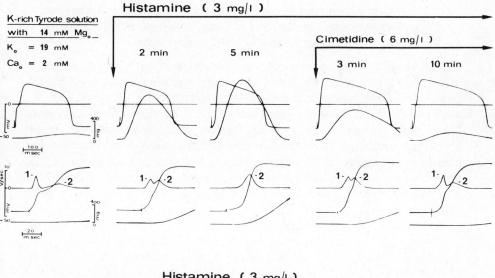

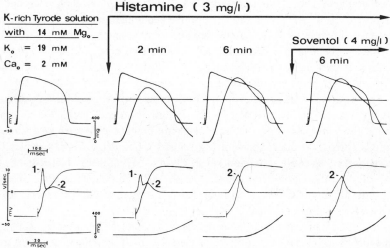

FIGURE 59. Reciprocal influence of histaminergic H_2-receptor stimulation on the Mg- and Ca-mediated bioelectric membrane activities of partially depolarized guinea pig papillary muscles. Decrease of the Mg peak, *1, pari passu* with augmentation of the Ca peak, *2*. These effects are responsive to H_2-receptor blockade with cimetidine (upper experiment), but refractory to the H_1-receptor blocking agent bamipine (Soventol®) as shown in the lower picture. Experimental procedures as in Figure 56. From Späh and Fleckenstein, unpublished.

2.8.5.   A Comprehensive Concept of Interaction of Calcium Antagonists and Calcium Promoters in Myocardial Excitation–Contraction Coupling; Particular Effects of Cardiac Glycosides

Since 1964 innumerable observations of our laboratory with sympathetic amines as well as our later studies with other Ca promoters (nicotine, histamine, dibutyryl cyclic AMP) have accumulated overwhelming evidence that the action of these drugs on myocardial transmembrane Ca conductivity contrasts diametrically with that of the Ca antagonists. Obviously, all Ca antagonists can be neutralized, under appropriate experimental conditions, by administration of adequate amounts of Ca promoters. Conversely, all Ca promoters can be rendered ineffective when the Ca antagonists are applied in high concentration. Thus it depends mainly on the actual dose ratio whether the promoters or the inhibitors of the myocardial slow inward Ca current prevail.

Nevertheless, the mode of action of the Ca promoters and the possibilities of interfering with them are much more complex than those of the Ca antagonists. Table 6 summarizes the various drug interactions and in Figure 60, the pertinent data are condensed to a functional scheme. This conception centers around the production of cyclic AMP and the presumptive accumulation of Ca at superficially located phosphoproteins in the sarcolemma membrane and the slow channels. We are inclined to believe that under the influence of high doses of Ca promoters, so many Ca ions may be accumulated by mediation of cyclic AMP in this superficial pool that Mg is completely displaced and consequently hindered from transsarcolemmal permeation. This could explain the reciprocal influence of the Ca promoters on the transmembrane Ca and Mg conductivities. It should, however, be kept in mind that the formation of cyclic AMP not only potentiates the transsarcolemmal inward Ca current (at the expense of Mg transfer), but also enhances intracellular Ca storage. As discussed in Section 1.4.2, cyclic AMP probably increases the Ca-uptake rate and the Ca-binding capacity of the SR. This latter effect is likely to augment the amount of Ca that is available for "Ca-triggered" intracellular Ca release from the SR in subsequent beats.

On the other hand, it has hitherto not been possible to interpret the actions of Ca antagonists in biochemical terms. For instance, the Ca antagonists tested so far were unable to interfere with the formation of cyclic AMP. Watanabe and Besch (1974b) have presented evidence that verapamil and D 600, unlike β-receptor blocking agents, do not inhibit the isoproterenol-induced rise in the cyclic AMP content of guinea pig ventricular myocardium although these Ca antagonists suppressed the slow Ca current. In confirmation of these findings, Hoeschen (1977) reported that adenylate cyclase in purified subcellular sarcolemma membrane fractions from rat and guinea pig ventricular muscle is also insensitive to verapamil. Moreover, the Ca antagonists lack any clear influence on catecholamine-stimulated intracellular Ca uptake or Ca release by the SR. In fact, all observations, particularly with verapamil and D 600, indicate that the negative inotropic effects of Ca antagonists are due to simple competition with Ca (see also Bristow and Green, 1977). This interaction seems to take place only at specific Ca-binding sites in the superficial

TABLE 6. Promoters[a] and Inhibitors of the Slow Ca Current in Isolated Ventricular Myocardium

Promoters of the slow Ca-current in isolated ventricular myocardium	Possible interference with the promoters of the slow Ca-current			
	(a) adrenergic β-receptor blockade	(b) previous catecholamine depletion with reserpine	(c) H_2-receptor blockade	(d) application of Ca-antagonists
Direct sympathomimetics (see Table 5)	inhibition	no interference	no interference	inhibition
Indirect sympathomimetics "Neurosympathomimetics" (see Table 5)	inhibition	inhibition	no interference	inhibition
Nicotine	inhibition	inhibition	no interference	inhibition
Histamine	no interference	no interference	inhibition	inhibition
Dibutyryl cyclic AMP	no interference	no interference	no interference	inhibition

[a]All promoters of the slow Ca current reciprocally restrict the myocardial transmembrane Mg-ion conductivity

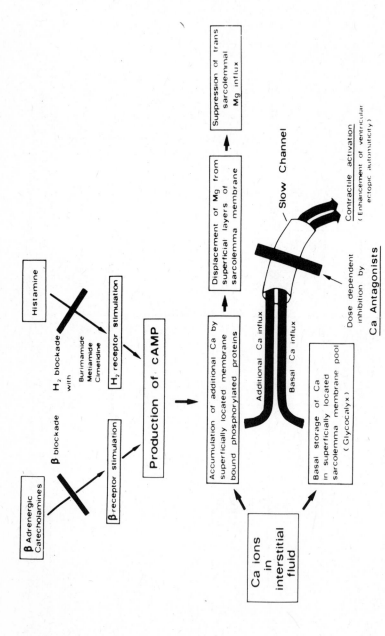

FIGURE 60. Mediator function of cyclic AMP between β- or H₂-receptor activation, and the consecutive membrane effects, i.e., promotion of transsarcolemmal Ca influx simultaneously with restriction of Mg uptake. As to the sequence of events, the scheme illustrates that the Ca antagonists interfere directly with the Ca influx across the slow channel without affecting the previous catecholamine- or histamine-induced production of cyclic AMP. The Ca antagonists probably inhibit the transsarcolemmal Ca inward movement by competing with Ca for specific binding sites in the carrier system. Moreover, the Ca antagonists seem to displace Ca ions from the superficially located sarcolemma membrane pools so that the availability of Ca to the slow channel is restricted. The latter effect is not visualized in the scheme. Besides intensifying contractile activation, an increase in the transsarcolemmal inward Ca current may also enhance ventricular ectopic automaticity (see sections 5.3.1, 5.3.4, and 5.3.5).

94

layers of the sarcolemma membrane and in the Ca-transport system of the slow channels, but spares Ca-dependent intracellular reactions.

In this context it also seems necessary to comment upon the Ca-synergistic influence of cardiac glycosides. As we have repeatedly demonstrated since 1964, contractile inhibition produced by Ca antagonists can also be reversed by ouabain, k-strophanthin, digoxin, proscillaridin, and so forth (see Figure 64). This was shown on isolated atria, papillary muscles, heart-lung preparations, and on the hearts *in situ* of rabbits, guinea pigs, cats, and rhesus monkeys. Apparently, the Ca-synergistic potency of cardiac glycosides, discovered by O. Loewi in 1917, enables them to overcome the negative inotropic effects of Ca antagonists. However, the restorative action of cardiac glycosides fundamentally differs from that of other Ca promoters, because cardiac glycosides only reinforce Ca-dependent contractile tension development, but are totally unable to resuscitate the electrogenic transsarcolemmal inward Ca current in partially K-depolarized mammalian ventricular myocardium (Tritthart, Weiss, Volkmann, and Späh, 1974). Similar results were obtained by Greenspan and Morad (1975) and McDonald, Nawrath, and Trautwein (1975) in voltage-clamp studies. Thus under the influence of cardiac glycosides, there is a complete dissociation of contractile activation from the strength of the slow electrogenic Ca current. In fact, cardiac glycosides even tend to *decrease* the Ca-dependent bioelectric membrane activity when they potentiate contractile force (see

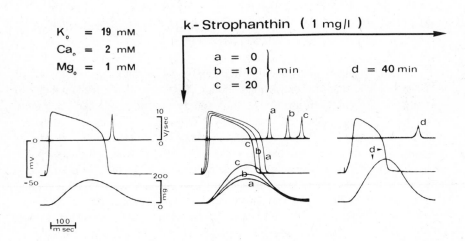

Partially depolarized guinea pig papillary muscle
Stimulation rate : 30 min^{-1} Temperature : 30 °C

FIGURE 61. Inverse effects of k-strophanthin on Ca-dependent action potential and contractility of a partially depolarized guinea pig papillary muscle. Whereas within 40 min, all Ca-dependent bioelectric parameters such as upstroke velocity ($= dV/dt_{max}$), height and duration of action potential are more and more decreased by k-strophanthin, isometric peak tension is potentiated. Strophanthin, by augmenting the intracellular free-Ca concentration in an electroneutral manner seems to lower the driving force of the electrogenic Ca inward current through the slow channel to the same extent as it enhances contractile strength. From Späh and Fleckenstein, unpublished.

Figure 61). In conclusion: There are two principal possibilities of neutralizing the negative inotropic action of Ca antagonists, namely:

1. Increasing the electrogenic transsarcolemmal Ca supply through the slow channel by β- or H_2-receptor stimulation, administration of dibutyryl cyclic AMP, or augmentation of the extracellular Ca concentration.
2. Increasing the cytoplasmic free-Ca concentration indirectly, in an electro-neutral way, probably by inhibition of transsarcolemmal Ca extrusion. This appears to be the mechanism of action of cardiac glycosides (see Section 1.4.4).

Regarding the medical implications, $CaCl_2$, β-adrenergic catecholamines (preferably isoproterenol or orciprenaline), and cardiac glycosides also proved to be excellent antidotes against overdoses of Ca antagonists on animal hearts *in situ* and in man. For instance, our toxicological studies on anesthetized guinea pigs under ECG control have shown that four to six times higher intravenous doses of nifedipine or verapamil are tolerated if given together with suitable amounts of $CaCl_2$ or isoproterenol. Similar results were obtained with intravenous k-strophanthin and proscillaridin.

2.9. INFLUENCE OF INHIBITORS AND PROMOTERS OF THE CALCIUM ACTION ON MYOCARDIAL HIGH-ENERGY-PHOSPHATE CONSUMPTION

The foregoing results demonstrate that there are many inhibitors and promoters of the Ca action in excitation–contraction coupling. By this basic mechanism they can intensify or restrict the utilization of high-energy phosphates in the contractile machinery, or even block it. Because less ATP is consumed in a Ca-deficient medium or under the influence of Ca-antagonistic inhibitors of excitation–contraction coupling, mechanical tension decreases while high-energy phosphates accumulate in the cardiac muscle. So the contractile failure produced by Ca-antagonistic drugs is generally accompanied by an elevated CP or ATP level and by a diminution in the orthophosphate fraction. Using paper chromatography we have analyzed more than 400 electrically driven isolated rabbit atria, 440 guinea pig left ventricles *in situ* (open-chest preparations) and 200 guinea pig heart-lung preparations for ATP, ADP, AMP, IMP, CP, and inorganic phosphate during the years 1963–1967 (Fleckenstein, 1964a, 1967, 1968b, c; Schildberg and Fleckenstein, 1965; Fleckenstein, Döring, and Kammermeier, 1967/1967; Fleckenstein, Kammermeier, Döring, and Freund, 1967). To assess cardiac contractile function in these studies, different techniques were used such as (1) measurement of isometric tension development of the isolated atria with mechanoelectric transducers, (2) continuous registration of the changes in ventricular diameter, heart rate, and arterial and central venous pressure on open-chest preparations, and (3) measurement of the cardiac systemic output of heart-lung preparations with bubble-flow meters at constant venous filling pressures and constant arterial resistance.

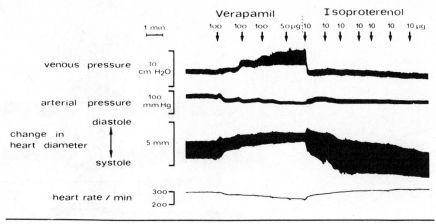

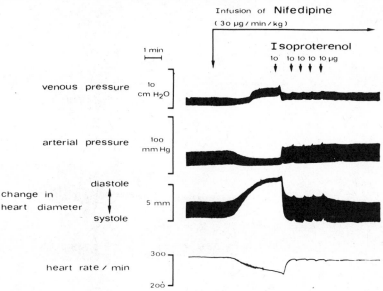

FIGURE 62. Acute contractile failure of 2 guinea pig hearts *in situ* produced by overdoses of verapamil (upper panel) or nifedipine (lower panel). Verapamil was intravenously injected in the form of single doses (total amount: 1.2 mg/kg body weight) until cardiac incompetence developed, whereas nifedipine was intravenously infused at a rate of 30 μg/min/kg during the whole course of the experiment. As indicated by the upward deflection of the records of heart diameter, verapamil and nifedipine produced large ventricular dilation in that they rapidly increased both the end-diastolic and particularly the end-systolic cross-diameters. Moreover, the contraction amplitude, as visualized by the difference between diastolic and systolic diameter, became smaller and smaller. In consequence of cardiac contractile failure, central venous pressure measured in the left jugular vein with the Statham element P 23 BB rose, whereas there was a simultaneous drop of arterial blood pressure measured with the Statham element P 23 Db in the right carotid artery. Heart rate also decreased. However, the first therapeutic dose of 10 μg isoproterenol (which corresponds to 30 to 35 μg/kg body weight) restored the contractile function of the verapamil- and nifedipine-treated hearts almost completely within 20 to 30 sec. The experiments were carried out on open-chest preparations under nembutal- ether- anesthesia and artifical respiration after the pericardium had been removed. The systolic and diastolic heart diameters were continuously registered using the method of Kammermeier and Döring (*Pflügers Arch. ges. Physiol.* **273**, 311, 1961). Ultrasensitive recordings of heart rate were done with an electronic device as indicated by Krause (*Z. Kreisl.-Forsch.* **52**, 128, 1963). The figures are taken from Fleckenstein (1964a) and Fleckenstein, Tritthart, Döring, and Byon (1972).

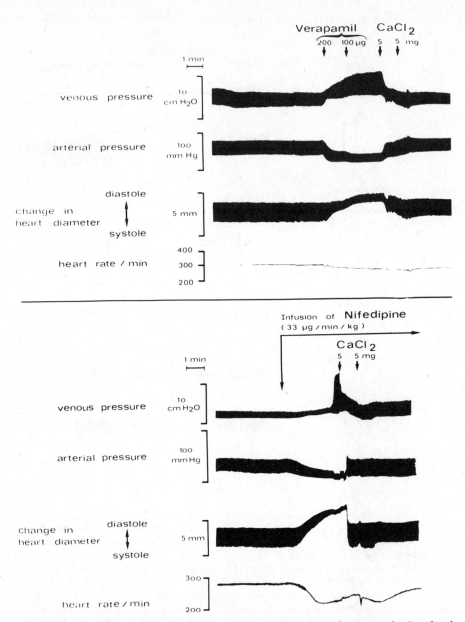

FIGURE 63. Acute contractile failure of 2 guinea pig hearts *in situ* (open-chest preparations) produced by overdoses of verapamil (upper panel) or nifedipine (lower panel) and registered with the same experimental techniques as in Figure 62. In the lower experiment, ventricular dilation led to transient tricuspid insufficiency. However, IV administration of $CaCl_2$ (15 to 30 mg/kg body weight) normalized cardiac contractile function as well as arterial and venous pressure within 2 min. From Fleckenstein (1970/1971a,b) and Fleckenstein, Tritthart, Döring, and Byon (1972).

98

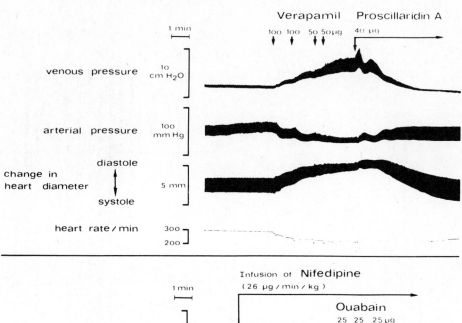

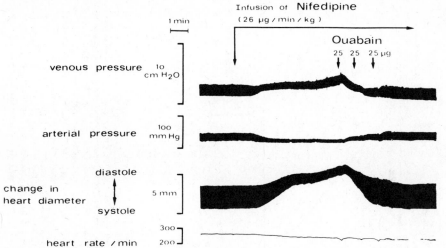

FIGURE 64. Acute contractile failure of 2 guinea pig hearts *in situ* (open-chest preparations) produced by overdoses of verapamil (1 mg/kg, upper panel) or nifedipine (26 µg/min/kg, lower panel). Following IV administration of proscillaridin A (0.13 mg/kg) or ouabain (0.23 mg/kg), complete recovery of the contractile cardiac function took place within 3 to 5 min. From Döring and Kammermeier, unpublished (1964), and Fleckenstein, Tritthart, Döring, and Byon (1972).

As expected, the concentrations of myocardial ATP and CP were always found to increase when contractile incompetence developed following extracellular Ca withdrawal or administration of Ca-antagonistic agents. As an example, some original experiments on guinea pig hearts *in situ* (open-chest preparations under artificial respiration; pericardium removed) are shown in Figures 62 to 64. Here acute contractile incompetence was produced by large intravenous overdoses of verapamil

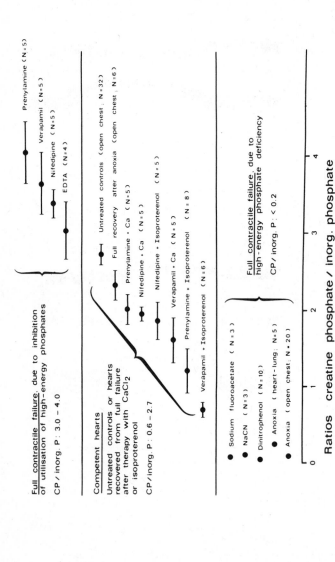

FIGURE 65. Increase of the CP: inorganic-phosphate ratio (up to a value of 3 to 4) in the left ventricular myocardium of guinea pig hearts *in situ* during contractile failure produced by inhibitors of excitation–contraction coupling. To cause this cardiac insufficiency large doses of specific Ca antagonists (6 to 12 mg prenylamine/kg; 0.4 to 1.0 mg verapamil/kg; 0.15 to 0.18 mg nifedipine/kg) were administered intravenously in open-chest experiments. Intravenous injection of EDTA (40 to 70 mg/kg) had a similar effect by simple chelation of Ca. If, however, the high-energy-phosphate utilization was restored by $CaCl_2$ (45 mg/kg) or isoproterenol (150 µg/kg), the CP: inorganic-phosphate ratio fell rapidly to the normal range *pari passu* with the recovery of the contractile tension. Identical results were obtained with epinephrine (300 µg/kg) or ouabain (150 to 300 µg/kg). For comparison, the graph also shows the very low ratios (0.1 to 0.2) found in the left ventricular myocardium of rats under the influence of anoxia or metabolic poisons (10 mg NaCN/kg; 15 mg sodium fluoroacetate/kg; 30 mg 2,4-dinitrophenol/kg) when contractile failure developed beause of a nearly complete high-energy-phosphate exhaustion. The absolute concentrations of the acid-soluble phosphate compounds in 32 untreated control hearts *in situ* (expressed as µmol/g blood-free tissue wet weight) were as follows: CP, 8.3 ($\pm$ 0.25);* inorganic phosphate, 3.2 ($\pm$ 0.11); ATP, 4.6 ($\pm$ 0.08); ADP, 0.8 ($\pm$ 0.03); total acid-soluble phosphorus, 1160 ($\pm$ 13) µg P/g. The corresponding control values for the left ventricular myocardium of 12 competent heart-lung preparations were: CP, 7.9 ($\pm$ 0.2); inorganic phosphate, 4.4 ($\pm$ 0.05); ATP 4.6, ($\pm$ 0.2); ADP, 0.8 ($\pm$ 0.03); total acid-soluble phosphorus, 1145 ($\pm$ 21) µg P/g. From Fleckenstein, Döring, and Kammermeier (1966/1967) and Fleckenstein, Tritthart, Döring, and Byon (1972). *SE of mean.

100

or nifedipine. There was a progressive ventricular dilation that did often lead to a transient insufficiency of the tricuspid valve (see Figure 63). Whereas central venous pressure rose (or even high positive venous pulses appeared in consequence of tricuspid dysfunction), contraction amplitude, stroke volume, arterial pressure, and heart rate declined. When the hearts were frozen in liquid nitrogen, propanol, or isopentane just at the climax of ventricular dilation and analyzed for their acid-soluble-phosphate fractions, peak values of ATP and CP appeared. Some of our data obtained on guinea pig hearts *in situ* under the influence of Ca antagonists (prenylamine, verapamil, nifedipine) or Ca deficiency (injection of EDTA) are shown in Figure 65. The graph represents the alterations of the ratio of CP to inorganic phosphate, a parameter that can serve as a most sensitive indicator of the intensity of high-energy-phosphate consumption in the beating hearts. In fact, supernormal ratios amounting to 3 to 4 were consistently observed when full contractile failure had occured following administration of overdoses of prenylamine, verapamil, nifedipine, or EDTA. If, however, the high-energy-phosphate utilization was restored by intravenous application of $CaCl_2$, β-adrenergic catecholamines such as isoproterenol, or cardiac glycosides, the myocardial CP:inorganic phosphate ratio rapidly fell to the normal range of 0.6 to 2.7 simultaneously with the recovery of contractile force. Isoproterenol normalized mechanical performance of the hearts in most cases within 30 sec, whereas intravenous injections of $CaCl_2$ were generally effective in the course of 2 min. Cardiac glycosides acted more slowly, within 3 to 5 min. The graph also shows the extremely low figures of 0.1 to 0.2 that occurred in anoxic hearts and after poisoning with sodium cyanide, sodium fluoroacetate, or 2,4-dinitrophenol. Needless to say, this latter form of cardiac incompetence, produced by high-energy-phosphate exhaustion, cannot be successfully treated with isoproterenol, $CaCl_2$, or cardiac glycosides that merely promote high-energy-phosphate utilization.

2.10. REDUCTION BY CALCIUM ANTAGONISTS OF THE MYOCARDIAL OXYGEN REQUIREMENT

As discussed in Section 1.2, not only the utilization of ATP for tension development but also the consequent rise in oxygen consumption of active cardiac muscle above resting level is necessarily Ca-dependent. Therefore, it is easily understood that Ca-antagonistic drugs in reducing high-energy-phosphate consumption in the contractile system also lower cardiac oxygen requirement per heart beat. The decrease in cardiac oxygen demand strictly parallels that of contractile force. Figure 66 demonstrates the proportional reduction of isometric tension and extra consumption of oxygen under the influence of increasing doses of verapamil. In this case a 50% decrease in contractile force and extra consumption of oxygen was produced in a rabbit papillary muscle by a dose as low as 0.1 mg verapamil/l. With 1 mg verapamil/l, both tension and oxygen consumption dropped almost to the resting level, since the persisting electric activity of the myocardial fibers influences the rate of respiration to a rather insignificant extent. The results of three other experiments on

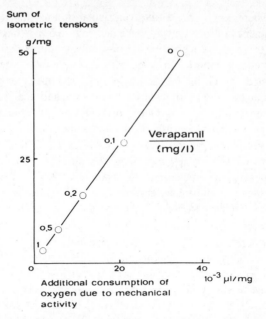

FIGURE 66. Linear reduction of isometric tension and additional consumption of oxygen due to mechanical activity under the influence of increasing doses of verapamil (0.1, 0.2, 0.5, and 1.0 mg/l) in Tyrode solution containing 2.0 mM Ca. The experiment was carried out on a rabbit papillary muscle (1.7 mg wet weight) that was incubated at rest in the different media each time for 20 min and then stimulated for 3 min at a frequency of 60/sec. Measurements of the rates of oxygen consumption with a platinum electrode and of mechanical tension with a mechanoelectronic displacement transducer were made throughout the experiment at 30°C. From Byon and Fleckenstein (1969) and Fleckenstein (1970/1971a,b).

rabbit papillary muscle with prenylamine, diltiazem, and nifedipine are shown in Figures 67, 68, and 69. As can be seen from Figure 69, only 0.01 mg nifedipine/l is required for an almost 50% inhibition of isometric tension and extra oxygen consumption. By increasing the extracellular Ca concentration up to 16 mM, mechanical activity and oxygen consumption were rapidly restored to normal even when the contractile system had previously been almost paralyzed.

In contrast with the Ca sensitivity of extra oxygen consumption during mechanical activity, the oxygen uptake of cardiac-tissue preparations at rest does not show any depression when the Ca-antagonistic inhibitors of excitation–contraction coupling are administered even in relatively big doses. So their oxygen-saving effect is due only to a restriction of the cardiac metabolic demands in consequence of diminished tension development, whereas all other ATP-consuming metabolic reactions that are not connected with Ca-dependent mechanical activity are not affected by these drugs (Byon and Fleckenstein, 1965; see Fleckenstein, Kammermeier, Döring, and Freund (1967).

The interrelationship between tension development and myocardial oxygen consumption is one of the most fundamental problems in heart physiology. In the past,

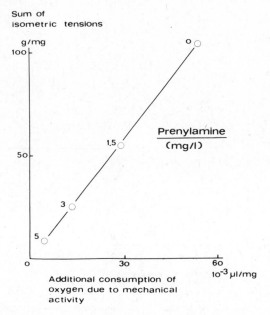

FIGURE 67. Linear reduction of isometric tension and additional consumption of oxygen due to mechanical activity under the influence of increasing doses of prenylamine (1.5, 3.0, and 5.0 mg/l) in Tyrode solution containing 2.0 mM Ca. The experiment was carried out on a rabbit papillary muscle (0.6 mg wet weight). Experimental procedure as in Figure 66. From Byon and Fleckenstein (1969) and Fleckenstein (1970/1971a,b).

two parameters have been postulated to determine the extra uptake of oxygen due to mechanical activity, namely (1) isometric peak tension attained, and (2) the rate of tension rise. However, during the course of our studies, a clear influence of changes in the rate of tension rise was in no case discernible. This led us to suppose that in reality, peak tension is the major determinant of cardiac oxygen requirement in isometric activity, whereas the rate parameter might be of minor or even no importance. To further elucidate this problem we did some crucial experiments, in which the amount of tension attained (T) was kept constant whereas large changes in the ratio dT/dt were allowed to occur (Byon and Fleckenstein, 1973). The changes in the maximum rate of tension development were not only produced by negative inotropic Ca antagonists but also by administration of positive inotropic agents such as extra calcium, adrenaline, or k-strophanthin. However, in order to equalize the amounts of developed tension, the isometric-contraction curves were always interrupted by quick releases at the same level of tension reached. The expectation was that under these conditions the oxygen consumption might also be equal regardless of the different rates of tension rise.

The experiments were carried out on very small rabbit papillary muscles excised from the right ventricle. The muscles were firmly placed into the measuring capillary of a conventional flow respirometer. The tendon side of the muscle was connected through an inextensible thin glass rod to an isometric-tension transducer, which

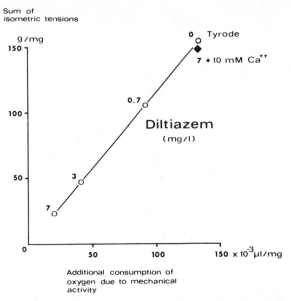

FIGURE 68. Linear reduction of the extra O_2 consumption and the sum of isometric peak tensions in a rabbit papillary muscle (wet weight 1.6 mg) by increasing doses (0.7, 3, and 7 mg/l) of diltiazem in Tyrode solution with normal Ca content of 2 mM. Complete restoration of original contractile tension development and height of oxygen consumption by raising the Ca content of the Tyrode solution, containing 7 mg diltiazem/l, from 2 to 12 mM[◆]. Experimental procedure as in Figure 66. From Fleckenstein, Fleckenstein-Grün, and Byon (1977).

was carried by the quick-release mechanism. The signal from the transducer was recorded and further differentiated electronically for the estimation of the rate in tension change. In addition, the output was also fed into a threshold feeler. This threshold feeler could activate an electromagnet at any preset level of active tension reached, so that a sudden downward movement of the tension transducer was produced, thus initiating a quick release. The distance over which the release was allowed to occur could be adjusted by a simple screw mechanism to avoid redevelopment of tension during release. The oxygen concentration was monitored in the flowing fluid using an oxygen cathode placed downstream to the muscle. The resulting current was displayed on a galvanometer. Special care was taken to ascertain a sufficient distance between muscle and electrode so that possible errors in oxygen measurements arising from unequal mixing of oxygen in the fluid could be eliminated. To avoid any oxygen deficiency during the course of the experiments, flow, total number, and rate of stimulations were adjusted so that the oxygen saturation in the measuring capillary never fell below 75%. The temperature was kept constant at 30°C.

Figure 70, for instance, shows an experiment on a rabbit papillary muscle in which the normal extracellular Ca concentration of 2 mM was increased by a factor of four up to 8 mM. Normally, a high Ca concentration causes a considerable augmentation of isometric peak tension and of the maximum rate of tension de-

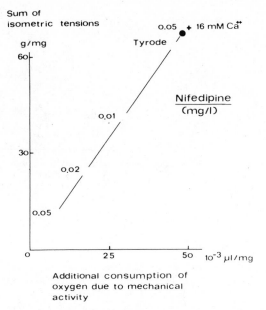

FIGURE 69. Linear reduction of isometric tension and additional consumption of oxygen due to mechanical activity under the influence of increasing doses of nifedipine (0.01, 0.02, and 0.05 mg/l) in Tyrode solution containing 2.0 mM Ca. With 0.05 mg/l, tension development and extraconsumption of oxygen were greatly depressed. This drug effect could be completely neutralized by increasing the extracellular Ca concentration up to 16 mM in the presence of 0.05 mg nifedipine/l [●]. Experiment on a rabbit papillary muscle (wet weight, 0.8 mg); procedure as in Figure 66. From Fleckenstein, Tritthart, Döring, and Byon (1972).

velopment. In this experiment, however, the high Ca concentration could only produce an increase in dT/dt, whereas the muscle was not allowed to develop more tension since in both normal and high Ca concentrations, a sudden relaxation was enforced at the same preset level of tension. Consequently, because the amount of tension was equal, the oxygen consumption also did not show any difference between the contraction in normal and high Ca concentrations, although the rates of tension rise were very different. The same type of experiment with the use of adrenaline is shown in Figure 71. Again, with or without adrenaline, the tensions attained were held equal by quick releases, whereas dT/dt differed widely. And again the rise in oxygen consumption was the same whether adrenaline had been added or not. Figure 71 represents a still further experiment of this type, which was carried out with the use of k-strophanthin. Here again no change in total oxygen consumption could be observed after the administration of strophanthin when the tension development was kept constant regardless of the large differences in dT/dt.

These results clearly contradict the widespread opinion that in addition to the absolute amount of tension produced, the rate parameter of tension rise also influences the oxygen consumption of active heart muscle. Our findings are at variance with the observations of Coleman (1967) on acetylstrophanthidin- or noradrenaline-

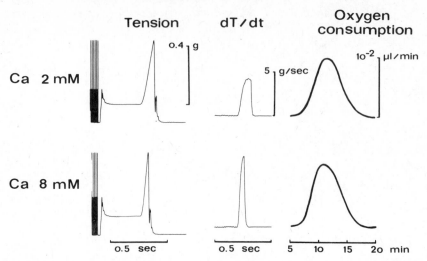

FIGURE 70. Constant relationship between active isometric tension and oxygen uptake unaffected by a Ca-induced increase in dT/dt. Rabbit papillary muscle (wet weight, 2.1 mg). Length of the muscle 4.6 mm. In the moment of quick release, the muscle was allowed to shorten over a distance of 1.5 mm. In each experiment 140 contractions were pooled at a stimulation frequency of 45/min, and the total oxygen consumption was measured for 20 min after the end of stimulation. From Byon and Fleckenstein (1973).

treated papillary muscles since in contrast to his statements, we were unable to realize an extra stimulation of cardiac respiration when dT/dt increased at constant peak tensions. Generally, in all our experiments on isolated myocardium, no indication of any oxygen-wasting effect of positive inotropic agents was detectable as long as the cells were not damaged. Accordingly, there was also no increase in the "efficiency" of tension development in relation to the oxygen requirement. In short: Cardiac activity metabolism—as indicated by the rise in oxygen consumption above resting level—is quantitatively determined by the tension attained, but not by the rate of tension development when studied on isolated myocardium under strictly controlled isometric conditions.

Interestingly enough, the duration of the contraction is also no determinant for the increase in respiration. This is evident from the fact that in quick-release experiments, an abbreviation of contraction did not alter the oxygen consumption when a sudden relaxation had been produced at the moment of peak tension reached or at any later moment during the relaxation phase (Byon, 1971). Hence, under isometric conditions, the duration or speed of relaxation does not significantly influence the intensity of oxidative activity metabolism. If, however, the quick release was applied during the rising phase of isometric contraction, again a strictly linear relationship between the tension attained at the moment of quick release and the extra uptake of oxygen could be demonstrated.

These results are fully consistent with the current concept concerning the fundamental mechanism of contraction (see Section 1.3). In fact, the height of isometric tension development in the cardiac myofibrils seems to be strictly correlated (1)

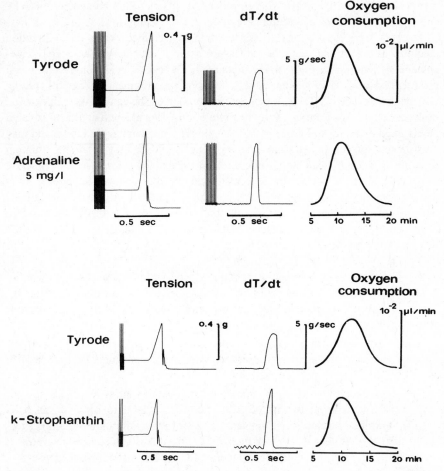

FIGURE 71. Constant relationship between active isometric tension and oxygen uptake unaffected by increases in *dT/dt. (Upper experiment with adrenaline)* Rabbit papillary muscle (wet weight, 2.1 mg; length of muscle, 4.6 mm; distance of quick release, 1.5 mm). *(Lower experiment with k-strophanthin)* Rabbit papillary muscle (wet weight, 1.7 mg; length of muscle, 5.0 mm; distance of quick release, 1.2 mm). Experimental procedure as in Figure 70. From Byon and Fleckenstein (1973).

with the number of cross bridges produced, (2) with the quantity of ATP split during the actin–myosin interaction, and (3) with the extra amount of oxygen consumed in connection with the subsequent ATP resynthesis. Therefore, all interventions that enhance or restrict the Ca supply to the myofilaments always produce proportional increases or decreases in contractile tension, ATP consumption, and oxygen requirement regardless of the speed of contractile activation or deactivation. All observations indicate that these mechanical and metabolic reactions are rigidly linked together and cannot be dissociated either by inotropic agents, by changes in the contraction rate, or by quick releases. This holds true as long as *no* myocardial membrane injury occurs that would produce an uncontrolled breakdown of ATP and thereby, possibly, an additional respiratory stimulation.

In conclusion, the Ca-antagonistic inhibitors of cardiac excitation–contraction coupling are direct opponents of the Ca promoters, particulary β-adrenergic cate-cholamines, with respect not only to myocardial Ca uptake, ATP consumption, and contractile tension development, but also to oxygen requirement. In fact, all specific Ca antagonists listed in Table 4 are capable of reducing the cardiac oxygen demand of the active myocardium in a fully reversible, dose-dependent manner. In isolated hearts, high experimental doses of Ca antagonists cause contractile failure and may even depress oxygen uptake almost to the resting level. Needless to say, the situation is totally different if small therapeutic doses of Ca antagonists are used systemically in humans. Here, of course, the administration of Ca antagonists is aimed only at a moderate reduction of heart work and oxygen demand as, for instance, in patients with a hyperkinetic heart function. In this respect, the Ca antagonists exert a beneficial influence similar to that of the β-receptor blocking agents, in spite of the fact that there are certain differences:

1. Ca-antagonistic substances interfere directly with Ca-dependent myocardial excitation–contraction coupling, whereas β-receptor blocking agents act indirectly by neutralizing the Ca-promoter effects of β-adrenergic catechol-amines.

2. β-Blockade renders the heart insensitive to the regulatory influence of sympathetic cardiovascular reflexes, whereas the Ca antagonists do not abolish the adrenergic cardiac reactivity.

3. Consequently, on hearts *in situ,* the cardiodepressant action of Ca antagonists, in contrast to that of β-blockers, is at least to some extent self-controlled, because each time an unproportionate fall in arterial blood pressure tends to occur, a reflex release of endogenous sympathetic neurotransmitters can still counteract exaggerated Ca-antagonistic drug responses.

Thus for the treatment of hyperkinetic cardiac disorders, the Ca antagonists represent a therapeutic alternative to the β-receptor blocking agents, however, with the advantage of a higher degree of safety (for more details see the clinical Chapter 7).

CHAPTER THREE

Prevention by Calcium Antagonists of Deleterious Calcium Overload: A New Principle of Cardioprotection

3.1. MYOCARDIAL HIGH-ENERGY-PHOSPHATE DEPLETION AND STRUCTURAL DECAY

The fundamental function of oxidative myocardial metabolism and the glycolytic substrate conversions is maintaining adequate stores of ATP and CP in the heart muscle cell. These high-energy-phosphate compounds are required mainly for two important energy-dependent tasks, namely:

1. To supply the energy for contraction and to drive the "ion pumps" (active transport of Na, K, and Ca ions connected with bioelectric and mechanical performance).
2. To cover the energy expenditure for the various synthetic reactions that are necessarily involved in the continuous cellular repair.

Of course, structural integrity can be maintained only by intense regenerative processes that need a permanent supply of ATP whether the heart is active or not. The myocardial fiber, like every other living structure, is in a state of dynamic equilibrium between spontaneous degradation and opposite recovery reactions that operate at the expense of phosphate-bond energy. For instance, the basal rate of oxygen consumption of the quiescent mammalian myocardium amounts to approximately 0.01 to 0.02 ml O_2/g tissue per minute at 37°C. At a P:O ratio of 3, these figures correspond to a quantity of 2.5 to 5 μmol high-energy phosphate/g myocardial tissue per minute metabolized under the conditions of cardiac arrest. Considering that the total high-energy-phosphate content does not exceed 15 to 20 μmol/g myocardial tissue, this rate of ATP consumption is surprisingly high. In case of a total blockade of ATP synthesis, the high-energy-phosphate stores would be completely exhausted within 4 to 8 min even in the absence of any mechanical activity. Because of glycolysis, this critical state is certainly somewhat postponed in the anoxic or ischemic myocardium (see Figure 2). Nevertheless, as shown by Büchner and Onishi (1968) in oxygen-deprived rat hearts, the first signs of degradation of the mitochondrial and myofibrillar structures appear as early as within 5 to 10 min.

Interestingly enough, the resting oxygen requirement of cardiac muscle is much greater than that of skeletal muscle. According to the classical studies of Clark and White (1929), the respiration rates of quiescent tortoise and frog atria exceed those of resting skeletal muscle by a factor of 10 to 20. Approximately the same ratio was found in our own experiments on rats. Similarly, the intracellular turnover rates of ATP and CP are considerably greater in cardiac muscle than in skeletal muscle (Fleckenstein and Janke, 1958, 1959; Fleckenstein, Janke, and Gerlach, 1959; Fleckenstein, 1961, 1963b). Figure 72 shows experiments in which ^{32}P-labeled orthophosphate was intravenously administered to anesthetized rats, and the ^{32}P-uptake into the ventricular and skeletal ATP and CP fractions measured. As can be easily seen, in the myocardium there was a 10 to 20 times faster incorporation

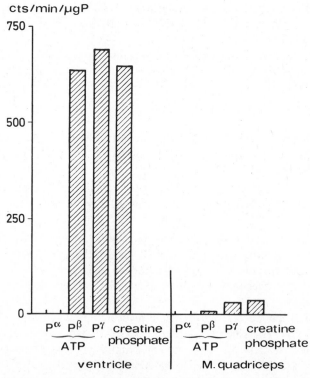

FIGURE 72.   Rate of ^{32}P incorporation into ATP and CP in cardiac and skeletal muscle of rats after IV injection of 0.2 mCi ^{32}P-labeled orthophosphate. The anesthetized animals were killed by immersion in liquid nitrogen 20 min after the ^{32}P injection. From Fleckenstein and Janke (1959).

of radiophosphorus into CP and the different phosphate groups of ATP than in the M. quadriceps of the same animals. These figures reveal large differences in the rates of oxidative phosphorylation that are probably due to the fact that the myocardial fibers—in contrast with skeletal muscle—contain an exceedingly great amount of mitochondria. The individual ^{32}P-uptake rates remain in the same order of magnitude whether cardiac and skeletal muscle preparations are stimulated or not, but are largely influenced by changes in temperature. When, for instance, the temperature was lowered from 30 to 0°C, the absolute concentrations of ATP and CP in quiescent rabbit auricles did not change, but the rate of ^{32}P uptake into these high-energy-phosphate fractions was reduced to approximately $^{1}/_{100}$ of the original value (see Figure 73). Because all "catabolic" reactions are considerably slower at low temperature, less ATP must be split and resynthesized in the cold to cover the energy expenses for cellular regeneration of the resting auricular tissue. Accordingly, at low temperature, the basal oxygen requirement declines in parallel with the high-energy-phosphate turnover. Therefore, as commonly known, the most effective way of protecting anoxic or ischemic hearts against rapid cellular disintegration consists of cooling in order to reduce their basic energy requirement.

Our results obtained with ^{32}P-labeled orthophosphate were accomplished by

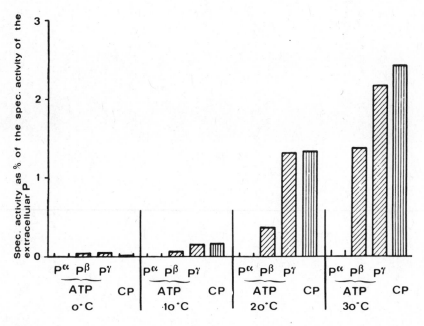

FIGURE 73. Influence of temperature on the cardiac high-energy-phosphate metabolism at rest. Quiescent rabbit auricles were exposed to a Tyrode solution containing 0.4 μmol/ml orthophosphate of an activity of about 100 μCi/ml for 15 min at 0, 10, 20, and 30°C. Then the ^{32}P-uptake rates into CP and the 3 phosphate groups of ATP were determined. The specific activities measured are expressed as percentage of the specific activity of the extracellular phosphate. From Fleckenstein, Janke, and Gerlach (1959).

TABLE 7. Uptake of ^{18}O from $H_2^{18}O$ into the Three Phosphate Groups of ATP According to Their Individual Turnover Rates at Different Temperatures[a]

Muscular Tissue	Temperature (°C)	Total Uptake (atom ^{18}O per molecule)	Distribution			Number of Experiments
			Adenosine·O–P$^\alpha$(=O)–OH	–O–P$^\beta$(=O)–OH	–O–P$^\gamma$(=O)–OH	
M. rectus ab-domin. (frog)	0	0.012	0	0	0.012 (100%)	5
	10	0.046	0	0	0.046 (100%)	8
	20	0.15	0	0.02 (13%)	0.13 (87%)	6
Isolated rabbit auricle	10	0.34	>0.01	0.06 (18%)	0.28 (82%)	5
	20	0.97	0.01 (1%)	0.13 (13%)	0.83 (86%)	5

[a]Fleckenstein, Janke, and Marmier (1965).

further turnover studies with ^{18}O-labeled water. The latter technique is based on the ^{18}O uptake from $H_2{}^{18}O$ into the inorganic-phosphate groups that are hydrolytically split off from intracellular organophosphate compounds. Thereby a rapid ^{18}O-labeling of the intracellular orthophosphate fraction occurs followed by incorporation of this ^{18}O-labeled orthophosphate into the organophosphate compounds in the course of their resynthesis. The quantitative evaluation of ^{18}O uptake into the different intracellular phosphate fractions allows an estimate of the *absolute turnover rates* of the individual phosphate fractions inside the cell (see Fleckenstein, Gerlach, Janke, and Marmier, 1959, 1960; Fleckenstein, 1961a, 1963b; Fleckenstein and Janke, 1964; Fleckenstein, Janke, and Marmier, 1965; Janke, Marmier, and Fleckenstein, 1965; Janke, Fleckenstein, Marmier, and Koenig, 1966). Measurements of ^{32}P uptake indicate only *relative turnover rates* of the intracellular organophosphate fractions because the orthophosphate transfer from the extracellular space to the internal compartments is not only restricted by a low sarcolemma membrane permeability but also influenced by the height of the transmembrane orthophosphate gradient. In contrast, $H_2{}^{18}O$ permeates freely toward all intracellular sites where organophosphate compounds are hydrolytically split and resynthesized.

Table 7 contains some data about the ^{18}O incorporation into the different phosphate groups of ATP both in resting frog skeletal muscle and in quiescent rabbit auricles. As shown by these figures, two principal findings, previously obtained with radiophosphorus, were confirmed with the more reliable ^{18}O technique:

1. The myocardial ATP turnover at rest is rather high, and changes with a factor of about 3 at a temperature variation of 10°C.
2. At a given temperature, the ATP turnover at rest is many times faster in the atrial myocardium than in skeletal muscle. According to the data of Table 7, the pertinent ratio is approximately 6 or 7:1. This applies to frogs as well as to mammals.

In conclusion, the great amount of metabolic energy required for basic maintenance reactions at 37°C renders the cellular structures of the mammalian myocardium particularly sensitive to any interruption of the high-energy-phosphate supply.

3.2. MYOCARDIAL-FIBER DAMAGE CAUSED BY EXHAUSTIVE HIGH-ENERGY-PHOSPHATE CONSUMPTION DUE TO CALCIUM OVERLOAD

As commonly known, high-energy-phosphate deficiency leading to structural decay, inevitably results from anoxia, ischemia, lack of metabolizable substrates, or toxic impairment of respiration, glycolysis, or oxidative phosphorylation. However, a negative myocardial energy balance is produced not only by an insufficient rate of ATP synthesis. Another important reason why the high-energy phosphates may be exhausted is excessive ATP consumption due to mechanical hyperactivity. This applies particularly to β-adrenergic overstimulation of the heart. As previously shown, sympathetic catecholamines increase cardiac contractile force by enhancing Ca-dependent utilization of high-energy phosphates in the contractile machinery. This effect is naturally harmless in a physiological concentration range. However, with increasing doses of catecholamines, Ca uptake and high-energy-phosphate breakdown may become so excessive that not enough ATP is left for the various anabolic processes that are involved in the regeneration of the living structures. In other words, overdoses of β-adrenergic catecholamines leading to an abundant Ca influx waste in useless mechanical reactions ATP that is necessary for the maintenance and survival of the myocardial cells.

The initiation of myocardial necrotization by excessive sympathetic-transmitter release or by administration of overdoses of natural adrenergic catecholamines has been studied by many researchers since the first decade of this century (see the reviews of Raab, 1953, 1963). However, as first shown by Rona, Chappel, Balazs, and Gaudry (1959), the most convenient way of producing disseminated or confluent myocardial lesions consists of a subcutaneous injection of a large dose of the synthetic β-receptor stimulant isoproterenol. But the etiology remained obscure until recently. As pointed out by Stanton and Schwartz (1967), the following hypotheses have been produced:

1. Cardiac hypoxemia may result from isoproterenol-induced hypotension accompanied by increased cardiac work and enhanced myocardial oxygen demands (Rona, Chappel, Balazs, and Gaudry, 1959).

2. Dilation of precapillary shunts may cause blood to bypass the capillary circulation and induce endocardial ischemia (Hanforth, 1962).

3. Hypoxia may result from direct, metabolic, oxygen-wasting actions of catecholamines on the heart (Raab, 1963).

4. Hyperlipidemia may elicit, in an unidentified manner, alterations in cell membrane permeability, which induce myocardial lesions (Rosenblum, Wohl, and Stein, 1965).

5. Cardiac necrosis may occur because of local potassium loss from the cardiac cell (Rosenmann, Gazenfield, Laufer, and Davies, 1964).

However, none of these hypotheses were satisfactory until in 1968 we were able to demonstrate the crucial role of myocardial Ca overload and consequent high-energy-phosphate depletion in the pathogenesis of isoproterenol-induced cardiac necrotization (Fleckenstein, 1968a). As an example, Figure 74 shows the increase in net ^{45}Ca uptake by the rat heart *in situ* as a function of time under the influence of a high subcutaneous dose of isoproterenol (30 mg/kg body weight). In the untreated control rat hearts, the ^{45}Ca incorporation was always small. Here the radioactivity of 1 g of fresh cardiac tissue, for instance, never exceeded 30% of the radioactivity that was simultaneously measured in 1 ml of the blood plasma. But after administration of 30 mg isoproterenol/kg, the radiocalcium incorporation into the myocardium was increased by a factor of 6 to 7 within a few hours.

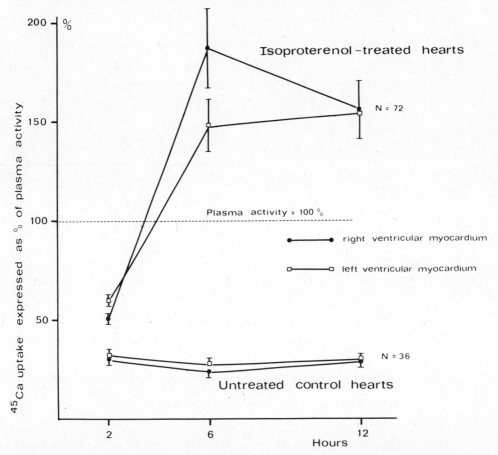

FIGURE 74.   Increase of the net radiocalcium uptake into the left and right ventricular myocardium of rats produced by subcutaneous injection of 30 mg isoproterenol/kg. The ^{45}Ca uptake into 1 g of fresh cardiac tissue is expressed as a percentage of the corresponding ^{45}Ca activity in 1 ml of blood plasma during an observation period of 12 hours after intraperitoneal administration of 10 μCi ^{45}Ca/kg body weight. From Fleckenstein (1970/1971a,b).

However, the labeled Ca is not evenly accumulated in the ventricular wall. As can be seen from the log dose–response curves in Figure 75, the isoproterenol-induced radiocalcium uptake into the inner layers of the left ventricular wall proved to be greater than that into the subepicardial cardiac tissue. Hence it is not surprising that the extent of high-energy-phosphate breakdown and the density of necrotic areas were generally more pronounced in the inner than in the superficial ventricular layers.

The average changes in the high-energy-phosphate concentrations of the left ventricular myocardium of 90 rats during an observation period of 24 hours following the injection of 30 mg isoproterenol/kg are shown in Figure 76. Because

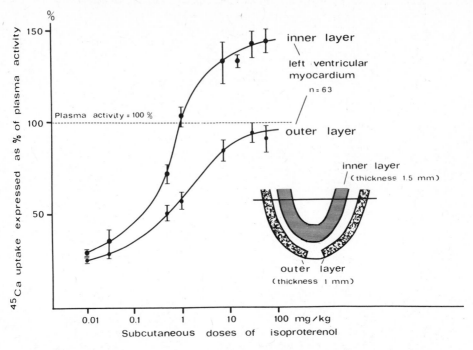

FIGURE 75. Log dose–response curves of the isoproterenol-induced net ^{45}Ca uptake into the inner and outer layer of the left ventricular myocardium of rats (apical region). The measurements were carried out 6 hours after injection of different subcutaneous doses of isoproterenol and of 10 μCi $^{45}Ca/kg$ intraperitoneally. From Fleckenstein, Janke, Döring, and Leder (1974).

of the excessive transmembrane Ca influx, a 50% loss of ATP and an 85% loss of CP occurred within 2 hours; but later there was a partial recovery. Nevertheless, disseminated myocardial-fiber necroses developed in all cases. The number and size of the isoproterenol-induced cardiac lesions are determined by the extent and particularly the duration of the Ca-mediated high-energy-phosphate deficiency. For instance, in our studies on rats, an increasing number of necroses were produced by raising the subcutaneous doses of isoproterenol from 0.5 and 1 mg to 30 mg/kg body weight. All these doses were practically equipotent with regard to the acute breakdown of ATP and CP they initiated. However, as can be seen from Figure 77, the lowest dose of 0.5 mg isoproterenol/kg, which produced only a small number of disseminated necroses, allowed a relatively rapid recovery of the high-energy-phosphate stores. On the other hand, the return to normal was more and more postponed when the higher doses were administered. In parallel, the myocardial lesions became much larger and more numerous. The most deleterious consequence of a prolonged energetic imbalance is a progressive degradation of cellular nucleotides. Earlier investigations from our laboratory on ischemic hearts have shown that the situation becomes critical when more than 60% of the myocardial ATP has definitely been broken down to the useless end products inosine, hypoxanthine, and xanthine (Gerlach, Deuticke, and Dreisbach, 1963; see Section 1.1). Therefore, it is interesting to note that according to recent observations of Zimmer, Ibel, Steinkopff, and Korb (1979) on rats, both isoproterenol-induced degradation of myocardial adenine nucleotides and necrotization can be counteracted by previous infusion of ribose. This prophylactic treatment apparently stimulates the biosynthesis of myocardial adenine nucleotides (Zimmer and Gerlach, 1978) so effectively that the dangerous fall in ATP and, consequently, structural damage is, to a great extent, prevented.

The intracellular sites where myocardial Ca overload induces exhaustive ATP consumption are situated in different structures (myofibrils, SR, mitochondria). The first reaction of the contractile system to an abundant splitting of ATP by the Ca-activated myofibrillar ATPase consists of a supercontraction. Tension development is often so vigorous that the connection of the myofilaments with the Z-line structures is disrupted, as can be seen from the electron micrograph of Figure 92. Then, within a few hours, the Z lines and myofibrils of the necrotizing cardiac cells totally disintegrate to an amorphous mass. Only some dispersed myofibrillar fragments may still be found enclosed in the intracellular detritus (see Figure 93). Apparently an abundant transsarcolemmal Ca influx produces a state of excitation–contraction "overcoupling" by which the myofilaments are eventually destroyed if the myo-

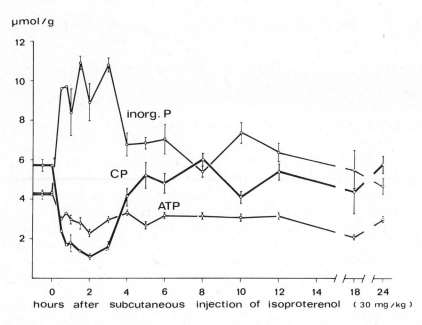

FIGURE 76. Isoproterenol-induced changes in the concentrations of ATP, CP, and orthophosphate in the left ventricular myocardium of 90 rat hearts after a single subcutaneous injection of 30 mg isoproterenol/kg during an observation period of 24 hours. From Fleckenstein, Döring, and Leder (1969).

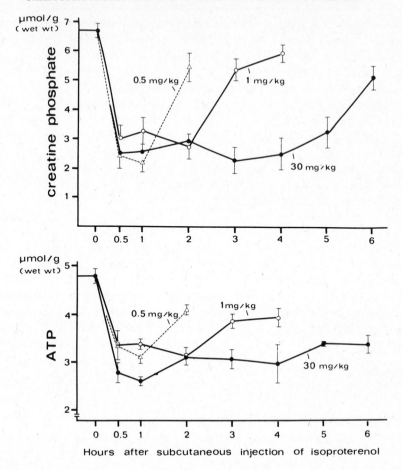

FIGURE 77. Prolongation of myocardial CP and ATP deficiency by increasing single subcutaneous doses of isoproterenol in rats. From Fleckenstein, Janke, Döring, and Leder (1975).

cardial fiber cannot get rid of the Ca overload in time. The lysis of Z lines is probably brought about by a special Ca-activated protease (Busch, Stromer, Goll, and Suzuki, 1972; Reddy, Etlinger, Fischman, Rabinowitz, and Zak, 1975).

Apart from myofibrillar destruction, intracellular Ca overload is most injurious to the mitochondria. It is a well-known fact that isolated mitochondria from heart muscle (Slater and Cleland, 1953) as well as from liver, kidney, or suprarenal cortex* can rapidly concentrate Ca by means of an ATP-driven active transport

*Concerning the influence of Ca on mitochondria from liver, see Rossi, C.S., and Lehninger, A.L. (*J. Biol. Chem.* **239,** 3971, 1964), Carafoli, E., and Rossi, S.C. (*Eur. J. Biochem.* **2,** 224, 1967), Azzi, A., and Azzone, G.F., (*Biochem. Biophys. Acta* **113,** 438, 1966; Cohn, D.V., Bawdon, R., Newman, R.R., and Hamilton, J.W., *J. Biol. Chem.* **243,** 1089, 1968), from kidney (Cohn, D.V., Bawdon, R., and Eller, G., *J. Biol. Chem.* **242,** 1253, 1967) and from suprarenal cortex (Whysner, J.A., Paule, W.J., Nelson, D.H., and Harding, B.W., *Clin. Res.* **14,** 180, 1966).

system, while the rates of oxygen uptake simultaneously rise (See Section 1.4.3). As a sign of Ca overload, even intramitochondrial calcium phosphate precipitates, probably consisting of hydroxyapatite (Greenawalt, Rossi, and Lehninger, 1964), may appear. But with increasing binding of Ca, the isolated mitochondria are severely damaged since they swell, and deteriorate in their respiratory control and phosphorylating capacity. Thus an excessive rise in the surrounding Ca concentration will spoil the most important mitochondrial function, that is to say, oxidative ATP synthesis. Mitochondria *in situ* undergo similar ultrastructural changes upon perfusion of isolated myocardial tissue with solutions containing high Ca (Legato, Spiro, and Langer, 1968).

Evidence exists that intracellular Ca overload of isoproterenol-treated rat hearts produces functional and morphological changes of the mitochondria *in situ* that are virtually identical with those brought about by direct application of excess Ca. In fact, cardiac mitochondria *in situ* also incorporate large amounts of Ca when overdoses of isoproterenol are administered. Simultaneously, mitochondrial swelling, vacuolization, and cristolysis occur, often followed by complete evacuation of all structured intramitochondrial constituents so that at the end, only empty mitochondrial "ghosts" remain (see Figure 93). Physiologically, the intramitochondrial sequestration of Ca has probably to be considered a myocardial self-defense mechanism ("Ca-buffer") against a disproportionate rise in the cytoplasmic free-Ca concentration that exaggerates ATP consumption. When, however, necrotizing doses of isoproterenol are administered, transsarcolemmal Ca inflow is so dramatically stimulated that the following are by far surpassed:

1. The maximum rate of Ca extrusion from the myocardial fiber.
2. The capacity of rapid Ca binding by the SR.
3. The physiological limits of innocuous mitochondrial Ca sequestration.

In this situation, the enormous Ca accumulation by the mitochondria becomes suicidal for these organelles, and consequently, for the whole myocardial fiber. Thus the toxic effects of Ca overload of the mitochondria may eventually be more disastrous for the isoproterenol-treated myocardium than is the Ca-dependent enhancement of ATP consumption.

In summary, our investigations have shown the following facts:

1. Calcium ions are highly cardiotoxic if they are taken up excessively into the myocardial fibers.
2. Intracellular Ca overload initiates a deleterious breakdown of the high-energy-phosphate fractions (ATP, CP) by a fatal coincidence of exhaustive ATP consumption with progressive impairment of mitochondrial ATP resynthesis.
3. Calcium-induced high-energy-phosphate exhaustion is the determinant factor in the etiology of noncoronarogenic myocardial fiber necroses by adrenergic catecholamines.

The significance of Ca uptake during necrotization of cardiac tissue is by no means a new problem. However, in the past, calcification of myocardial lesions has usually been considered a phenomenon that is secondary to inflammatory or toxic tissue alterations (see Hart, 1909; Fischer, 1911; Gore and Arons, 1949; Selye, 1960). Nevertheless Katase, as early as 1913, called attention to the fact that administration of Ca salts to healthy animals may act as a primer for the development of calcified cardiac fiber necroses. Similarly, overdoses of parathyroid (Collip) hormone or vitamin D were shown to produce myocardial damage that was also directly attributable to specific effects on Ca metabolism (Herzenberg, 1929). It is now clear from our results, depicted in this and the following chapters, that intracellular Ca overload is indeed responsible for the development of myocardial necroses following administration of excessive doses of Ca salts, dihydrotachysterol, vitamin D, cardiac glycosides, direct or indirect catecholamines, and other Ca promoters. Furthermore, it turned out in our studies that the myocardial lesions that ensue from alimentary K or Mg deficiency in rats are also primarily due to excessive intracellular Ca accumulation (Section 3.5.3). As shown in collaboration with other research groups, Ca overload is also the decisive pathogenetic factor in the spontaneous development of myocardial necroses in hereditary cardiomyopathy of Syrian hamsters (Section 3.6). Moreover even in anoxic or ischemic hearts, intracellular Ca overload, by additionally damaging the mitochondria, accelerates and aggravates the inevitable structural decay (Section 3.5.4). All these observations indicate that Ca-overload is a causative principle in cardiac pathophysiology rather than a concomitant or subsequent phenomenon.

3.3.   PARALLEL POTENTIATION OF EXCESSIVE CALCIUM UPTAKE AND MYOCARDIAL-FIBER DAMAGE BY FLUOROCORTICOSTEROIDS, DIHYDROTACHYSTEROL, VITAMIN D, AND INORGANIC PHOSPHATES

In their investigations of the factors that enhance myocardial necrotization, Selye (1960) and Bajusz (1963) discovered that rats can be sensitized for the production of cardiac necroses by pretreatment with certain corticosteroids, dihydrotachysterol, or monosodium phosphate. According to the observations of Rona, Chappel, and Kahn (1963), the same substances aggravate the cardiotoxicity of isoproterenol. Therefore, we have also examined how these sensitizing substances can influence cardiac Ca uptake. As shown in Figure 78, the pretreatment with 9 α-fluorocortisol acetate, dihydrotachysterol, and NaH_2PO_4 apparently had no appreciable effect per se on ^{45}Ca incorporation (black columns) under the actual experimental conditions. But if isoproterenol was administered after pretreatment with these sensitizing agents, a tremendous increase in ^{45}Ca uptake occurred (striped columns). For instance, in the hearts of dihydrotachysterol-pretreated rats, a radiocalcium accumulation was found 6 hours after administration of isoproterenol that was 36 times greater than the control value. After sensitization with 9 α-fluorocortisol acetate or monosodium

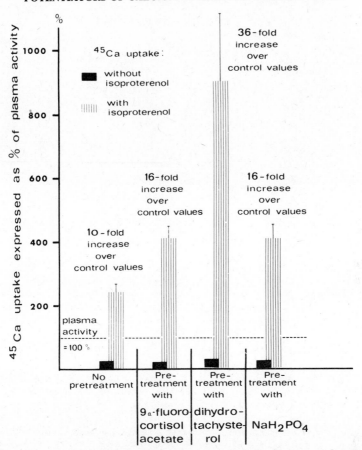

FIGURE 78. Potentiation of isoproterenol-induced ^{45}Ca uptake in the myocardium of the right ventricle of rats by pretreatment with 9 α-fluorocortisol acetate, dihydrotachysterol (AT 10), or NaH$_2$PO$_4$. The following dosages were used: 9 α-fluorocortisol acetate, 10 mg/kg subcutaneously per day for 7 days; dihydrotachysterol, 3 mg/kg orally per day for 3 days; NaH$_2$PO$_4$, 10 mmol/kg orally twice per day for 7 days. Radioactivity was measured 6 hours after the intraperitoneal injection of 10 μCi ^{45}Ca/kg and 6 hours after the subcutaneous isoproterenol injection (30 mg/kg). Data from Janke and Fleckenstein, see Fleckenstein (1970/1971a,b).

phosphate, the increase was 16-fold. Simultaneously, dramatic changes took place in the absolute myocardial Ca concentration (see Figure 79). Again, the control value, amounting to about 2 mEq Ca/kg heart tissue, was not markedly influenced by pretreatment with the sensitizing agents. But as soon as isoproterenol was administered, the myocardial Ca concentration rose steeply. In the hearts of dihydrotachysterol-pretreated rats, a Ca accumulation up to 52 mEq/kg wet weight was found 24 hours after the administration of isoproterenol. This concentration exceeds the control value of 2 mEq Ca/kg by a factor of 26. After sensitization with 9 α-

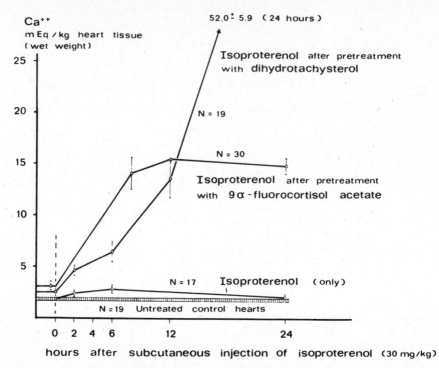

FIGURE 79. Massive isoproterenol-induced Ca overload of the myocardium of rats pretreated with dihydrotachysterol or 9 α-fluorocortisol acetate. In order to sensitize the animals for the production of myocardial lesions, daily oral doses of dihydrotachysterol (3 mg/kg for 3 days) or daily subcutaneous doses of 9 α-fluorocortisol acetate (10 mg/kg for 7 days) were administered prior to subcutaneous injection of 30 mg isoproterenol/kg. From Fleckenstein, Janke, Döring, and Leder (1971).

fluorocortisol acetate, the increase was eightfold. Most of this Ca was found to be concentrated in severely injured mitochondria.

As to the concomitant changes in the high-energy-phosphate fractions, it is not surprising that pretreatment with the sensitizing agents leads to a further augmentation and prolongation of the isoproterenol-induced fall in the myocardial ATP and CP concentrations. As can be seen from Figure 80, isoproterenol lowered the cardiac ATP level in the fluorocortisol-pretreated rats to less than 50% of the normal ATP content, with no sign of recovery. The simultaneous potentiation of the isoproterenol-induced CP breakdown is also shown in Figure 80. The magnitude of this myocardial high-energy-phosphate deficiency is critical and could not be survived in many cases for more than a few hours after the isoproterenol administration. The hearts of such animals exhibited infarctlike confluent necrotic areas as described previously by Rona, Chappel, Balazs, and Gaudry (1959); Rona, Chappel, and Kahn (1963); and Rona, Kahn, and Chappel (1963). It is obvious that the energetic state of the myocardium of isoproterenol-treated animals, especially after sensiti-

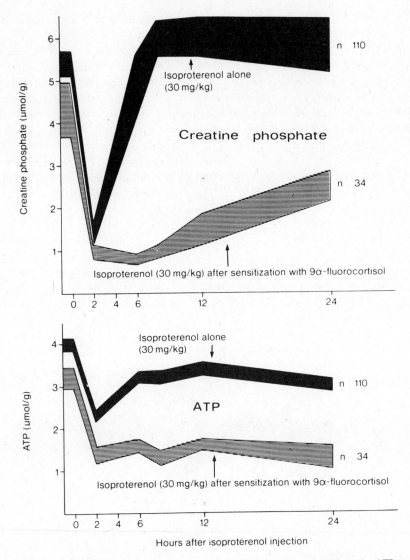

FIGURE 80. Accentuation and prolongation of the isoproterenol-induced fall in the ATP and CP content of the left ventricular myocardium of rats by pretreatment with 9 α-fluorocortisol acetate. The rats sensitized with this steroid (10 mg/kg/day for 7 days) not only reacted to the test dose of isoproterenol (30 mg/kg) with a greater decrease in their high-energy-phosphate fractions but also lost to a greater extent their capacity to regenerate their myocardial energy reserves (especially ATP) within 24 hours. Data from Döring and Fleckenstein; see Fleckenstein (1970/1971a,b).

zation, is comparable to the metabolic situation of the heart muscle in anoxia and ischemia, or under the influence of metabolic poisons such as cyanide or 2,4-dinitrophenol, insofar as in all these cases, cardiac function and structural integrity cannot be maintained because the high-energy-phosphate pool is exhausted. The experiments reveal that not only dihydrotachysterol but also fluorinated corticosterols greatly enhance catecholamine-induced myocardial transsarcolemmal Ca influx. This effect potentiates the positive inotropic action of β-adrenergic catecholamines as well as their necrotizing power if they are applied in excessive doses.

3.4. CARDIOPROTECTIVE ACTIONS OF CALCIUM ANTAGONISTS AGAINST CALCIUM OVERLOAD, ATP WASTING, AND NECROTIZATION

Definite evidence for the crucial role of Ca overload in the production of noncoronarogenic cardiac necroses could be obtained in a most obvious way with the help of specific Ca antagonists. Thus we were able to show that verapamil, D 600, and prenylamine are capable of protecting isoproterenol-treated rat hearts *in situ* against Ca overload, high-energy-phosphate exhaustion, and subsequent necrotization (Fleckenstein, 1968a, 1969/1971, 1970/1971a,b; Fleckenstein, Döring, and Leder, 1969; Fleckenstein, Janke, Döring, and Leder, 1971, 1974, 1975; Fleck-

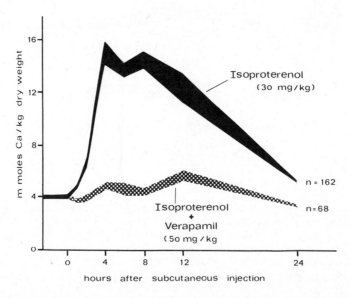

FIGURE 81. Protection by verapamil of the right ventricular myocardium of rats against isoproterenol-induced Ca overload during an observation period of 24 hours. Administration of 30 mg isoproterenol/kg with and without verapamil (50 mg/kg) at separate subcutaneous injection sites. From Janke, Frey, and Fleckenstein, unpublished.

enstein, Janke, Döring, and Pachinger, 1973). By their inhibitory action on trans-sarcolemmal Ca uptake, the Ca antagonists apparently can neutralize even the effects of overdoses of sympathomimetic catecholamines on the Ca channel without influencing the adrenergic β-receptors. For instance, Figure 81 shows the changes in the absolute Ca content of the right ventricular myocardium during an observation period of 24 hours following subcutaneous administration of the necrotizing standard dose of isoproterenol (30 mg/kg). Here the absolute Ca content rose from 4 to 16 mmol/kg dry weight within 4 hours. When, however, verapamil (50 mg/kg) was subcutaneously administered together with the isoproterenol, the Ca concentration was only slightly increased up to a peak value of 5.5 mmol/kg dry weight after 12 hours. Figure 82 represents log dose–response curves of the isoproterenol-induced net radiocalcium uptake into the right ventricular myocardium of rats. The measurements were made 6 hours after subcutaneous injection of different amounts of isoproterenol. The rise in Ca uptake above the control level began with a dose as

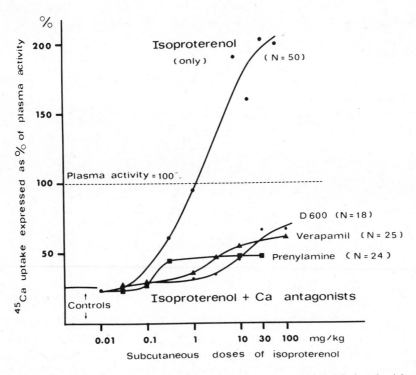

FIGURE 82. Prevention of excessive isoproterenol-induced uptake of labeled Ca into the right ventricular myocardium of rats by three Ca-antagonistic compounds. Log dose–response curves of the isoproterenol-induced radiocalcium incorporation obtained with or without simultaneous administration of D 600 (10 mg/kg), verapamil (17 mg/kg), or prenylamine (250 mg/kg). All measurements were made 6 hours after subcutaneous injection of the drugs. From Janke and Fleckenstein; see Fleckenstein (1970/1971a,b).

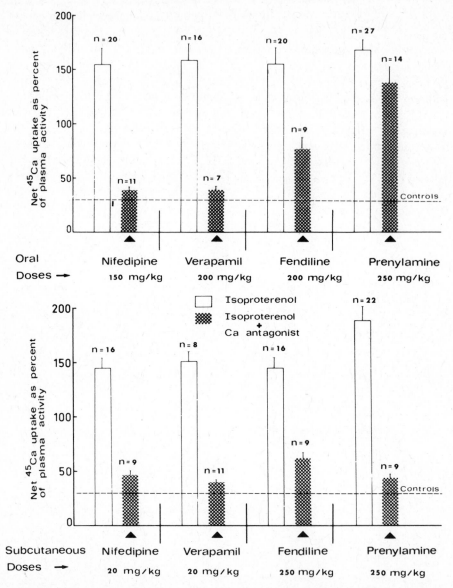

FIGURE 83. Prevention of excessive isoproterenol-induced uptake of labeled ^{45}Ca into the right ventricular myocardium of rats by administration of certain Ca antagonists such as nifedipine, verapamil, fendiline, or prenylamine. Comparison of the prophylactic potency of subcutaneous and oral application of the Ca antagonists. The drugs were given twice 24 hours and 30 min prior to the subcutaneous injection of 30 mg isoproterenol/kg and the simultaneous intraperitoneal administration of 10 μCi Ca/ kg. All radioactivity measurements were carried out 6 hours later. From Frey, Janke, and Fleckenstein, unpublished.

small as 0.1 mg/kg and proceeded steeply to a maximum that was beyond the high dose of 30 mg/kg. Again, the Ca-antagonistic compounds verapamil, D 600, or prenylamine inhibited the isoproterenol-induced radiocalcium uptake to a rather impressive degree when they were injected simultaneously with the isoproterenol. Small doses of isoproterenol were completely neutralized, whereas the effects of higher doses were greatly diminished. Figure 83 represents the results of a further study on rats in which the two ways of subcutaneous and oral administration of nifedipine, verapamil, fendiline, and prenylamine were compared with respect to their efficacy in restricting isoproterenol-stimulated cardiac radiocalcium incorporation. Nifedipine and verapamil exhibited the strongest cardioprotective action in these experiments. Oral doses of prenylamine acted only weakly. A further series of observations, carried out with the use of diltiazem, is shown in Figure 84. As could be expected, this Ca antagonist too counteracted the isoproterenol-induced promotion of myocardial Ca uptake very effectively on both ventricles. Regarding the strength of inhibition of isoproterenol-stimulated myocardial Ca uptake by different Ca antagonists, our studies on rats revealed the following order of increasing potency: prenylamine < fendiline < diltiazem < verapamil, nifedipine < D 600.
The same doses of Ca-antagonistic compounds that prevent the rat hearts from

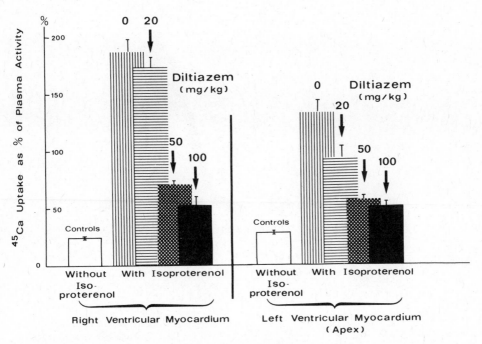

FIGURE 84. Inhibition by diltiazem of excessive isoproterenol-induced uptake of radiocalcium into the right and left ventricular myocardium of rats. Subcutaneous administration of different doses of diltiazem (20 to 100 mg/kg), according to the scheme of Figure 83.

isoproterenol-induced Ca overload are also effective in stabilizing the ATP and CP contents of the myocardial fibers at a sufficiently high level to maintain structural integrity. The results of a parallel study (1) on the preservation by Ca antagonists of the myocardial CP stores and (2) on the prevention by Ca antagonists of myocardial necrotization are shown in Figures 85 and 86. In both series of experiments the same doses of isoproterenol (30 mg/kg) and the Ca antagonists D 600 (20 mg/kg), verapamil (50 mg/kg), or prenylamine (250 mg/kg) were subcutaneously administered. With isoproterenol alone, the CP content of the left ventricular myocardium fell almost immediately from 5.4 to approximately 1.5 μmol/g cardiac tissue wet weight and stayed at this low level for nearly 3 hours (Figure 85). However, with the help of D 600, verapamil, or prenylamine, the precipitous CP breakdown could be completely or almost completely prevented. The corresponding histological data in Figure 86 indicate the proportion of necrotic myocardial tissue, as measured with the Zeiss "integration plate 1," after a time lapse of 6 hours following the injection of isoproterenol alone or of isoproterenol plus the Ca an-

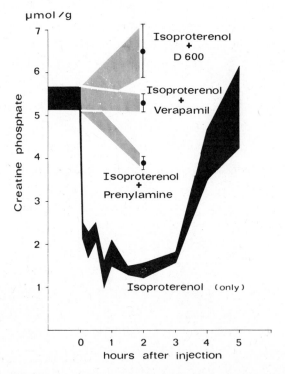

FIGURE 85. Inhibition of the isoproterenol-induced CP breakdown in the left ventricular myocardium of rats by three Ca-antagonistic compounds. The drugs were applied simultaneously by single subcutaneous injections at separate sites. The following doses were administered: isoproterenol (30 mg/kg), verapamil (50 mg/kg), compound D 600 (20 mg/kg), prenylamine (250 mg/kg). From Fleckenstein, Döring, and Leder (1969).

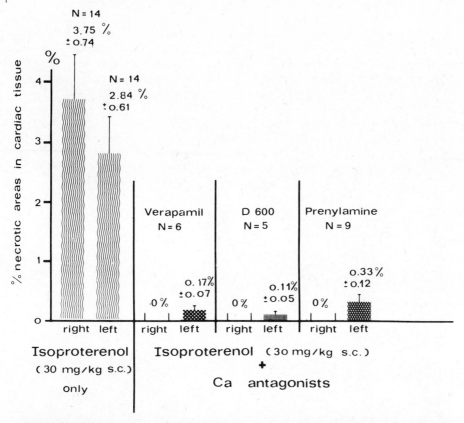

FIGURE 86. Proportion of necrotic myocardial tissue 6 hours after isoproterenol with or without prophylactic administration of Ca-antagonistic compounds. Evaluation was carried out with the use of the Zeiss integration plate number 1 on the right and left ventricular myocardium of rats. From Fleckenstein, Janke, Döring, and Leder (1974).

tagonists. In fact, D 600, verapamil, and prenylamine in the given dosage range not only stabilized the myocardial CP content, but also provided full protection against isoproterenol-induced right ventricular tissue damage. In the left ventricular wall some sparse necrotic fibers were still discernible. But even here, the efficacy of the Ca antagonists was highly significant, since the extent of tissue damage was reduced to 6% (verapamil), 4% (D 600) and 12% (prenylamine) of that found in the unprotected left control ventricles (= 100). Similarly, fendiline was also shown to maintain structural integrity and mitochondrial enzyme activity in isoproterenol-treated rat hearts (Ciplea and Bock, 1976).

Histological evidence of the cardioprotective potency of Ca antagonists was obtained with different techniques. For instance, Figure 87 shows reproductions of hematoxylin-eosin–stained sections from the right ventricular myocardium of two

Isoproterenol

Isoproterenol
+
Verapamil

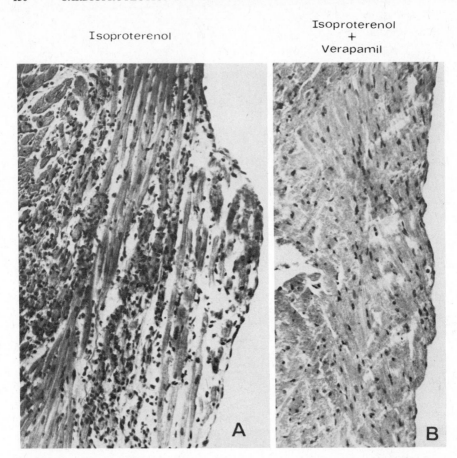

FIGURE 87. (A) Myocardial-fiber necroses, infiltrated with numerous leukocytes, in the right ventricle of a rat 24 hours after subcutaneous injection of 30 mg isoproterenol/kg (hematoxylin-eosin stain). (B) Prevention of the isoproterenol effect shown in (A) by the simultaneous administration of isoproterenol (30 mg/kg) + verapamil (50 mg/kg) at different subcutaneous injection sites (neck, abdominal region). Experiments of Fleckenstein and Leder; see Fleckenstein (1968a).

Wistar rats. In this early study (Fleckenstein, 1968a), rat A, following one single subcutaneous dose of 30 mg isoproterenol/kg, developed within 24 hours many disseminated necroses, infiltrated by a large number of leukocytes. Rat B, on the other hand, had been given isoproterenol (30 mg/kg) plus verapamil (50 mg/kg). In consequence, the right ventricular myocardium of animal B remained completely intact. The same type of experiment is shown in Figure 88. In this case, compound D 600 was successfully applied for cardioprotection.

The rapid incorporation of Ca into the hearts of isoproterenol-treated rats was also demonstrated histochemically with the help of v. Kossa's (1902) method. This

Isoproterenol

Isoproterenol
+
D 600

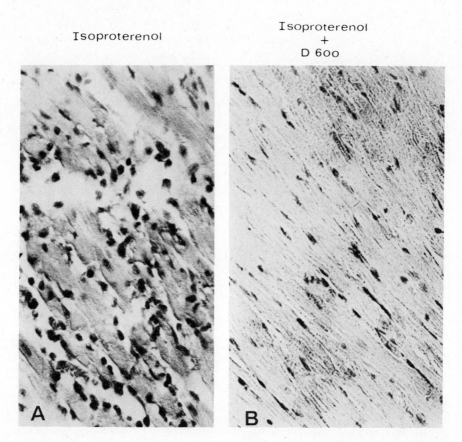

FIGURE 88. (*A*) Myocardial necroses produced by 30 mg isoproterenol/kg in the right ventricular wall of a rat 24 hours after subcutaneous injection (hematoxylin-eosin stain). (*B*) Prevention of isoproterenol-induced myocardial necroses by D 600 (20 mg/kg) simultaneously administered with 30 mg isoproterenol/kg, however at separate subcutaneous injection sites. From Fleckenstein, Döring, and Leder (1969).

technique visualizes Ca deposits as black spots. Thereby cardiac calcification could be revealed as early as 3 hours after the isoproterenol injection (see Figure 89*A*). However again, no calcified necroses developed when the cardiotoxic dose of isoproterenol (30 mg/kg) was injected simultaneously with 20 mg/kg of compound D 600 (Figure 89*B*).

Cardiac necroses in rats were also produced in the course of our studies by intraperitoneal injection of high doses of Ca salts. In addition, the animals were subjected to strong physical exercise (swimming stress) in order to elicit endogenous sympathetic transmitter release. Under these conditions, again multiple calcified

Isoproterenol

Isoproterenol
+
D 600

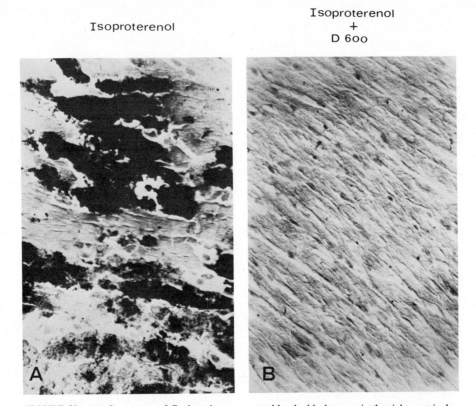

FIGURE 89. (*A*) Occurrence of Ca deposits, represented by the black areas, in the right ventricular wall of a rat 3 hours after the subcutaneous injection of 30 mg isoproterenol/kg. (v. Kossa's stain for Ca salts.) (*B*) Protection from the isoproterenol effect shown in (*A*) by the simultaneous subcutaneous administration of 20 mg D 600/kg. From Fleckenstein, Döring, and Leder (1969).

left ventricular fiber necroses appeared within 1 hour after the Ca administration (Rat A in Figure 90*A*). However, in most cases only minor or no calcified lesions were discernible when the rats had received a prophylactic dose of verapamil (50 mg/kg) 10 min before the Ca administration (Rat B in Figure 90*B*).

Another particularly reliable method of producing within 3 days severe calcified myocardial lesions in rats consists, according to our observations, of the injection of one single intramuscular dose of 300,000 to 500,000 IU vitamin D_3/kg in the form of water-soluble cholecalciferol (Vi-De$_3$-Hydrosol®, Wander AG, Bern, Switzerland). This type of myocardial Ca overload is also highly responsive to certain Ca antagonists. For instance, with verapamil (two daily subcutaneous doses of 30 mg/kg for 4 days) the promoter effect of vitamin D_3 on myocardial Ca uptake was inhibited by approximately 85 to 90% regarding the absolute amount of incorporated

Calcium   Overdose

Calcium   Overdose
+
Verapamil

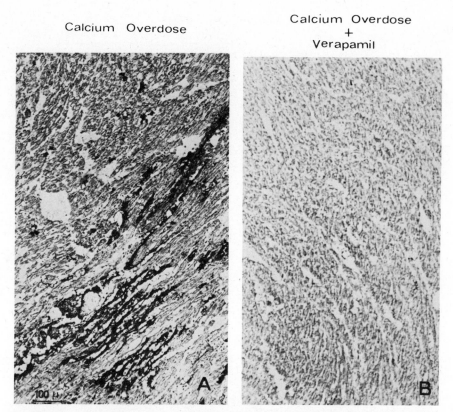

FIGURE 90.   (A) Occurrence of Ca deposits in necrotic cardiac tissue, represented by black areas ·
Kossa's stain). Left ventricular wall of a rat 60 min after intraperitoneal injection of 540 mg Ca/kg
the form of a 20% solution of "Calcium-Sandoz," ie., a mixture of Ca gluconate and Ca lactobionate.
In addition, the rat was subjected to swimming stress for 15 min between the 30th and 45th min after
the Ca administration. (B) Complete protection against Ca-induced left ventricular necroses by intraperitoneal injection of 50 mg verapamil/kg 10 min before intraperitoneal administration of 540 mg Ca/
kg. All other experimental conditions were exactly the same as in experiment A.

Ca, and by 90 to 95% regarding the accumulation of ^{45}Ca. Complete protection
against D_3-stimulated myocardial Ca overload has also been provided by diltiazem
(for more details see Figure 185 and Tables 16 and 17 in Section 6.2.4).

However the most impressive demonstration of the cardioprotective efficacy of
Ca antagonists such as verapamil and D 600 was achieved, apart from using v.
Kossa's method, by electron microscopy (Figures 91 to 94), ^{45}Ca autoradiography
(Figure 95), and with the fuchsinophilic reaction (Figure 96). As an example, Figure
91 shows the normal ultrastructure of the right ventricular myocardium of a control

Control rat heart

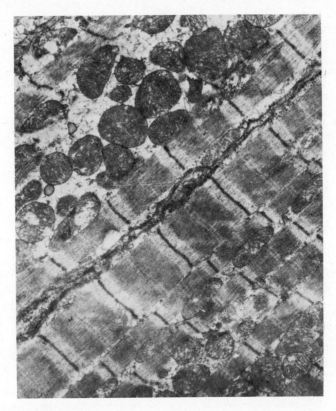

FIGURE 91.   Normal ultrastructure of right ventricular myocardium of a control rat. From Fleckenstein, Janke, Döring, and Leder (1975).

rat without isoproterenol. Figures 92 and 93 illustrate severe ultrastructural damage of two right ventricles 6 hours after subcutaneous injection of 30 mg isoproterenol/ kg. The latter pictures are characterized by the well-known degradation of myofibrils and mitochondria as has been already discussed. In contrast to this, the same dose of 30 mg isoproterenol/kg produced (Figure 94) only slight ultrastructural changes when given simultaneously with 50 mg verapamil/kg. In addition, Figure 95A represents an autoradiogram of the left ventricular myocardium of a rat examined 6 hours after injection of 30 mg isoproterenol/kg subcutaneously and 100 μ Ci ^{45}Ca/ kg intraperitoneally. Here many radioactive spots are distributed over the ventricular wall with a certain preference for the inner layer. However, in the same type of experiment, simultaneous administration of 50 mg verapamil/kg prevented the formation of radiocalcium deposits completely (Figure 95B). There is no other his-

Isoproterenol

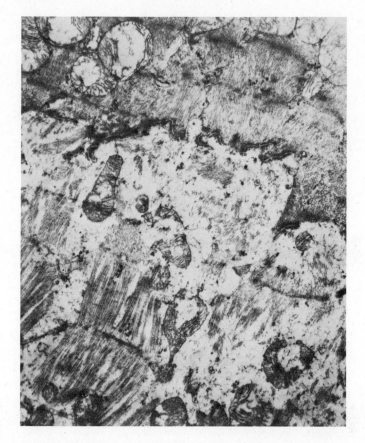

FIGURE 92.   Ultrastructural lesions of myofibrils and mitochondria in the right ventricular myocardium of a rat 6 hours after subcutaneous injection of 30 mg isoproterenol/kg. Note the disruption of internal texture resulting from myofibrillar supercontraction following cytoplasmic Ca overload. From Fleckenstein, Janke, Döring, and Leder (1975).

tological method that marks necrotizing cardiac tissue in such a colorful manner as the fuchsinophilic reaction. The principle is that the damaged fibers appear in red or pink, whereas the intact myocardium is blue or green-blue. As an example, Figure 96A shows that following subcutaneous injection of the cardiotoxic standard dose of 30 mg isoproterenol/kg to a rat, relatively great proportions of the right ventricular wall took up the red color, indicative of tissue damage, whereas after administration of isoproterenol plus verapamil, only the green-blue color of intact myocardial tissue appeared (Figure 96B). However, the fuchsinophilic reaction is positive not only in definitely necrotic areas but also in myocardial fibers that are

Isoproterenol

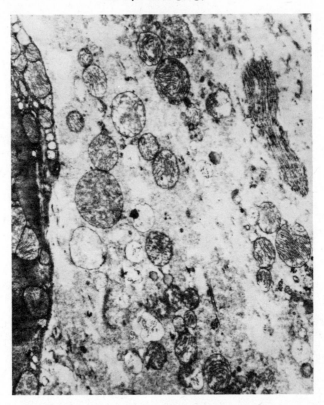

FIGURE 93.   Severe ultrastructural damage, consisting of myofibrolysis and mitochondrial degradation in the right ventricular myocardium of a rat 6 hours after subcutaneous injection of 30 mg isoproterenol/ kg. From Fleckenstein, Janke, Döring, and Leder (1975).

in a subnecrotic state, possibly with a chance to recover. Accordingly, the red-colored regions are usually larger than the irreversibly damaged parts of the tissue, marked with ^{45}Ca autoradiography or with v. Kossa's technique.

The isoproterenol-induced lesions are evenly distributed over the right ventricular wall and do not exhibit any relation to the vascular topography. It should be remembered in this context that one of the early hypotheses had incriminated the hypotensive action of isoproterenol as being the primary cause of a decrease in coronary blood flow and consequently of hypoxic myocardial damage. However, in the light of our actual results, this old concept is no longer tenable because it does not account for other types of cardiac necrotization that are also due to Ca overload, but are lacking concomitant hypotensive reactions. Moreover, the cardioprotective action of Ca antagonists certainly does not depend on the neutralization

Isoproterenol + Verapamil

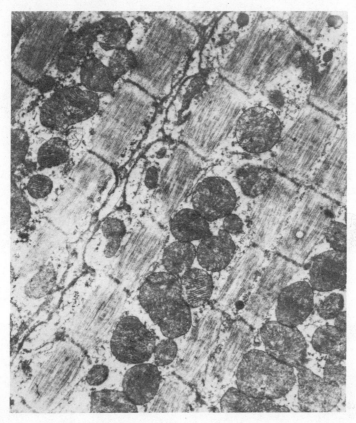

FIGURE 94. Prevention by verapamil of considerable ultrastructural alterations in the right ventricular myocardium of a rat. Picture was taken 6 hours after simultaneous administration of 30 mg isoproterenol/ kg + 50 mg verapamil/kg at separate injection sites. From Fleckenstein, Janke, Döring, and Leder (1975).

of isoproterenol-induced hypotension (or tachycardia). For instance, verapamil could completely prevent cardiac necrotization without attenuation of the isoproterenol-induced fall in coronary perfusion pressure and without normalization of the increase in heart rate (Fleckenstein, Janke, Döring, and Leder, 1974). Thus hemodynamic factors do not seem of major etiological importance either in the development of isoproterenol-induced cardiac necrotization or in the cardioprotection provided by Ca antagonists. This was also shown in a detailed study of Strubelt and Siegers (1975) on rat hearts *in situ*. Moreover, both necrotization produced by β-adrenergic overstimulation as well as cardioprotection by verapamil was demonstrated to occur

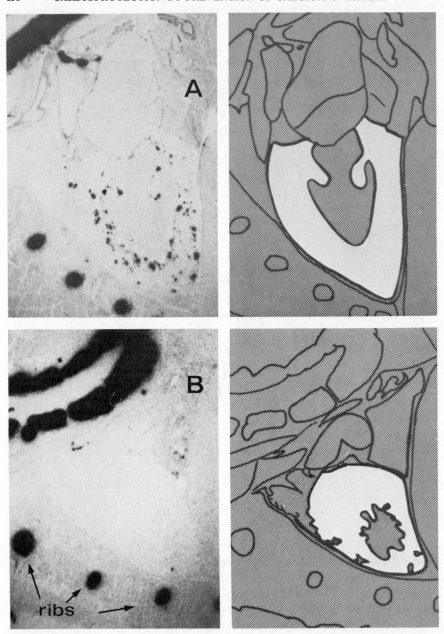

FIGURE 95.   (*A*) Autoradiogram of 30-μm-thick section of rat thorax taken 6 hours after subcutaneous injection of 30 mg isoproterenol/kg; 100 μCi ^{45}Ca/kg administered intraperitoneally at the same time as isoproterenol. Note accumulation of activity, particularly in inner layer of left ventricle. Position of heart (white area) marked on the right side. (*B*) Same as in (*A*), except for simultaneous injection of 50 mg verapamil/kg subcutaneously. Note prevention by verapamil of isoproterenol-induced radiocalcium deposition. Exposure of films (Kodak Regulix), 8 months at −20°C; ×4.8. From Fleckenstein, Janke, Döring, and Leder (1975).

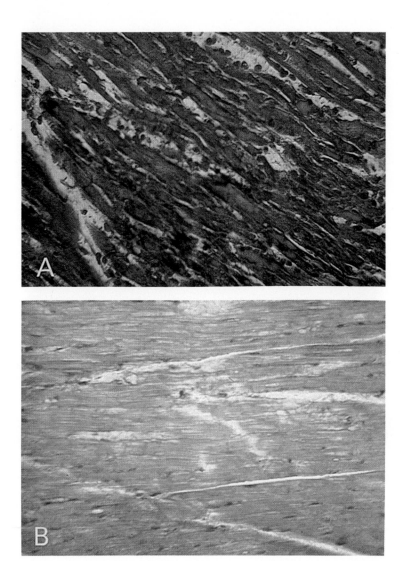

FIGURE 96. Fuchsinophilic reaction. Demonstration of the cardioprotective action of verapamil. (*A*) Disseminated structural lesions in the right ventricular myocardium of a rat 24 hours after subcutaneous administration of 30 mg isoproterenol/kg only. Necrotic and prenecrotic fibers are visualized by their positive fuchsinophilic reaction (red or pink color), whereas normal myocardial tissue appears blue or green-blue. (*B*) Prevention of isoproterenol-induced necrotization by simultaneous administration of isoproterenol (30 mg/kg) + verapamil (50 mg/kg) at different subcutaneous injection sites. The absence of red-colored necrotic tissue, 24 hours later, is obvious. The pink-colored material in the cross-sectioned capillaries consists merely of erythrocytes. From O. Leder in Fleckenstein, Döring, Janke, and Byon (1975).

in vitro in tissue cultures of fetal human heart muscle, that is to say, completely independent of any vascular circulatory influence (Hofmann, Schleich, Schroeter, Weidinger, and Wiest (1977)).

3.5. PROMOTION OR INHIBITION OF MYOCARDIAL CALCIUM OVERLOAD AND NECROTIZATION BY CHANGES IN THE EXTRACELLULAR CATION CONCENTRATIONS

3.5.1. Modifications of Cardiotoxicity Following Alterations of the Plasma Calcium Level

The new concept of Ca overload implies that the susceptibility of the myocardium to necrotization varies in parallel with the availability of extracellular Ca. This means that the extracellular Ca concentration plays a most important role in determining the magnitude of myocardial Ca overload, and consequently the number and size of cardiac lesions. For instance, Table 8 shows that daily oral doses of 3.0 mg dihydrotachysterol/kg increased the Ca concentration in the rat plasma within 3 days from the control value of 4.77 up to 7.13 mEq/l. Conversely there was a fall down to 2.30 mEq Ca/l 6 hours after injection of suitable doses of calcitonin. Such changes in plasma Ca concentrations fundamentally alter the extent of Ca uptake in isoproterenol-treated hearts. Thus dihydrotachysterol, by improving the Ca supply, tremendously potentiated the isoproterenol-induced Ca incorporation, as already demonstrated in Figures 78 and 79. Calcitonin, on the other hand, by reducing the availability of Ca, restricted the promoter effect of isoproterenol on myocardial Ca uptake considerably (see Figure 97). Thereby the production of necroses was significantly inhibited (Fleckenstein, Pachinger, Leder, Hein, and

TABLE 8. Increase or Decrease of Extracellular Ca Supply to Rat Hearts Following Administration of Dihydrotachysterol or Calcitonin, Respectively[a]

Treatment	Plasma Ca Concentration (mEq Ca/ℓ)
Control rats	4.77 (± 0.09)
Treatment with dihydrotachysterol (daily oral dose of 3.0 mg/kg for 3 days)	7.13 (± 0.23)
Treatment with calcitonin (6 hours after subcutaneous injection of 2 $\times$ 40 units/kg)	2.30 (± 0.10)

[a]From Fleckenstein, Janke, Döring, and Leder (1974).

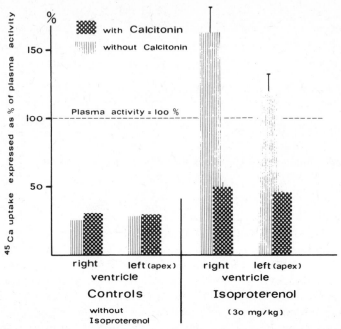

FIGURE 97. Restriction by calcitonin of the isoproterenol-induced radiocalcium accumulation in the myocardium of rats. Subcutaneous application of calcitonin (each time 4 units/100 g body weight) 2 hours before and 2 hours after administration of isoproterenol. The net ^{45}Ca uptake into the right and left ventricular wall was measured after a time lapse of 6 hours following the simultaneous injection of isoproterenol (30 mg/kg subcutaneously) and radiocalcium (10 μCi ^{45}Ca/kg intraperitoneally). From Fleckenstein, Janke, Döring, and Leder (1974).

Janke, 1972). Similarly Urbanek, Vasku, Bednarik, and Urbankova (1969) observed a prophylactic effect of EDTA against necroses in corticosteroid-cardiomyopathic rats. This action was obviously due to inhibition of Ca overload by means of chelation of interstitial free Ca ions. Nevertheless, the quantity of accumulated Ca and the number and size of myocardial lesions also depend on the actual concentrations of K, Mg, and H ions, which are capable of interfering with the mechanisms of Ca uptake or storage.

3.5.2. Cardioprotection Due to the Natural Calcium-Antagonistic Efficacy of Potassium and Magnesium Ions

A beneficial cardioprotective effect of K and Mg salts against corticosteroid cardiomyopathy and isoproterenol-induced myocardial necroses was early recognized by Selye (1960), Bajusz (1963), Rona, Kahn, and Chappel (1965), and others. But at this time, a loss of myocardial K simultaneously with a gain of Na was the only ion shift that was considered as being pathogenetically important. Thus for a while, the prophylactic efficacy of K and Mg salts remained unexplained. When, however, the decisive role of Ca overload had been established in the course of our studies, the question arose whether, for instance, KCl or $MgCl_2$ act as antidotes against necrotizing agents by way of inhibiting myocardial Ca accumulation. In fact, the results shown in Figure 98 demonstrate surprisingly strong Ca-antagonistic potencies of the K and Mg salts. Even one single oral dose of KCl or $MgCl_2$ (10 mmol/kg) could greatly depress the isoproterenol-induced ^{45}Ca uptake in the wall of both ventricles. The isoproterenol-induced rise of the absolute myocardial Ca content was also lowered by the oral KCl or $MgCl_2$ administration (see Figure 99). In parallel, the occurrence of disseminated fiber necroses was considerably rarified (Figure 100). However, when compared with the outstanding cardioprotection by verapamil or D 600 (see Figure 86), the prophylactic efficacy of the K or Mg salts is less pronounced. Interestingly enough, the sites of action of K and Mg ions seem to be different from those of verapamil and other organic Ca antagonists, since the K and Mg ions do not block the transsarcolemmal Ca channels. Presumably, the K and Mg ions restrict only the capacity for intracellular Ca accumulation, probably

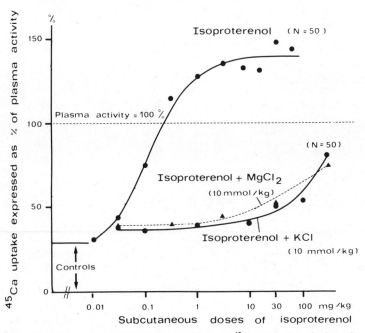

FIGURE 98. Prevention of excessive isoproterenol-induced ^{45}Ca uptake into the inner layer of the left ventricular myocardium of rats by a single oral standard dose of KCl (10 mmol/kg) or $MgCl_2$ (10 mmol/kg). The log dose–response curves were obtained 6 hours after simultaneous injection of 10 μCi ^{45}Ca/kg (intraperitoneally) and the different amounts of isoproterenol (subcutaneously), with and without KCl or $MgCl_2$. The salt solutions were always given with a stomach tube just before the isoproterenol and ^{45}Ca administration. From Janke and Fleckenstein, see Fleckenstein (1970/1971a,b).

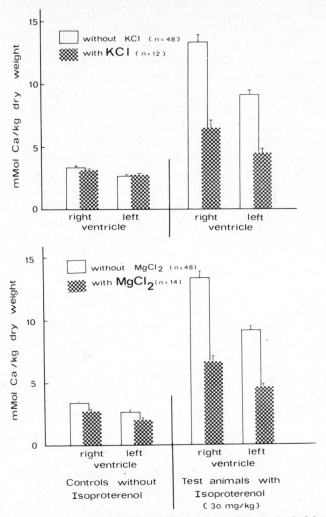

FIGURE 99. Marked diminution of the isoproterenol-induced Ca overload of the right and left ventricular myocardium of rats by one single oral dose of 10 mmol KCl/kg or 10 mmol MgCl$_2$/kg. The salt solutions were given with a stomach tube just before the subcutaneous injection of 30 mg isoproterenol/kg. The absolute Ca contents of the ventricular walls were determined 6 hours later. From Frey, Janke, and Fleckenstein, unpublished.

by competing with Ca for certain intracellular binding sites. Confirmatory evidence of the proposed type of cardioprotection, that is, prevention of intracellular Ca overload via displacement of Ca by Mg and K ions, has subsequently been presented by other investigators at the Meeting of the International Study Group for Research in Cardiac Metabolism 1973 in Freiburg (see the contributions of Urbanek, Vasku, Bednarik, Praslicka, and Pospisil, 1975; Fedelesova, Ziegelhöffer, Luknarova, and Kostolansky, 1975; Slezak and Tribulova, 1975 in the Proceedings).

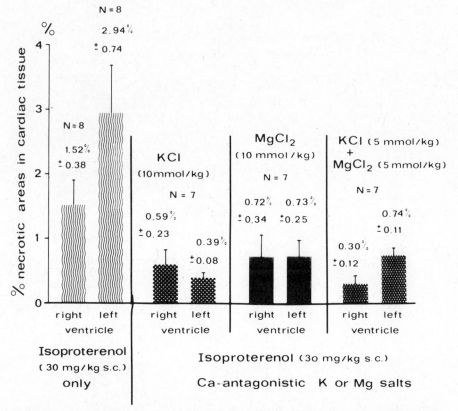

FIGURE 100.   Proportion of necrotic tissue 6 hours after subcutaneous injection of 30 mg isoproterenol/ kg with or without prophylactic administration of the Ca-antagonistic Ca or Mg salts. Experimental procedure as in Figure 99. From Leder and Fleckenstein, unpublished.

3.5.3.   Facilitation of Myocardial Calcium Overload and Necrotization by Potassium or Magnesium Deficiency; Prevention by Calcium Antagonists of Excessive Calcium Uptake in Potassium-deficient Hearts

In contrast with cardioprotection by high K or Mg intake, a tremendous sensitization to Ca-induced myocardial damage takes place in the state of K or Mg deficiency. Thus diets of low K or Mg content render the rat hearts extremely responsive to all promoters of myocardial Ca accumulation and their cardiotoxic influences. Thus in our experiments, there was a striking potentiation of the isoproterenol-induced net ^{45}Ca uptake into the rat ventricular myocardium after the animals had been fed a K-deficient diet for 7 days. During this period the K content of the blood plasma declined from 4.62 ($\pm$ 0.07) mEq/l to 2.80 ($\pm$ 0.1) mEq/l. Simultaneously the sensitivity to isoproterenol was raised in the right ventricular myocardium by a factor of 100 and in the left ventricular wall by a factor of nearly 1000. For instance, the log dose–response curves in Figure 101 demonstrate that in K-deficient rats the

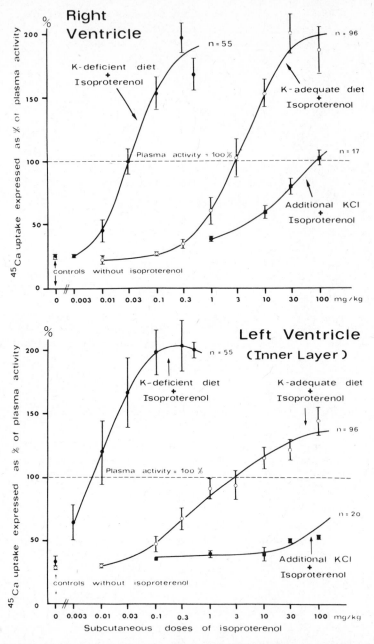

FIGURE 101. Tremendous potentiation by alimentary K deficiency of the net isoproterenol-induced radiocalcium uptake into the right and left ventricular myocardium of rats. The test animals were fed a K-deficient diet containing 0.005% K for 7 days, whereas the control animals were kept on a K-adequate diet with 0.9% K. The responsiveness to isoproterenol-induced ^{45}Ca uptake in the right and left ventricular myocardium of K-deficient rats is 100 and 1000, respectively, times greater than that of the control rats kept on a K-adequate regime. Conversely, the radiocalcium incorporation was reduced to an intensity far below the control level if additional KCl (one single oral dose of 10 mmol/kg) was administered together with the isoproterenol. All radioactivity measurements were carried out 6 hours after simultaneous injection of 10 μCi ^{45}Ca/kg intraperitoneally and the different doses of isoproterenol subcutaneously. From Frey, Janke, and Fleckenstein, unpublished.

small quantity of 0.03 mg isoproterenol/kg increased the right ventricular radiocalcium uptake to the same extent as the big dose of 3 mg/kg did in the control rats fed a K-adequate diet. Moreover, in the left ventricular wall of the K-deficient rats, the isoproterenol dose of 0.01 mg/kg proved to be equivalent to 10 mg/kg in the control animals.

A decrease in the plasma K concentration, similar to that produced by a K-deficient diet, can also be obtained in rats by administration of certain corticosteroids (desoxycorticosterone acetate, 9 α-fluorocortisol acetate, etc.). The sensitizing effects of 9 α-fluorocortisol acetate on isoproterenol-induced Ca accumulation was described in Section 3.3. In fact, the enormous potentiation of myocardial Ca uptake by this corticosteroid can now easily be related to the decrease in plasma K concentration the drug produces. The same explanation applies to an observation of Guideri, Barletta, and Lehr (1975). These authors found that the cardiotoxicity of isoproterenol was increased about 17,000 times in rats pretreated for 3 weeks with desoxycorticosterone acetate and saline. Even pretreatment of rats with this corticosteroid for 6 days potentiated the isoproterenol-induced ultrastructural lesions considerably (Bier and Rona, 1979).

It is a well-known fact that a diet of low K content, with or without additional administration of corticosteroids and saline, produces multiple cardiac necroses in rats (Follis, Orent-Keiles, and McCollum, 1942; Kornberg and Endicott, 1946; Grundner-Culemann, 1952; Selye and Bajusz, 1959; Nickerson, Karr, and Dresel, 1961; Tucker, Hanna, Kaiser, and Darrow, 1963). The K content of such hearts was reduced by 30% (Orent-Keiles and McCollum, 1941). There is no doubt that such a K deficit largely facilitates Ca overload and consequential necrotization, particularly under stress conditions when the endogenous sympathetic catecholamine release is intensified. However, even in this special situation of K deficiency, verapamil proved to be capable of completely neutralizing, in our experiments on rats, the exaggerated Ca uptake and the greater susceptibility to necrotizing agents such as isoproterenol (see Figure 102) and other Ca promoters. And $MgCl_2$ also effectively counteracted the excessive deposition of Ca in the myocardium of rats fed a low-K diet (Figure 103). Apparently the Mg ions occupy free intracellular binding sites in the K-deficient heart muscle fibers where otherwise a deleterious accumulation of Ca would take place. On the other hand, the effects of alimentary Mg deficiency in rats, dogs, and calves closely resemble those of a K-deficient diet, because in all these cases, calcified myocardial necroses develop (Schrader, Prickett and Salmon, 1937; Moore, Hallman, and Sholl, 1938; Lowenhaupt, Schulman, and Greenberg, 1950; Vitale, Hellerstein, Nakamura, and Lown, 1961; for more pertinent references see Heggtveit, Herman, and Mishra, 1964). The latter authors presented a detailed study on the ultrastructure of Mg-deficient rat hearts and emphasized as the most obvious alterations (1) mitochondrial damage (swelling, vacuolization, cristolysis, calcification) and (2) myofibrillar destruction (disruption of Z-line structure, fragmentation of myofilaments, myofibrolysis), that is to say, ultrastructural changes of striking similarity to those produced by Ca overload under the influence of cardiotoxic doses of isoproterenol (see Figures 92 and 93).

In this connection Lehr, Chau, and Irene (1975) put forward the interesting

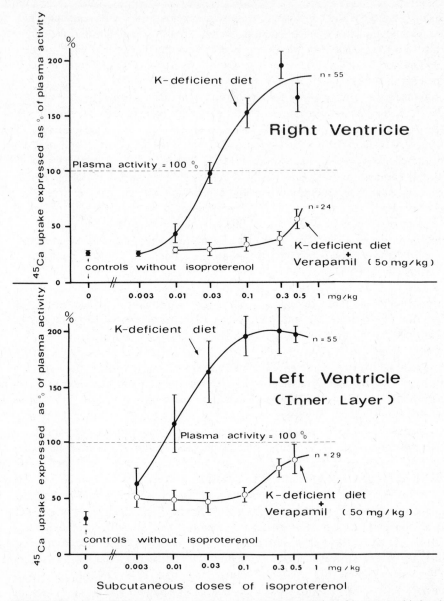

FIGURE 102. Neutralization by verapamil of the tremendous potentiation of isoproterenol-induced myocardial radiocalcium uptake in K-deficient rats (kept on a diet with 0.005% K for 7 days). The log dose–response curves were obtained using the same principal procedures as in Figure 101. From Frey, Janke, and Fleckenstein, unpublished.

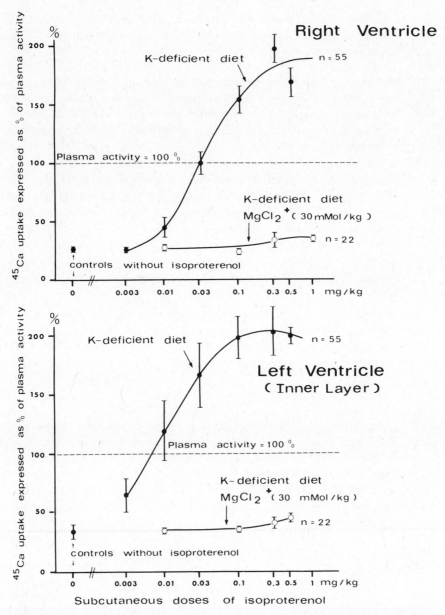

FIGURE 103. Neutralization by $MgCl_2$ of the tremendous potentiation of isoproterenol-induced myocardial radiocalcium uptake in K-deficient rats (kept on a diet with 0.005% K for 7 days). Administration of a single oral dose of 30 mmol MgCl/kg, using a stomach tube, simultaneously with the subcutaneous injection of the different amounts of isoproterenol. All other experimental procedures were identical with those in Figures 101 and 102. From Frey, Janke and Fleckenstein, unpublished.

question whether, even in the etiology of isoproterenol-induced cardiac lesions, Mg losses from the myocardium might play a decisive role. Pertinent studies on rats carried out in our laboratory have since then led to the following results:

1. The onset of high-energy-phosphate breakdown, as the most fundamental step in the course of necrotization, temporally coincides, during the first 2 hours after isoproterenol administration, with the acute gain of Ca. At this early stage, myocardial Ca overload is the absolutely dominant intracellular electrolyte shift.

2. Nevertheless, a negative myocardial Mg balance slowly develops in the isoproterenol-treated rats as a regular phenomenon. A quantity of up to 20% of the normal cardiac Mg content may be lost within 12 hours after subcutaneous injection of 30 mg isoproterenol/kg (Janke, Fleckenstein, Hein, Leder, and Sigel, 1975).

3. Both potentiation of Ca influx and inhibition of Mg uptake through the sarcolemma membrane have to be considered integral consequences of adrenergic β-receptor stimulation by isoproterenol (Späh and Fleckenstein, 1979).

4. At an advanced stage of the isoproterenol intoxication, Ca sequestration and Mg losses, probably attributable to large mitochondrial cation shifts (Sordahl and Silver, 1975), became closely linked, so that the myocardial Ca and Mg movements approach reciprocal magnitude.

The results confirm the general conclusion that myocardial Ca overload is the primary event in the production of cardiac necroses by isoproterenol. However, the simultaneous restriction of transsarcolemmal Mg supply to the myocardium may act as an auxiliary factor in facilitating isoproterenol-induced myocardial Ca overload, and thereby functional and structural decay. On the other hand, Mg deficiency is certainly not an indispensible prerequisite of necrotization . For instance, as recently shown by Barzu, Dam, Cuparencu, Dancea, and Böhm (1979), an even sevenfold increase in the cardiac Ca concentration, leading to high-energy-phosphate breakdown and ultrastructural alterations, could be obtained in rats by intravenous infusion of a 2.5% $CaCl_2$ solution; but there was no change in the global Mg content of the hearts. Again, prophylactic administration of verapamil stabilized the myocardial structures.

3.5.4. Prevention of Myocardial Calcium Overload by Hydrogen Ions; Cardioprotective Effects of Acidosis and Organic Calcium Antagonists in Hypoxic and Ischemic Hearts

The cardiotoxicity of isoproterenol not only changes in response to variations of the myocardial Ca, K, or Mg supply, but also exhibits a clear pH dependency. Thus we have found in the course of our studies on rat hearts *in situ* that H ions are able to antagonize the isoproterenol-induced myocardial Ca overload, whereas alkalization promotes the Ca uptake (Janke, Döring, Hein, and Fleckenstein, 1972; Fleckenstein, Janke, Döring, and Leder, 1974). Accordingly, acidification by oral doses of NH_4Cl or by an increase in the CO_2 content of the respiration mixture restricts the radiocalcium incorporation considerably. Figures 104 and 105 show the results using rats pretreated with oral doses of NH_4Cl, which were so adjusted that the arterial blood pH dropped from an initial value of 7.4 to a final value between 7.1 and 7.2 before the different doses of isoproterenol were subcutaneously administered. A preventive efficacy of NH_4Cl against isoproterenol-induced myocardial injury has also been observed by Lehr, Chau, and Kaplan (1972). But these authors postulated that the beneficial effect of NH_4Cl was primarily based upon the removal of Na. However, our results from the experiments in which rats were kept in a respiration mixture containing 10% CO_2 show that in fact it is the increased concentration of H ions that is responsible for the limitation of radiocalcium uptake (Figure 104). These results are fully consistent with observations of other researchers, who also demonstrated a direct inhibition of the myocardial radiocalcium uptake by acidosis (Morgenstern, Noack, and Köhler, 1972; Poole-Wilson, 1978). Conversely, as also shown in Figure 104, alkalization by oral doses of $NaHCO_3$ led to

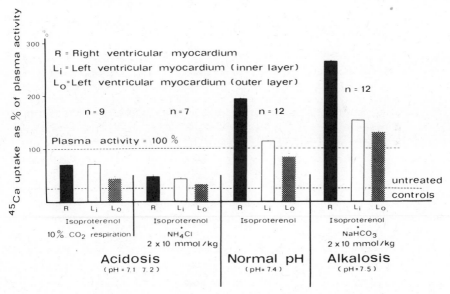

FIGURE 104. Influence of plasma pH on isoproterenol-induced net radiocalcium uptake into the ventricular myocardium of rats: inhibition by acidosis, potentiation by alkalosis. The net ^{45}Ca uptake was always measured 6 hours after simultaneous injection of 30 mg isoproterenol/kg (subcutaneously) and 10 μCi ^{45}Ca/kg (intraperitoneally). *Acidosis* was produced either by keeping the rats in an artificial atmosphere of 10% CO_2, 40% O_2, and 50% N_2 for 6 hours after the isoproterenol administration or by oral pretreatment with NH_4Cl. In the latter case, two doses of 20 mmol NH_4Cl/kg each were fed with a stomach tube 24 and 12 hours before and a third dose immediately before the isoproterenol administration. For *alkalization* two oral doses of 10 mmol $NaHCO_3$ each (12 hours and immediately before the isoproterenol injection) were applied. From Fleckenstein, Janke, Döring, and Leder (1974).

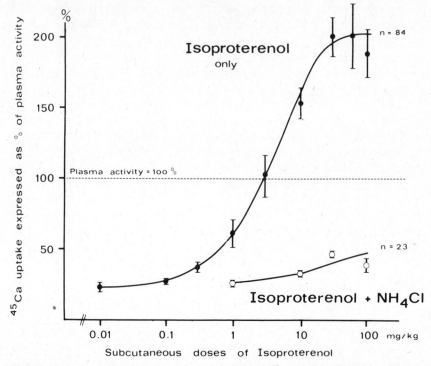

FIGURE 105.   Prevention of excessive isoproterenol-induced ^{45}Ca uptake into right ventricular myo-cardium of rats by oral pretreatment with NH_4Cl. Two doses of 20 mmol NH_4Cl/kg each were admin-istered 24 and 12 hours prior to the experiments. A third dose was given simultaneously with subcutaneous injection of different amounts of isoproterenol and 10 μCi ^{45}Ca/kg intraperitoneally. Net ^{45}Ca uptake into 1 g of fresh cardiac tissue was measured 6 hours later and expressed as percentage of corresponding ^{45}Ca activity in 1 ml of plasma. From Janke, Fleckenstein, Hein, Leder, and Sigel (1975).

a potentiation of the isoproterenol effect. This applies to the incorporation of labeled Ca as well as to the high-energy-phosphate breakdown and the subsequent pro-duction of myocardial lesions.

The decrease in transsarcolemmal Ca influx by H ions was visualized in our laboratory also with electrophysiological techniques (Kohlhardt, Haap, and Figulla, 1976). Thus in voltage-clamp experiments on trabeculae and small papillary muscles from the right ventricle of cats, the slow inward Ca current was found to be shifted by acidosis to considerably lower values over a wide voltage range. Consequently, after partial depolarization, the upstroke velocity (dV/dt_{max}) of the Ca-mediated action potentials was also clearly diminished. There is no doubt that the well-known negative inotropic effect of a lowered pH (see Brown and Miller, 1952; Nahas, 1957; McElroy, Gerdes, and Brown, 1958; Bendixen, Lauer, and Flacke, 1963; and others) can be explained, to a great extent, by this inhibitory action of H ions on the transmembrane Ca conductivity. Probably acidosis, by protonation of struc-tural proteins, reduces the number of negatively charged binding sites that temporarily store Ca at the myocardial fiber surface and subsequently deliver it to the slow channel (see Section 1.4.1).

However, there are still two other possibilities of proton interference with Ca-dependent excitation–contraction coupling, that is to say, (1) a reduction by acidosis of the release of Ca from the cardiac SR and (2) a competition of H ions with Ca at the myofibrils. Concerning the first effect on the SR, optimal Ca binding takes place, according to observations of Schwartz (1970/1971), at a pH around 6.5 to 6.7. At this pH the delivery of Ca from isolated SR is minimal. If, however, the pH is normalized, bound Ca is rapidly liberated. Therefore, Schwartz suggested that the intracellular proton concentration might act as a physiological controller in that acidosis, naturally occurring in hypoxia, reduces the availability of Ca to the contractile system and thereby spares ATP. There is also ample evidence of the second effect, that is, competitive inhibition by H ions of the Ca-activated myofibrillar ATPase itself (for details see Schädler, 1967). Thus acidosis reduces transsarcolemmal Ca incorporation as well as the physiological and pathological effects of Ca ions in the intracellular space. Hence cardioprotection by H ions is pluricausal in its nature, but in any case consists of preventing excessive Ca-dependent high-energy-phosphate breakdown and its deleterious functional and structural consequences. Alkalosis exerts the opposite effects. All our findings about the influence of Ca, Mg, K, and H ions on the development of cardiac lesions can be reduced to the following simple scheme (Fleckenstein, Döring, Janke, and Byon, 1975):

$_{Ca}$	Ca	Ca
Mg, K, H	Mg, K, H	$_{Mg, K, H}$
Prevention	Normal	Production
of	cationic	of
necroses	balance	necroses

As indicated on the right, necrosis will be facilitated when the cationic ratio changes in favor of Ca. This occurs in consequence of a large increase in the extracellular Ca concentration or because of a deficiency of Ca-antagonistic K, Mg, or H ions, as well as under the influence of excessive doses of β-adrenergic catecholamines or other promoters of transsarcolemmal Ca influx. Conversely, as shown on the left, myocardial necrotization can be prevented if Mg, K, or H ions predominate. Any measure that counteracts abundant intracellular Ca uptake (decrease in plasma Ca; greater availability of Mg, K, or H ions; inhibition of transsarcolemmal Ca influx by organic Ca antagonists) will accordingly stabilize the reserves of high-energy phosphates and thus help to prevent myocardial damage. There is no doubt that the H ions, among these cardioprotective factors, deserve particularly high interest because they alone are capable of spontaneously multiplying their concentration by many times in case of natural acidosis. Hence lowering of pH is an especially powerful means of myocardial self-defense.

The present results, originally obtained from studies on noncoronarogenic cardiac necroses, may also help to understand a series of interesting observations that were made on hypoxic and ischemic hearts. It has turned out in recent years that myocardial hypoxia or ischemia is usually complicated by an increase in transsarcolemmal Ca permeability that favors the occurrence of dangerous intracellular Ca accumulation, particularly in the mitochondria (Shen and Jennings, 1972a,b; Henry, Shuchleib, Davis, Weiss, and Sobel, 1977). Thus in hypoxic or ischemic hearts, the consequences of simple depression of ATP synthesis may be seriously aggravated by superimposed symptoms of Ca overload such as excessive splitting of ATP, rise in resting tension, rapid development of rigor, mitochondrial destruction, myofibrolysis, and so forth. Due to this fatal coincidence, necrotization of the hypoxic or ischemic myocardium is precipitated. On the other hand, elimination of these Ca-dependent accessory factors should result in a considerable attenuation of the detrimental influence of anoxia or ischemia. This is in fact true since it was demonstrated that verapamil (Nayler, Grau, and Slade, 1976; Reimer, Lowe, and Jennings, 1977; Nayler, Fassold, and Yepez, 1978; Robb-Nicholson, Currie, and Wechsler, 1978; Nayler, Ferrari, and Slade, 1978/1980), as well as nifedipine (Henry, 1976; Henry, Shuchleib, Borda, Roberts, Williamson, and Sobel, 1978; Henry, Clark, and Williamson, 1978/1980) and diltiazem (Weishaar, Ashikawa, and Bing, 1979; Nagao, Matlib, Franklin, Millard, and Schwartz, 1980) can improve the rate and extent of postanoxic or postischemic recovery by preventing additional damage resulting from Ca overload. A similar prophylactic affect is exerted by lowering the pH. Several authors have noted the beneficial influence of acidosis in maintaining myocardial structure and functional resuscitability of ischemic hearts (Bing, Brooks, and Messer, 1973; Greene and Weisfeldt, 1977). In the light of the present results, cardioprotection by acidosis now has to be attributed to the interference with intracellular Ca overload. Recent studies of Lakatta, Nayler, and Poole-Wilson (1979) and Nayler, Ferrari, Poole-Wilson, and Yepez (1979) have further substantiated this conclusion. The most critical phase at which an "avalanche" of Ca ions invades the ischemic myocardium is the moment of onset of reperfusion after previous circulatory standstill. In consequence, an explosionlike destruction of the myocardial mitochondria and myofibrils takes place. Certainly, with restoring the blood perfusion of the previously ischemic region, an unlimited Ca supply is reestablished, possibly comparable with the "calcium-paradox" described by Zimmerman and Hülsmann (1966). But in our opinion, the instantaneous disruption of the intracellular texture is also a "wash-out effect" in that local acidosis is reversed. Thereby the natural self-defense of the ischemic myocardium against Ca overload is abolished. In this situation, only the organic Ca antagonists of the verapamil-nifedipine type may afford a sufficient cardioprotective action. Moreover reoxygenation seems to be another factor that possibly contributes to the Ca-dependent myocardial self-destruction (Ruigrok, Boink, Spies, Blok, Maas, and Zimmerman, 1978). This is because the excessive uptake of Ca into the mitochondria, which eventually leads to functional and structural disintegration of these organelles, is an active respiration-supported process that instantaneously recommences when the oxygen supply is restored (see Section 1.4.3).

3.6. PROPHYLACTIC EFFICACY OF CALCIUM ANTAGONISTS AGAINST SPONTANEOUS MYOCARDIAL NECROTIZATION IN HEREDITARY CARDIOMYOPATHIC SYRIAN HAMSTERS

The results of our studies in the years 1968 to 1970 could be condensed, as schematically shown in Figure 106, to three essential statements (see Fleckenstein, 1968a, 1970/1971; Fleckenstein, Döring and Leder, 1969):

1. Calcium ions destroy the myocardium both functionally and structurally in case their intracellular concentration surpasses a critical level.

2. Intracellular Ca overload, leading to high-energy-phosphate exhaustion, is a decisive factor in the etiology of noncoronarogenic cardiac necrotization produced by β-adrenergic catecholamines, dihydrotachysterol, vitamin D, and so forth.

3. Calcium antagonists such as verapamil, D 600, or prenylamine exert cardioprotective actions and inhibit necrotization by preventing deleterious Ca overload.

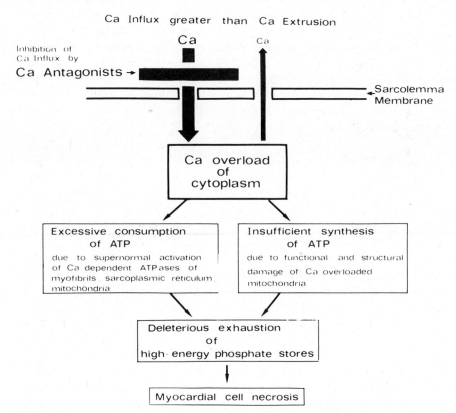

FIGURE 106. Scheme of myocardial necrotization produced by intracellular Ca overload and of prevention by Ca antagonists.

This concept attributed to intracellular Ca overload the distinct pathophysiological role of a "killer," whereas at that time most pathologists still considered Ca overload a cellular postmortem phenomenon, leading to the production of "calcic tombstones." However, in the early 1970s, an ideological change came about *pari passu* with a better understanding of one of the most fascinating disease models that experimental pathology has ever studied: the hereditary cardiomyopathy of the Syrian hamster. Since 1966, thanks to the effort of Dr. Eörs Bajusz, this disease, characterized by a spontaneous development of multifocal myocardial necroses, had rapidly become a subject of worldwide interdisciplinary research. Interestingly enough, one of the first significant observations of Bajusz, Baker, and Nixon (1966) was that cardiomyopathic hamsters in the prenecrotic phase responded to epinephrine with severe calcifying myocardial necroses, whereas similarly treated hearts from normal hamsters remained unaffected. Thus at the meetings of the International Study Group for Research in Cardiac Metabolism in London (1970) and Cape Town (1972), it was suggested that a joint study by three laboratories (Bajusz, Lossnitzer, Fleckenstein) be undertaken to clarify the possibly causative role of Ca overload in the hamster cardiomyopathy and to study the eventual responsiveness to a prophylactic treatment with Ca antagonists. Although Dr. Bajusz's death on February 24, 1973, meant the end of this common research project, he was still successful in demonstrating, together with Jasmin, that a long-term treatment with verapamil for 30 to 40 days prevented the development of disseminated myocardial necroses in cardiomyopathic hamsters up to 100% (personal communications of Dr. Bajusz dated December 14, 1972, and February 19, 1973).

According to the findings of Lossnitzer on cardiomyopathic hamsters of the strain BIO 8262, three age-dependent histopathological phases of the disease can be differentiated (Lossnitzer, 1975):

I.   Prenecrotic phase at the age of 27 to 36 days with no discernible cardiac lesions.

II. Phase of progressive multifocal myocardial necrotization at the age of 54 to 84 days.

III. Late phase at the age of 237 to 291 days, characterized by a smaller number of new lesions, but an increased occurrence of calcified scars.

The corresponding myocardial Ca contents of the left ventricular and septal myocardium at the different stages of the disease are shown in Table 9. During the prenecrotic phase there is obviously no spontaneous increase in Ca content above the control level found in healthy animals (about 8 mEq/kg dry weight). On the other hand, myocardial tissue with progressive necroses, obtained from phase II animals, exhibited a roughly 30 times higher Ca concentration (about 240 mEq/kg dry weight as an average). The particularly interesting changes in the myocardial Ca content during transition from the prenecrotic to the necrotizing phase are shown in Figure 107. Here in several cases peak values of approximately 1000 mEq Ca/kg dry weight were found around the 65th day of life. After this climax, the

TABLE 9. Myocardial Ca Content[a] in Different Age Groups of Myopathic Hamsters (BIO 8262) and Healthy Controls[b]

	Ca (mEq/kg)		
	Group I 27–31 Days	Group II 61–82 Days	Group III 237–264 Days
BIO 8262	7.90 ± 1.84	241.70 ± 180.81[c]	167.25 ± 140.00[c]
Controls	7.93 ± 1.09	8.85 ± 1.10	8.94 ± 1.58

[a]Values are expressed as the mean in mEq/kg dry tissue (left ventricle and septum) ± standard deviation (N = 13 in each group).
[b]Lossnitzer, Steinhardt, Grewe, and Stauch (1975).
[c]$p < 0.01$ (Student's t-test).

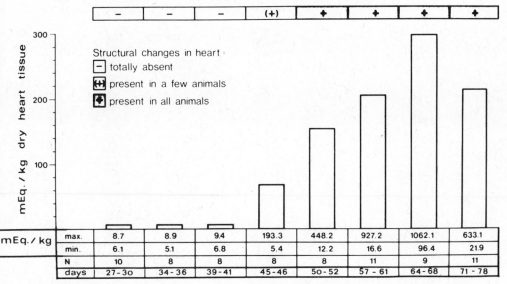

Myocardial calcium during transition from prenecrotic to necrotizing phase of cardiomyopathy in BIO 8262 hamsters

mEq./kg	max.	8.7	8.9	9.4	193.3	448.2	927.2	1062.1	633.1
	min.	6.1	5.1	6.8	5.4	12.2	16.6	96.4	21.9
	N	10	8	8	8	8	11	9	11
	days	27–30	34–36	39–41	45–46	50–52	57–61	64–68	71–78

FIGURE 107. Parallelism between the onset of spontaneous myocardial Ca overload around the 45th day of life and the development of fresh myocardial lesions in the left ventricular wall and the intraventricular septum of cardiomyopathic hamster hearts. The columns indicate the averages of Ca content of the left ventricular myocardium + septum at the different ages between the 27th and 78th day of life. N = number of animals in each age group. The maximum and minimum values indicate the extreme variations of Ca content (mEq/kg dry heart tissue) in each age group. Unpublished observations of Lossnitzer on a total of 73 cardiomyopathic animals of the strain BIO 8262.

155

myocardial Ca content seemed to decline, but the animals of age group III still contained in their hearts 15 to 20 times more Ca than normal.

The underlying changes in the net Ca-uptake rates, measured with labelled ^{45}Ca by Lossnitzer, Janke, Hein, Stauch, and Fleckenstein (1975), can be seen from Figure 108. During the first age period of 27 to 36 days, the ventricular myocardium of healthy and cardiomyopathic hamsters did not differ with respect to the intensity of ^{45}Ca incorporation. Then, in the age group II, with the onset of necrotization, the rate of net uptake of labeled Ca into the left ventricular myocardium (including the septum) of myopathic hamsters increased 10- to 15-fold in comparison with the controls. On the other hand, the cardiomyopathic hamsters of age group III exhibited a rate of ^{45}Ca incorporation that was only three times that of healthy animals. Thus the increase in the myocardial Ca uptake rate and the consequent rise in myocardial Ca content followed approximately the same time course as the development of fresh myocardial necroses did. However, this occurred only in the left ventricular myocardium and septum, since the musculature of the right ventricle is apparently

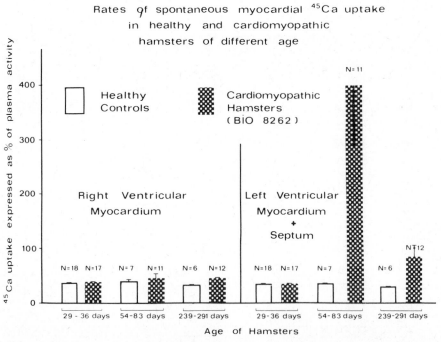

FIGURE 108.   Rates of net uptake of labeled Ca into the right and left ventricular myocardium of healthy and cardiomyopathic hamsters at various ages. The measurements were carried out 6 hours after intraperitoneal injection of 50 μCi ^{45}Ca/kg body weight. The ^{45}Ca uptake into 1 g of fresh cardiac tissue is expressed as a percentage of the corresponding ^{45}Ca activity in 1 ml of blood plasma (plasma activity = 100%). Values are expressed as mean ± SEM. Apparently ^{45}Ca incorporation is most intense in the left ventricular myocardium and septum of 54- to 83-day-old cardiomyopathic hamsters (age group II) that develop progressive multifocal cardiac necroses. The right ventricular myocardium of BIO 8262 hamsters is exempt from the disease. From Lossnitzer, Janke, Hein, Stauch, and Fleckenstein (1975).

exempt from the disease. The Ca concentration in the serum of BIO 8262 hamsters did not differ from that of healthy control animals and remained at the same value of approximately 5.5 to 6.0 mEq/l in the three age groups.

Regarding the dramatic increase in Ca content, it is not surprising that the necrotizing foci in the left ventricular myocardium of cardiomyopathic hamsters (strain BIO 14.6 and BIO 8262) exhibit practically the same ultrastructural manifestations of myocardial Ca overload that are also discernible after high doses of isoproterenol, alimentary K or Mg deficiency, or direct exposure to excess Ca. This applies, for instance, to the functional and structural alterations of the myofibrils that in diseased cardiac cells display supercontraction in the form of so-called contraction bands, lysis, and homogenization of the myofilaments with disappearance of the I bands and Z-line structures (Büchner and Onishi, 1970; Onishi, Bajusz, Büchner, and Rickers, 1970; Nakao, Oka, Chen, Bajusz, and Angrist, 1970). In fact, all these myofibrillar changes may be considered common features of intracellular myocardial Ca overload. The same is true of the characteristic appearance of mitochondrial damage (cristolysis, swelling, vacuolization, clarification of the matrix) that the necrotizing hamster myocardium also shares with other types of abundant myocardial Ca incorporation. As can be seen from Figure 109B, the spontaneous ultrastructural changes in a myocardial cell of a 280-day-old BIO 14.6 hamster are nearly identical with those resulting from isoproterenol-induced Ca overload (Figures 92 and 93). In addition, the frequent occurrence of granular Ca precipitates in the mitochondria of the diseased hamster myocardium is also indicative of excessive Ca engulfment. The precipitates closely resemble those produced by exposure of isolated mitochondria or cardiac tissue to high environmental Ca concentrations (Greenawalt, Rossi, and Lehninger, 1964; Legato, Spiro, and Langer, 1968). In both experimentally Ca-overloaded and cardiomyopathic hearts (Mohr, Hersener, and Lossnitzer, 1973) the mineral deposits are composed of Ca and phosphate as principal constituents, probably in the form of hydroxyapatite.

The average Ca content of mitochondria isolated from cardiomyopathic hamster hearts also proved to be abnormally high (Wrogemann, Blanchaer, Thakar, and Mezon 1975; Wrogemann and Nylen, 1978). Nevertheless, the demonstrable augmentation of the mitochondrial Ca in the diseased hearts was considerably smaller than under the influence of cardiotoxic doses of isoproterenol. This is presumably for the following reasons. The florid necrotizing phase, with excessive uptake of Ca into the mitochondria, is a transient stage that is rapidly terminated by the Ca-dependent self-destruction of these organelles. Administration of one single necrotizing dose of isoproterenol affects the whole mass of myocardial fibers *synchronously*. This means that even if only a minor fraction of the cardiac tissue perishes definitely in the form of multifocal lesions, all myocardial fibers and their mitochondria react simultaneously, so that an easily discernible peak of their Ca content is reached within 4 to 8 hours after the isoproterenol injection (see Figure 84). Contrarily, in cardiomyopathic hamster hearts, Ca-dependent necrotization of the individual fibers is totally *asynchronous*. Accordingly, fresh necroses can be observed in all cardiomyopathic hamster hearts of the age groups II and III (strain BIO 8262), that is, over a period of roughly 200 days. Hence the number of cells

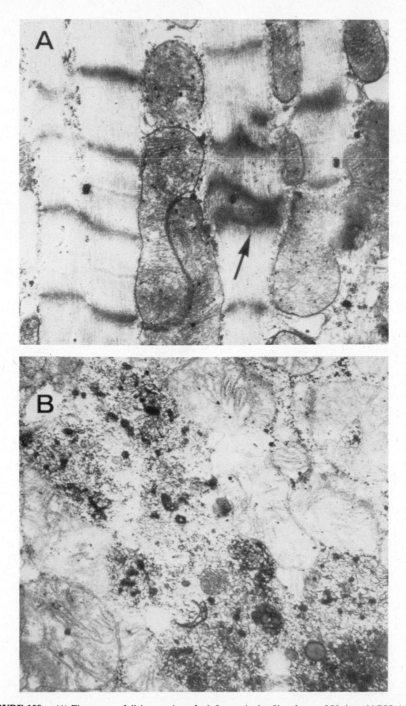

FIGURE 109. (*A*) First stage of disintegration of a left ventricular fiber from a 250-day-old BIO 14.6 cardiomyopathic hamster. As a typical response to intracellular Ca overload, local myofibrillar super-contraction with distortion of the Z lines and myofibrolysis sets in. The ultrastructure of the mitochondria is still intact. From Büchner, Onishi, and Wada (1978). (*B*) Advanced stage of disintegration of a left ventricular fiber from a 280-day-old BIO 14.6 cardiomyopathic hamster. Calcifying detritus originating from totally dissipated myofibrils fills the intermitochondrial space. The mitochondria too are badly damaged and show swelling, vacuolization, and cristolysis. From Büchner and Onishi (1970).

that just undergo acute necrotization do not constitute, at any moment of the disease, more than a small fraction in comparison with the overwhelming mass of ventricular fibers that have not yet been entangled by the pathogenic process. Therefore, during the usual procedure of isolation, the small amount of Ca-rich mitochondria that originates from acutely necrotizing cells always becomes strongly "diluted" with normal mitochondria from hitherto intact fibers. Thereby the true extent of mitochondrial Ca overload in fresh cardiomyopathic foci (and the repercussive defect in oxidative phosphorylation) is concealed to a great extent from assessment. Nevertheless, Wrogemann and Nylen (1978), studying the isolated mitochondria from 21- to 412-day-old cardiomyopathic hamster hearts, found a nearly twofold increase in Ca concentration on the average. On the other hand, the Mg content remained virtually unaffected. These functional data and the ultrastructural findings cited above certainly fit quite well into our concept of *necrotization by Ca overload*. However, to establish this causality, more than merely circumstantial evidence was required.

3.6.1. Acute Normalization of Prenecrotic Disorders of Ca Metabolism by Ca Antagonists

Needless to say, the hard facts that have brought understanding of the hamster cardiomyopathy into line with other forms of Ca-dependent myocardial necrotization originated almost exclusively from pertinent studies with Ca antagonists. The ability of Ca antagonists to overcome the exaggerated uptake of Ca could be demonstrated in our studies as early as the prenecrotic phase of the disease. In fact, as shown by Lossnitzer, Janke, Hein, Stauch, and Fleckenstein (1975), the first sign of the genetic abnormality consists of an increase in responsiveness of the left ventricular myocardium to isoproterenol-induced Ca uptake. Thus in 27- to 32-day-old cardiomyopathic hamsters (BIO 8262), a single subcutaneous dose of 1 mg isoproterenol/kg body weight produced, within 6 hours, an approximately 40% increase in the Ca content of the left ventricular myocardium, whereas healthy hamsters did not respond to this dose. Similar results were obtained on such young animals regarding the uptake rates of ^{45}Ca. In the absence of isoproterenol, no differences were discernible between 29- to 36-day-old healthy and cardiomyopathic hamsters. When, however, 1 mg isoproterenol/kg body weight was injected, the 28- to 33-day-old cardiomyopathic hamsters incorporated the labeled Ca much faster into the prenecrotic left ventricular and septal myocardium than the healthy controls of the same age did (see Figure 110). In other words, there is a latent facilitation of myocardial Ca uptake or an insufficiency of Ca extrusion that clearly precedes the spontaneous development of cardiomyopathic lesions. It is only under the influence of β-adrenergic catecholamines that this early inclination to excessive Ca incorporation manifests itself and even leads to a precipitous development of premature calcified necroses, as first shown with epinephrine by Bajusz, Baker, and Nixon (1966). Our attempts to counteract these early disorders of Ca metabolism with the Ca antagonist verapamil led promptly to satisfactory results. As reported on the occasion of the sixth annual meeting of the International Study Group for Research

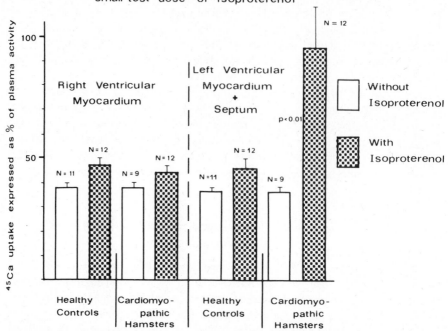

FIGURE 110. Influence of a small test dose of isoproterenol on ^{45}Ca uptake by the right and left ventricular myocardium of healthy and cardiomyopathic hamsters during the prenecrotic stage (age 28 to 33 days). Measurements were carried out 6 hours after subcutaneous administration of 1 mg isoproterenol/kg and intraperitoneal injection of 50 μCi ^{45}Ca/kg. Values are expressed as mean $\pm$ SE. Even before spontaneous cardiac lesions develop, the prenecrotic left ventricular myocardium and interventricular septum of cardiomyopathic hamsters respond to isoproterenol with a much larger incorporation of labeled Ca than normal. Thus the tendency to Ca overload clearly precedes the morphological manifestation of the disease. From Lossnitzer, Janke, Hein, Stauch, and Fleckenstein (1975).

in Cardiac Metabolism in 1973 in Freiburg, one single subcutaneous dose of verapamil (5 to 10 mg/kg) was fully effective in normalizing the exaggerated responsiveness of the prenecrotic hamster hearts to isoproterenol (Lossnitzer, Janke, Hein, Stauch, and Fleckenstein, 1975). Thus with the help of verapamil, the uptake rate of labeled Ca and the absolute Ca content of the left ventricular and septal myocardium of the prenecrotic hearts could be kept in the normal range (Figure 111). However, the ability of a single dose of verapamil to acutely normalize the myocardial Ca-uptake rates declined beyond the fortieth day of life, when the spontaneous production of overt necroses had started. The results obtained with verapamil resemble the observations with other Ca antagonists as, for instance, fendiline (Lossnitzer, Konrad, and Jakob, 1980).

Normalization by verapamil of exaggerated isoproterenol - induced
[45]Ca uptake into left ventricular and septal myocardium of
cardiomyopathic hamsters during the prenecrotic phase

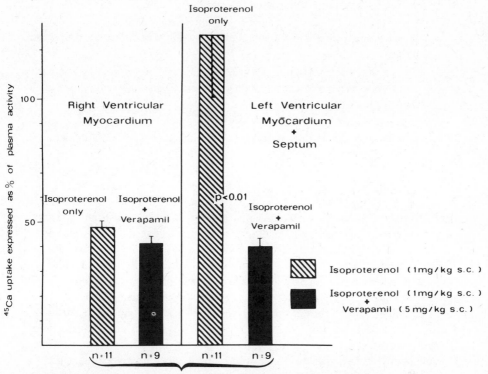

FIGURE 111. As shown in Figure 110, cardiomyopathic hamsters (BIO 8262) develop a supernormal susceptibility to β-adrenergic stimulation of myocardial Ca uptake during the prenecrotic stage as a prodromal symptom of the disease. Accordingly, in these experiments on 29-to-35-day-old cardiomyopathic animals, a small single test dose of 1 mg isoproterenol/kg body weight increased the net uptake of [45]Ca into the prenecrotic left ventricular myocardium and septum from 35% up to 125% in relation to the radioactivity of the blood plasma (= 100%). If, however, verapamil (5 mg/kg) and isoproterenol (1 mg/kg) were given at the same time at different subcutaneous injection sites, the radioactivity of the left ventricular myocardium + septum was kept in the normal range of about 40%. This value nearly corresponded to the [45]Ca uptake of healthy control hamsters without isoproterenol in Figure 108. All measurements were carried out after a time lapse of 6 hours following administration of the drugs and intraperitoneal injection of 50 μCi [45]Ca/kg. From Lossnitzer, Janke, Hein, Stauch, and Fleckenstein (1975).

3.6.2. Prevention of Ca Overload and Necrotization of Cardiomyopathic Hamster Hearts by Long-Term Administration of Ca Antagonists

The chronic treatment of cardiomyopathic hamsters with Ca antagonists also proved to be fully successful under the following conditions:

1. It is necessary that the Ca-antagonistic therapy begins in the prenecrotic phase.
2. The therapy has to be protracted over a period of 30 to 40 days in order to interfere with the asynchronous development of cardiac lesions over a sufficiently long time.
3. The single doses, twice daily, must correspond to those that are capable of acutely normalizing the isoproterenol-stimulated excessive Ca uptake in the prenecrotic phase.

These prerequisites were, in fact, fulfilled in the studies of Jasmin and Bajusz, when they demonstrated the outstanding cardioprotective efficacy of chronically applied verapamil. According to Jasmin's report, also presented at the sixth International Study Group meeting in 1973 in Freiburg, their investigations were carried out on cardiomyopathic hamsters from a subline (UM - X 7.1) of the BIO 14.6 strain. Without therapy, these animals developed particularly severe cardiac and skeletal muscle lesions with 100% incidence. When, however, verapamil was administered beginning at an age of 28 to 30 days for subsequent 30 days in doses of twice daily, 0.5 mg during the first week and 0.75 mg during the following weeks, cardiac necrotization no longer occurred (see Jasmin and Bajusz, 1975). The hearts treated with verapamil exhibited intact histological structures. Out of 20 animals of this group, only 1 showed a small focus of myocardial necrosis, whereas in the remaining 19 cardiomyopathic hamsters, there were no detectable lesions. The normal growth-dependent gain in weight of the verapamil-treated animals was not affected by this long-term therapy. The doses applied were roughly equivalent to 10 mg verapamil/kg body weight twice daily.

Pertinent electrolyte data originating from a study on chronically verapamil-treated cardiomyopathic BIO 8262 hamsters were first reported by Lossnitzer and Mohr (1973). They also injected the drug, beginning with the thirtieth day of life, at a dose of 10 mg/kg body weight subcutaneously twice daily for 15 days and continued with 15 mg/kg twice daily for a further period of 15 days. Untreated hamsters from the same litters served as controls. The results are shown in Table 10.

Without the verapamil treatment, multifocal necrotization occurred as usual, and the myocardial Ca content was found to be elevated in the 60-day-old cardiomyopathic hamsters up to 127 mEq/kg dry weight. With verapamil, on the other hand, the rise in Ca content and myocardial damage were almost completely prevented. Thus under the influence of verapamil, the Ca concentration in the musculature of the left ventricle and the septum remained at a value of 10 mEq/kg dry tissue. This figure nearly corresponds to the Ca level in the myocardium of healthy 60- to 80-

TABLE 10.   Myocardial Electrolyte Content[a] in 60-Day-Old Myopathic Hamsters (BIO 8262) after Long-Term Treatment with Verapamil over 30 Days, as Compared with Diseased Controls not Receiving Verapamil[b]

	Ca	Mg	K	Na
Verapamil	10.42 ± 0.39^c	82.21 ± 1.62	304.37 ± 7.71	175.33 ± 4.79
Controls	127.45 ± 26.43	87.83 ± 3.16	292.43 ± 8.27	170.43 ± 4.10

[a]Values are expressed as the mean in mEq/kg of dry tissue $\pm$ SE ($N = 16$).
[b]From Lossnitzer and Mohr (1973).
[c]$P < 0.001$ (Student's t-test).

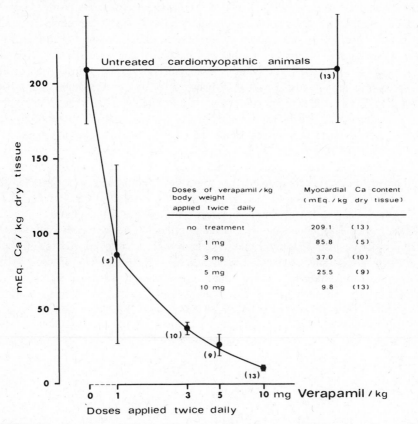

FIGURE 112.   Ca content of left ventricular myocardium and septum of 60-day-old cardiomyopathic hamsters after long-term treatment during 30 days with different doses of verapamil (1, 3, 5, and 10 mg/kg body weight twice daily). The degree of cardioprotection against Ca overload clearly improves with increasing dosage. The small dose of 1 mg verapamil/kg twice daily inhibited excessive Ca uptake by nearly 60%. With 10 mg verapamil/kg twice daily, deleterious Ca overload and necrotization were prevented by practically 100%. The study was carried out on a total of 50 cardiomyopathic hamsters. The number of animals used in each series is given in brackets. Values are expressed as mean $\pm$ SE Data from Lossnitzer, Mohr and Stauch (1975), Lossnitzer, Mohr, Konrad and Guggenmoos (1978), and Lossnitzer, Konrad, and Jakob (1978/1980).

day-old hamsters ($=$ 8.85 $\pm$ 1.10 mEq Ca/kg dry tissue). Differences in myocardial Mg, K, and Na content could not be found between treated and untreated animals. A subsequent series of experiments on cardiomyopathic BIO 8262 hamsters showed that the inhibition of Ca overload sets in with 1 mg verapamil/kg twice daily and proceeds in a strictly dose-dependent manner when greater amounts (3, 5, or 10 mg/kg twice daily) are administered (see Figure 112).

Verapamil shares, of course, its cardioprotective effects on cardiomyopathic hamster hearts with other Ca-antagonistic compounds tested so far. This applies to prenylamine (Jasmin and Solymoss, 1975), D 600 (Jasmin and Proschek, 1978/1980), and fendiline (Lossnitzer, Konrad, and Jakob, 1978/1980). Cinnarizine, another Ca-antagonistic drug, also counteracts both isoproterenol-induced myocardial damage (Godfraind and Sturbois, 1975) and the spontaneous necrotization in cardiomyopathic hamster hearts (Jasmin and Solymoss, 1975). Moreover, Mg salts are not only useful antidotes against the cardiotoxic effects of isoproterenol but also exert a beneficial influence on the hamster cardiomyopathy (Lossnitzer, Konrad, and Jakob, 1978/1980). The chronic administration of Ca antagonists was equally effective whether the cardiomyopathic hamsters originated from the strains BIO 14.6, UM-X 7.1, or BIO 8262. Propranolol (2 $\times$ 30 mg/kg daily for 30 days) also proved to prevent spontaneous myocardial Ca overload and necrotization in cardiomyopathic BIO 8262 hamsters (Heine and Lossnitzer, 1976; Lossnitzer, Konrad, and Jakob, 1978/1980). However, such high doses of propranolol exert strong Ca-antagonistic side effects. Thus the cardioprotective influence of propranolol in cardiomyopathic hamsters probably has to be attributed to the Ca-antagonistic side action of this drug rather to than to a β-receptor blockade (see Section 2.1.1). Accordingly, atenolol, which in comparison with propranolol is a more specific β-blocker but a weaker Ca antagonist, lacked a sufficient cardioprotective action even when excessive doses (300 mg atenolol/kg body weight twice daily during 30 days) were applied (Lossnitzer, Konrad, and Jakob, 1978/1980). The efficacy of Ca antagonists in the treatment of human cardiomyopathy is discussed in Section 7.6.2.

In summary, all our pertinent observations with Ca antagonists clearly demonstrate that Ca overload has to be considered the keystone of a comprehensive concept of Ca-dependent myocardial necrotization, according to the scheme of Figure 106. This notion obviously covers the pathogenesis of spontaneous cardiomyopathic lesions in hamster hearts as well.

CHAPTER FOUR

Influence of Calcium Antagonists on Normal Calcium-Dependent Pacemaker Activity

4.1. GENERAL INVOLVEMENT OF CALCIUM IONS IN SINOATRIAL OR ATRIOVENTRICULAR AUTOMATICITY AND IN INTRANODAL IMPULSE CONDUCTION; DIFFERENTIATION BETWEEN FAST- AND SLOW-CHANNEL-MEDIATED EXCITATORY EVENTS

Although the spectacular involvement of Ca in myocardial contraction has for a while overshadowed other Ca-dependent functions, extensive studies during the last two decades have clearly shown that the Ca ions play an equally important key role in cardiac pacemaker activity. Thus the spontaneous impulse discharge from the sinoatrial (SA) node and the impulse conduction in the atrioventricular (AV) node also require Ca. An exemplary experiment on a spontaneously beating frog ventricle is shown in Figure 113. The recordings visualize three facts simultaneously:

1. As could be expected, withdrawal of Ca impaired excitation–contraction coupling in that contractile force declined, whereas the action potentials persisted.
2. Ca deficiency, in parallel with inhibiting mechanical performance, also reduced the pacemaker activity of the preparation. Indeed, withdrawal of Ca slowed the heart rate and finally led to cardiac standstill.
3. Adrenaline, by virtue of its function as a Ca promoter, restored both contractile force and automaticity of the Ca-deprived myocardium.

However, in our studies, adrenaline and other β-adrenergic substances proved to be effective only as long as traces of Ca were still available. If Ca had been completely withdrawn, the β-adrenergic agents lost their power. The results justified the conclusion that β-receptor stimulation enhances both cardiac contractility and

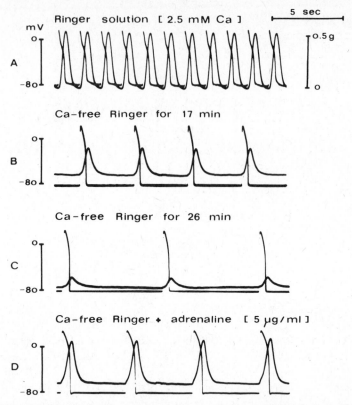

FIGURE 113. Simultaneous impairment of excitation–contraction coupling and pacemaker activity of a spontaneously beating isolated frog ventricle upon Ca withdrawal during an observation period of 26 min (*A*) to (*C*). Thereafter, a considerable recovery of excitation–contraction coupling and heart rate took place within 6 min following addition of adrenaline to the Ca-deficient solution [see (*D*)]. This restitution of contractile force and pacemaker activity by adrenaline or by other β-mimetic agents proved to occur only as long as at least traces of extracellular (or membrane-bound) Ca are available. From Antoni, Engstfeld, and Fleckenstein (1960).

pacemaker function in a basically similar way, namely with the help of Ca ions as transmitters.

In fact, not only the initiation of contraction but also the fundamental process of SA- and AV-node automaticity (as well as AV conduction) are necessarily linked with a transmembrane influx of Ca ions. Moreover, the Ca-transport systems that operate in the nodal cell membranes closely resemble the "slow membrane channels" of ordinary myocardial fibers as shown by extensive studies of Paes de Carvalho, Hoffman, and de Paula Carvalho (1969); Vassort, Rougier, Garnier, Sauviat, Coraboeuf, and Gargouil (1969); Zipes and Mendez (1973); Zipes and Fischer (1974); Wit and Cranefield (1974), and Cranefield (1975). Accordingly, in both nodal cells and ordinary myocardial fibers, these channels respond to virtually the same activators and inhibitors of the inward Ca current. Hence β-adrenergic agents, by

TABLE 11. Resting Potentials (or Maximal Diastolic Potentials) and Maximal Upstroke Velocities (dV/dt_{max}) of Different Cardiac Tissues

Cardiac Tissues	Resting or Maximum Diastolic Potential (mV)	Authors	dV/dt_{max} V/s	Authors
SA node	−50 to −60 −55 to −60 (Rhesus monkey)	Cranefield (1975) Fleckenstein (1963 b)	2 to 3	Brooks and Lu (1972)
Atrium	−78 (Rabbit) −80 to −90 (Guinea pig) −85 (Dog)	West (1955) Fleckenstein (1963b) Hoffman and Suckling (1952)	340 (dog)	Trautwein and Schmidt (1960)
AV node (N cells)	−53 (Dog)	Sano (1976)	6.7	Paes de Carvalho
Purkinje fibers	−96 (Dog) −85 (Rhesus monkey)	Trautwein and Zink (1952) Kotowski, Antoni, Vahlenkamp and Fleckenstein (1961)	400 (guinea pig, cat, rhesus monkey)	Tritthart, Grundy, Haastert, and Herbst (1972)
Ventricle (papil-lary muscles)	−85 (Dog) −88 (Cat) −90 (Rhesus monkey) −78 (Guinea pig)	Hoffman and Suckling (1952) Trautwein, Gottstein, and Dudel (1954) Antoni and Engstfeld (1961) Engstfeld, Antoni, and Fleckenstein (1961)	170 to 180 (guinea pig, cat, rhesus monkey)	Tritthart, Grundy, Haastert, and Herbst (1972)

promoting the transfer of Ca through the slow channels, not only cause an increase in contractile force, but also produce an analogous rise in heart rate and AV conduction velocity. Conversely, organic Ca antagonists exert negative inotropic, chronotropic, and dromotropic influences altogether. The Ca-antagonistic divalent Co, Ni, and Mn ions act similarly in that they also suppress, by inhibiting Ca inflow across the slow membrane channels (see Section 2.4), contractility as well as pacemaker excitation (Lenfant, Mironneau, Gargouil, and Galand, 1968; Zipes and Mendez, 1973; Zipes and Fischer, 1974; Iijima and Taira, 1976; Kohlhardt, Figulla, and Tripathi, 1976). The same functional impairment ensues from simple Ca withdrawal. On the other hand, tetrodotoxin (TTX), known to block the fast Na channels, does not inhibit SA- and AV-node automaticity or AV conduction (Yamagishi and Sano, 1966; Zipes and Mendez, 1973; Urthaler and James, 1973). But TTX slows or suppresses Na-dependent excitation and impulse propagation in the ordinary myocardium and in the normal His-Purkinje-fiber system.

As to the biophysical characterization of the carrier systems involved, it has previously been pointed out that the fast Na channels only work at a high membrane potential (see Section 2.5, Figure 34). This prerequisite is apparently fulfilled in

TABLE 12. Normal Conduction Velocities in Different Cardiac Tissues

Cardiac Tissues	Velocity (cm/sec)	Species	Authors
SA node	2–6	Rabbit	Sano and Yamagishi (1965)
Atrium	80	Rabbit	Sano and Yamagishi (1965)
	50–100	Rabbit	Paes de Carvalho, de Mello, and Hoffman (1959)
	90–120	Dog	Goodman, van der Steen, and van Dam (1971)
	80	Dog	Hogan and Davis (1971)
AV node (N cells)	2–5	Cow	van der Kooi, Durrer, van Dam, and van der Tweel (1956)
		Dog	Scher, Rodriguez, Liikane and Young (1959) Alanis, Lopez, Mandoki, and Pilar (1959)
		Rabbit	Pruitt and Essex (1960)
His bundle (and branches)	100–150	Different Species	Sano (1976)
Purkinje fibers	200	Dog	Draper & Weidmann (1951)
	80	Rhesus monkey	Antoni and Zerweck (1967)
Ventricle (papillary muscle)	60	Rhesus monkey	Antoni and Zerweck (1967)

the atrial and ventricular myocardium as well as in the His and Purkinje fibers. Here the resting potentials are normally in the range of -80 to -90 mV. Contrarily, the Ca inflow through the slow channels requires a reduced level of membrane polarization. Accordingly, the pacemaker cells of the SA and AV nodes operate at a rather low membrane potential since the maximal diastolic potential only amounts to -50 to -60 mV (see Table 11). Moreover, the slow-channel-mediated excitation is characterized by an extremely slow onset and propagation of the action potential. Thus the maximal upstroke velocities ($dV/dt_{\max}$) of the Ca-dependent action potentials were reported to be 2 to 3 V/sec in the SA node (Brooks and Lu, 1972) and 6.7 V/sec in the central part (N cells) of the AV node (Paes de Carvalho, 1961). These low figures sharply differ with the much higher upstroke velocities of the Na-dependent, fast-channel-mediated action potentials of atrial or ventricular myocardium and Purkinje fibers, which are generally in a range of between 170 (papillary muscle) and 400 V/sec (Purkinje fibers). An analogous gap exists with respect to the velocities of impulse propagation, that is, 2 to 6 cm/sec in SA and AV nodes, versus 60 to 200 cm/sec in ordinary atrial or ventricular myocardium, and in the fibers of the His-Purkinje system. More particular data are compiled in Tables 11

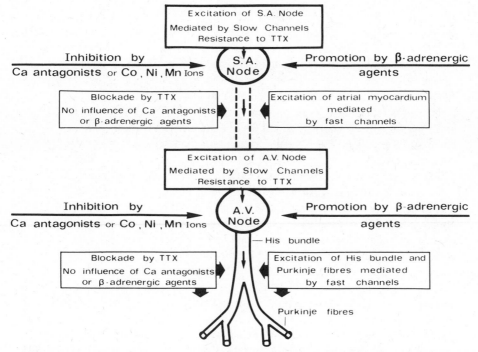

FIGURE 114. Opposite effects of Ca antagonists and Ca promoters (β-adrenergic agents) on slow-channel-mediated, TTX-insensitive SA-node automaticity and AV-node conductivity. Refractoriness to Ca antagonists and β-adrenergic catecholamines of normal TTX-sensitive impulse propagation in atrial, His-bundle, and Purkinje fibers. From Fleckenstein (1980/1981).

and 12. Hence there are two contrasting types of cardiac excitation that can be easily distinguished by their different sensitivities to drugs and by other criteria:

1. The fast, obviously Na-dependent, excitatory events in atrial myocardium, His bundle, Purkinje fibers, and ventricular myocardium.
2. The slow, obviously Ca-dependent, impulse generation and impulse conduction in the SA and AV nodes.

The scheme of Figure 114 summarizes the principal results on which this dualistic concept of cardiac excitation is based.

4.2.   DAMPING EFFECTS OF CALCIUM ANTAGONISTS ON SINOATRIAL-NODE AUTOMATICITY AND ATRIOVENTRICULAR CONDUCTION

4.2.1.   Observations on Isolated Preparations and on Hearts in Situ after Intravenous Application of Calcium Antagonists

The actual knowledge of the peculiarities of SA-node automaticity and AV conduction originates to a great deal from the research work with Ca antagonists. Early reports about the depressant effects of verapamil on the nodal functions were presented by Melville, Shister and Huq (1964) and by Fleckenstein (1964a). Melville and his colleagues found that high doses of verapamil induced sinus bradycardia and AV block together with cardiac contractile incompetence in isolated perfused rabbit hearts and in cat hearts *in situ*. However, Melville suggested that these inhibitory effects of verapamil might result from a β-receptor blocking activity of the drug. Fleckenstein (1964a) also recognized a simultaneous depression of sinus-node automaticity and myocardial contractility by verapamil and prenylamine in guinea pig hearts *in situ* (see Figures 62 to 64, which also include later experiments with nifedipine). But Fleckenstein, Kammermeier, Döring, and Freund (1967) showed that verapamil and prenylamine in exerting negative inotropic and negative chronotropic effects left the cardiac β-receptors unaffected. Isolated rat and guinea pig auricles exposed to increasing concentrations of verapamil, D 600, or nifedipine also responded with a parallel decline of SA-node automaticity and contractile performance (Refsum and Landmark, 1975; Refsum, 1975; Haastert and Fleckenstein, 1975). In a study of Landmark and Amlie (1976) on dog hearts *in situ*, verapamil injected intravenously did not influence the rates of intraatrial, His-Purkinje, and intraventricular conduction, but markedly impaired the passage of the impulse through the AV node. As could also be seen from simple ECG recordings on anesthetized guinea pigs, intravenous infusion of verapamil, D 600, nifedipine, or niludipine typically slows sinus discharge rate and AV conduction but does not alter Na-dependent intraventricular impulse propagation as reflected by a constant duration of QRS (see Figures 115 and 123). These findings are consistent with

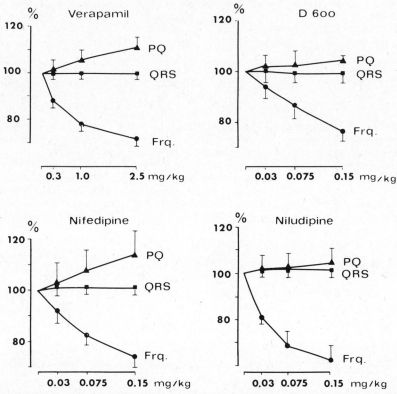

FIGURE 115.   Effects of intermittent intravenous infusion of increasing doses of Ca antagonists on the PQ and QRS intervals and on sinus frequency of guinea pig hearts. The characteristic responses to Ca antagonists consist of an increase in the PQ interval, due to the retardation of AV conduction, and a depression of spontaneous sinus rhythmicity, whereas Na-dependent intraventricular impulse propagation, represented by QRS, remains unchanged. Experiments on anesthetized guinea pigs using subcutaneous leads. The resulting data, on the ordinate, are expressed as percentages of the respective initial control values (= 100%) before drug administration. The doses marked on the abscissa were given into the right jugular vein each time over a period of 2 min with an interval of 7 min between the infusions. From Fleckenstein (1978/1980).

many observations concerning the influence of verapamil on cardiac impulse conduction in man (Bender, 1967; Bender and Zimmerhof, 1967; Neuss and Schlepper, 1971; Gleichmann, Seipel, and Loogen, 1973; Husaini, Kvasnicka, Ryden, and Holmberg, 1973; Roy, Spurrell, and Sowton, 1974; Heng, Singh, Roche, Norris, and Mercer, 1975; Seipel and Breithardt, 1978/1980). Some typical data obtained in humans with verapamil are shown in Table 13. However, the situation is somewhat different with respect to nifedipine (Taira, Motomura, Narimatsu, and Iijima, 1975; Raschack, 1976a; Ekelund and Orö, 1976), because in dogs and humans the negative chronotropic and dromotropic potency of this drug proved to be weaker than could be expected from the observations on guinea pigs and rats. Consequently,

TABLE 13.   Peak Effects of IV Verapamil[a,b] on the Electrocardiogram in Patients with Sinus Rhythm[c]

Interval (msec)	Before Verapamil	After Verapamil	N	Significance
R-R	743 ± 38	738 ± 27	15	NS
P-R	186.1 ± 6.2	205.4 ± 8.1	13	$P < 0.001$
QRS	65.5 ± 4.1	66.1 ± 4.6	13	NS
Q-T	457.8 ± 9.9	451.0 ± 6.6	12	NS

[a]Abbreviations: msec = milliseconds; N = number of patients; NS = not significant.
[b]A single dose of 10 mg verapamil was given intravenously over a period of 2 min. For assessment of the peak effects, complete sets of data were obtained between 3 and 5, 10, and 20 min after the completion of administration of the drug. At least five complexes were analyzed in order to obtain the mean value for each parameter that was measured. The absence of a discernible negative chronotropic effect is due to the compensatory influence of baroreceptor-dependent sympathetic responses to the acute verapamil-induced fall in arterial blood pressure.
[c]From Heng, Singh, Roche, Norris, and Mercer (1975).

nifedipine is also less suited than verapamil for the interruption of reentry pathways through the AV node in patients with the Wolff–Parkinson–White (WPW) syndrome (see Section 7.5.2).

4.2.2.   Topical Administration of Calcium Antagonists on Perfused Sinoatrial and Atrioventricular Nodes

Garvey (1969) as well as Lupi, Urthaler, and James (1979) cannulated the nutrient arteries of the SA and AV nodes of dogs, so that verapamil could be delivered directly to the pacemaker regions. Under these circumstances minute amounts of verapamil given through the SA-node artery produced negative chronotropic effects without concomitant systemic reactions. On the other hand, verapamil perfused through the AV-node artery during sinus rhythm selectively impaired AV conduction. However, with larger doses, in cases of AV junctional rhythm, the automaticity of the AV node was also suppressed. The highest degree of technical perfection was reached in perfusion experiments of Japanese researchers on isolated cross-circulated AV-node preparations of the dog (Hashimoto, Iijima, Hashimoto, and Taira, 1972; Taira and Narimatsu, 1975; Narimatsu and Taira, 1976). Interestingly enough, in dog hearts the upper and the central parts (N zone) of the AV node are perfused through the posterior septal artery (PSA). In this particular region, the excitatory process is mainly Ca-dependent, so that changes in AV conduction time obtained with injection of drugs into the PSA reflect primarily effects on the slow Ca channel. On the other hand, the more distal sections of the conducting system such as the lower part of the AV node, His bundle, and Purkinje fibers in the ventricular septum are supplied by the anterior septal artery (ASA). Excitation of this part of the heart is clearly Na-dependent. Therefore, changes in conduction time produced by application of drugs via the ASA are indicative of an effect on the fast Na channel. In fact, verapamil, nifedipine, and diltiazem, which have to be considered rather pure inhibitors of the slow Ca current in ventricular muscle, only increased AV conduction time, and in high doses produced a complete AV block when they were injected into the PSA. Manganese ions and both enantiomers of verapamil, that is, (−)-verapamil and (+)-verapamil, in these experiments also exerted purely Ca-antagonistic actions (Iijima and Taira, 1976; Satoh, Yanagisawa, and Taira, 1979). In contrast, when these drugs were administered through the ASA, none of them impaired AV conduction (Taira, Motomura, Narimatsu, Satoh, and Yanagisawa, 1978/1980). By injecting noradrenaline into the PSA, the inhibitory effects of the Ca-antagonistic drugs on AV conduction could be overcome.

4.2.3.   Interactions of Calcium Antagonists and β-Adrenergic Neurotransmitters

Regarding the positive influence of β-adrenergic catecholamines on sinus automaticity and AV conduction, it is easily understood that the height of the endogenous sympathetic tone is a decisive factor in determining the magnitude of the nodal responses to Ca antagonists. Thus the Ca-antagonistic drug effects manifest themselves most intensely if the natural sympathetic drive is low. Accordingly, as shown by Taira, Motomura, Narimatsu, and Iijima (1975) on dog hearts *in situ,* the negative dromotropic influence of verapamil and diltiazem on AV conduction is potentiated by sympathetic denervation (bilateral stellectomy). For the same reason the negative chronotropic and dromotropic (and inotropic) influences of Ca antagonists are always most obvious in isolated hearts or in isolated nodal tissues that are cut off from normal sympathetic impulse supply, or in topically perfused preparations where counteractions of the sympathetic system are also negligible. However, even more important is that a similar accentuation of the Ca-antagonistic drug effects takes place if the sympathetic drive has previously been suppressed by pharmacological interventions such as reserpinization, β-receptor blockade, or deep anesthesia. This applies particularly to patients who have previously been given a β-blocker. Under these circumstances serious troubles of SA automaticity and AV conduction, sometimes resulting in ventricular asystole, were observed upon intravenous injection of usual therapeutic doses of verapamil (see Benaim, 1972; Boothby, Garrard, and Pickering, 1972; Sacks and Kennelly, 1972; Vaughan-Neil, Snell, and Bevan, 1972; Krikler and Spurrell, 1972). Caution is also advisable when using verapamil or D 600 in patients with suspected sinus-node dysfunction or overt sick-sinus syndrome (Breithardt, Seipel, Wiebringhaus, and Loogen, 1976, 1978; Beck, Witt, Lehmann, and Hochrein, 1978). In these cases too, a hyperresponsiveness of the SA node to acetylcholine may coincide with a diminished level of resting sympathetic tone (Mandel, Hayakawa, Allen, Danzig, and Kermaier, 1972).

Conversely, in normal hearts a spontaneous reflex release of endogenous sympathetic transmitters may partially neutralize or even completely mask the Ca-antagonistic drug actions. As is generally known, the most significant reflex stimulation of the sympathetic system occurs in response to a fall in blood pressure. In fact, verapamil, D 600, diltiazem, and nifedipine as well as other Ca antagonists are able to reduce arterial tension not only by their cardiodepressant effects, but also by lowering Ca-dependent contractile tone of the peripheral resistance vessels in the systemic circulation (see Section 6.2.7 to 6.2.9).

In consequence, after acute intravenous administration of Ca antagonists, compensatory sympathetic reflex reactions are elicited that diminish, abolish, or even reverse the primary cardiac inhibition. Then the direct negative chronotropic influence of verapamil may even be turned into sinus tachycardia. However, as shown by Rowe, Stenlund, Thomsen, Corliss, and Sialer (1971), such paradoxical responses to intravenous verapamil disappear following β-blockade or catecholamine depletion. Similarly, Newman, Leroux, Peterson, Bishop, and Horwitz (1976) observed that a sinus rate increase of 64% after intravenous verapamil resulted in a net negative chronotropic response of 21% after dual autonomic neural blockade. Nifedipine is even more hypotensive than verapamil and therefore evokes particularly strong sympathetic repercussions (Kroneberg, 1975; Raschack, 1976a). In short, the positive chronotropic responses caused by acute systemic administration of Ca antagonists are due to a baroreceptor-mediated increase in sympathetic tone, whereas the negative chronotropic action is a direct effect on the nodal cells. It depends on circumstantial factors such as mode of application, dose, and individual sensitivity whether the direct or the indirect influence on the pacemaker function preponderates. As a rule, the direct effects of Ca antagonists distinctly prevail if the drugs are chronically administered.

4.3. ELECTROPHYSIOLOGICAL ANALYSIS OF THE CALCIUM-ANTAGONISTIC DRUG EFFECTS ON THE CARDIAC PACEMAKER FUNCTIONS

4.3.1. Subthreshold Automaticity and Propagated Pacemaker Action Potentials

One of the most perspicuous differences between the transmembrane potentials of ordinary myocardial fibers and pacemaker cells consists of the fact that automaticity is intimately linked with an instability of resting potential. Or in other words, ordinary nonautomatic atrial and ventricular fibers maintain a steady level of resting potential during the diastolic pause. The pacemaker cells, on the other hand, undergo a *slow diastolic depolarization* (see Figures 116 and 117). This means that the membrane potential of nodal cells, after a transient culmination in the early diastole, progressively declines. This spontaneous fall of membrane potential is usually large enough to reach the *threshold potential*. Then the slow diastolic depolarization gives rise to the upstroke of a propagated pacemaker action potential. If, however, the slow diastolic depolarization fails to reach this critical level, it remains confined to the primary pacemaker region. Then the intrinsic automaticity of the nodal cells appears unmasked in the form of continuous local oscillations of membrane potential.

The intrinsic pacemaker automaticity proved to be extremely insensitive to de-

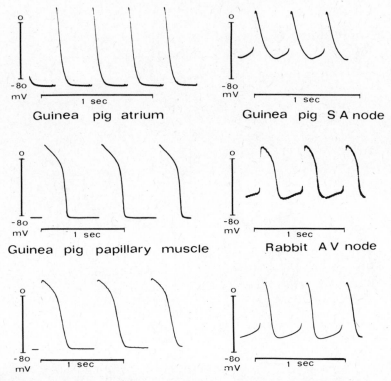

FIGURE 116. Comparison of transmembrane action potentials of electrically stimulated nonautomatic myocardial fibers from atrial or papillary muscles with those of spontaneously discharging SA- or AV-nodal cells. The characteristic feature of spontaneously active nodal cells is a slow diastolic depolarization that initiates a propagated pacemaker action potential as soon as the membrane potential is lowered to a critical level (threshold potential). The vertical calibrations of each record represent the zero potential and a membrane potential of −80 mV. The time calibrations indicate an interval of 1 sec each. From a collection of transmembrane action potentials recorded by Antoni, Herkel, and Fleckenstein (1961); see Fleckenstein (1963b).

polarization (Kotowski, Antoni, Vahlenkamp, and Fleckenstein, 1961). As shown on K-depolarized pacemaker cells of the frog AV node, there were still persistent bioelectric oscillations at a membrane potential of less than −20 mV (see Figure 118). The same local vacillation of membrane potential appeared in largely depolarized SA nodes of rabbits (Antoni, Herkel, and Fleckenstein, 1963). Also in these studies, the isolated pacemaker tissue was exposed to a K-rich (23 mM) Tyrode solution. Consequently, at a level of membrane potential of about −35 mV, the production of propagated pacemaker action potentials ceased. Instead, permanent local subthreshold oscillations signified the persistence of intrinsic nodal automaticity. The middle record in Figure 119 shows that in a series of four successive swings there was, by chance, an increase in amplitude so that the

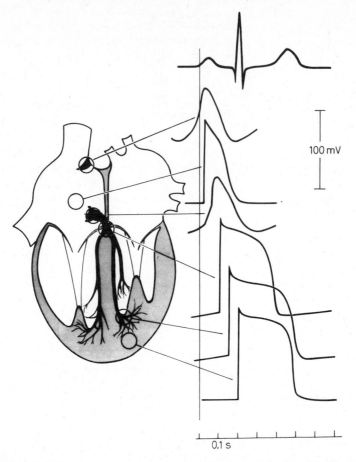

FIGURE 117. Typical transmembrane action potentials recorded from the following sites (from top down): SA node, atrium, AV node, bundle of His, Purkinje fiber, ventricular muscle fiber. Note the obvious peculiarities of the nodal action potentials such as (1) spontaneous depolarization leading to an extremely slow upstroke, (2) low amplitude, (3) obtuse shape of the peak, and (4) no clear plateau. Arrangement of drawings according to an original scheme of Hoffman and Cranefield (1960) modified by Antoni (1972).

depolarizing phase of the fourth oscillation reached the threshold. Thereby a single propagated pacemaker action potential was elicited.

All these observations indicated that the SA-node action potentials, shown in Figures 116 and 117, consist of two components, namely (1) a rhythmic local depolarization (slow diastolic depolarization) of the pacemaker cells that is part of an intrinsic oscillation of membrane potential, and (2) a superimposed propagated action potential in response to this local impulse. At a very low level of membrane potential (-20 to -35 mV), the propagation may fail, whereas the local oscillations continue. *Nevertheless, both components of the SA-node action potentials occur within a low range of membrane potential in which only the slow channel is*

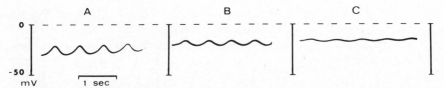

FIGURE 118. Persistence of rhythmic oscillations of membrane potential in a largely depolarized AV node of frog. The records were obtained (*A*) 2 min, (*B*) 7 min, and (*C*) 10 min after exposure of isolated AV tissue to a K-rich Ringer solution (20.4 m*M* K). Since no propagated action potentials can normally arise from a membrane potential of less than -30 mV, the intrinsic pacemaker automaticity, consisting of steady local vacillations of the membrane potential, appeared under these conditions in its pure form. Slow rhythmic oscillations of a very small amplitude were still discernible at a membrane potential of between -15 and -20 mV. From Kotowski, Antoni, Vahlenkamp, and Fleckenstein (1961).

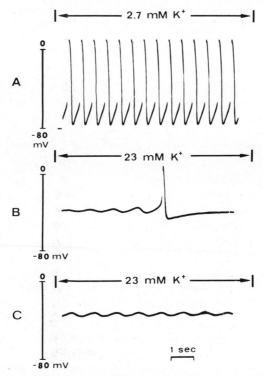

FIGURE 119. Persistence of rhythmic oscillations of membrane potential in a largely depolarized rabbit SA node after transfer from a normal (2.7 m*M* K) to a K-rich Tyrode solution containing 23 m*M* K. In (*B*) at a membrane potential of around 40 mV, one of the spontaneous rhythmic oscillations still elicited a small propagated action potential. In (*C*) at a membrane potential of about 30 to 35 mV, the pacemaker activity was reduced to local oscillations only. Temperature, 36°C. Observations of Antoni, Herkel, and Fleckenstein, see Fleckenstein (1964b).

177

operative. The same is true of the action potentials of isolated AV nodes. Therefore, the oscillations as well as the propagated nodal responses are TTX-insensitive, but highly susceptible to all agents that promote or, conversely, inhibit the slow-channel-mediated inward Ca fluxes.

4.3.2. Opposite Effects of Calcium Promoters (β-Adrenergic Agents) and Calcium Antagonists

Adrenaline and other β-adrenergic substances stimulate or even resuscitate the intrinsic pacemaker automaticity at a very low level of membrane potential. Figure 120 represents an experiment of Antoni, Herkel, and Fleckenstein (1963) on an isolated sinus node of a rhesus monkey. The upper line shows the progressive depolarization of a primary pacemaker cell by a Tyrode solution with an excessively high K content (26 and 33 m*M* respectively). After the membrane potential had

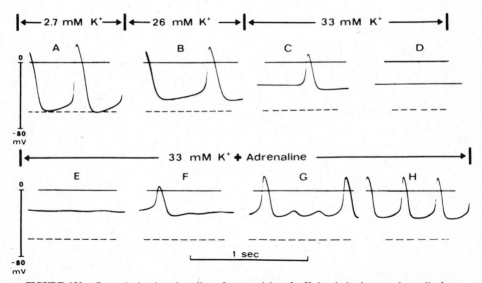

FIGURE 120.   Resuscitation by adrenaline of automaticity of a K-depolarized pacemaker cell of an isolated SA node from a rhesus monkey. (*A*) Regular pacemaker action potential in Tyrode solution with normal K content (2.7 m*M*). (*B*) Depolarization and slowing of pacemaker rate 2 min after exposure to K-rich Tyrode solution (26 m*M* K). (*C*) Last spontaneous action potential 14 min after increasing extracellular K concentration up to 33 m*M*. (*D*) Standstill of automaticity. (*E*) Commencement of slow oscillations of membrane potential 45 sec after addition of adrenaline (5 μg/ml) to the K-rich (33 m*M*) Tyrode solution. (*F*) First propagated action potential 1 min after administration of adrenaline. (*G*) Occurrence of local subthreshold oscillations and propagated action potentials in the ratio 2:1 after a time lapse of 1.5 min following the addition of adrenaline. (*H*) Restoration of a quasi-regular pacemaker function in the K-rich Tyrode solution 4 min after administration of adrenaline, although the maximal diastolic potential, compared with its original height in (*A*), remains persistently reduced by 25 mV. Intracellular recordings from one and the same nodal cell throughout the experiment at 36°C From Antoni, Herkel, and Fleckenstein (1963).

fallen below -30 mV within 14 min, not only the production of propagated action potentials but also the oscillatory pacemaker activity ceased. Then, in the experiment shown in the lower part of Figure 120, adrenaline (5 μg/ml) was added to the K-rich Tyrode solution. In consequence, after a time lapse of only 45 sec, again small rhythmic oscillations of membrane potential became discernible. The amplitude of these oscillations progressively increased until after 60 sec the first propagated action potential reappeared. After 90 sec, regular pacemaker activity was restored, but the occurrence of local oscillations, compared with that of propagated impulses, was still in the ratio of 2:1. Lastly, 4 min after the administration of adrenaline, all local impulses reached the threshold. Thus adrenaline is capable of maintaining a quasi-regular automaticity in largely K-depolarized nodal cells at a steady low level of membrane potential. Needless to say, the restoration of the Ca-dependent pacemaker function is basically identical with the ability of adrenaline to maintain Ca-dependent action potentials in largely K-depolarized myocardial fibers (see Figure 50 and the Section 2.8).

The influence of Ca antagonists, on the other hand, has to be considered the reverse of the adrenaline action. Whereas adrenaline resuscitates or potentiates the intrinsic local oscillations and enhances the upstroke of the nodal action potentials by virtue of its promoter effects on transmembrane Ca influx, the Ca antagonists operate in an exactly opposite direction. This means that Ca antagonists:

1. Suppress the Ca-dependent subthreshold oscillations that occur at a low nodal membrane potential.

2. Decrease the slope of the slow diastolic depolarization, thus retarding the initiation of propagated impulses.

3. Reduce upstroke velocity and overshoot of the nodal action potentials without affecting the resting potential.

4. May thereby counteract the positive chronotropic and dromotropic influence of β-adrenergic catecholamines (and vice versa).

The first preliminary report about the typical effects of verapamil on the transmembrane bioelectric activity of isolated rabbit AV nodes was presented by Tritthart, B. Fleckenstein, and A. Fleckenstein in 1970/1971 (see Figure 121). Further studies of other research groups confirmed and extended these findings. The most important contributions were those of Cranefield, Aronson, and Wit (1974), Wit and Cranefield (1974), and Cranefield (1975), who extensively analyzed the actions of verapamil and D 600 on the slow-channel-mediated automaticity of canine SA or AV nodes (and on that of Purkinje fibers exposed to a Na-free solution containing 16 mM Ca). The results of these researchers were fully consistent with the observations of our own laboratory on isolated SA and AV nodes of rabbits. Thus Cranefield and his group also came to the cogent conclusion that verapamil and D 600 exert their inhibitory influence on the nodal functions by interference with the slow electrogenic inward Ca current.

A. Isolated Sinoatrial Node (Rabbit)

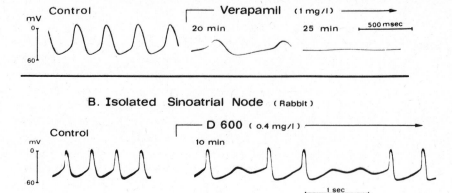

B. Isolated Sinoatrial Node (Rabbit)

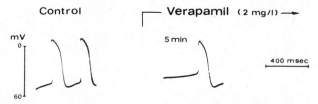

C. Isolated Atrioventricular Node (Rabbit)

FIGURE 121. Inhibition by verapamil and D 600 of the pacemaker function of isolated SA and AV nodes from rabbits. Verapamil and D 600 reduce both the steepness of the slow diastolic depolarization, thereby producing a negative chronotropic effect, and the velocity of upstroke of the propagated nodal action potentials. The height of the overshoot also decreases upon prolonged exposure to the drugs, whereas there is a growing tendency of hyperpolarization during diastole. As shown in (*B*), a nodal cell treated with the Ca antagonist D 600 more and more fails to elicit propagated pacemaker action potentials. This is due to (1) a reduction in the amplitude of the intrinsic oscillatory potential changes and (2) a shift of threshold potential toward zero. Thus an increasing number of spontaneous local depolarization waves remain unanswered. Each record in the experiments A, B, and C was taken by steady impalement of a single cell. Record A from Kohlhardt, Figulla, and Tripathi (1976); record C from Tritthart, B. Fleckenstein, and A. Fleckenstein (1970/1971); record B from Tritthart, Kohlhardt, and Fleckenstein; see Fleckenstein (1980/1981).

4.3.3. Participation of Sodium Besides Calcium Ions in the Slow Inward Current of Nodal Cells

Although the decisive role of Ca in maintaining cardiac pacemaker automaticity is above any doubt, a number of observations point to an additional participation of Na. For instance, it is still a pending problem whether the fast Na channel really does not exist in the nodal cell membranes or whether it is simply inactivated in consequence of the low level of membrane potential at which the pacemaker cells usually operate. Pertinent findings of Kreitner (1975) suggested that the second alternative is more likely than the first because the ascending phase of the SA-pacemaker action potential, which is normally irresponsive to the fast-channel inhibitor TTX, became partially sensitive to this agent after artificial hyperpolarization. Moreover, canine AV nodes *in situ,* well perfused with blood and therefore enjoying the most advantageous conditions of keeping their membrane potential at a maximal height, were also found to be not totally refractory to TTX if large doses were directly injected into the AV-node artery (Iijima, Motomura, Taira, and Hashimoto, 1974). Hence under certain conditions, a minor involvement of the fast TTX-sensitive Na channel in the initial phase of the nodal cell action potentials cannot be completely ruled out.

However, much more important was the question concerning to what extent Na ions participate as electric-charge carriers in the slow transmembrane inward current. The problem was studied in our laboratory by Kohlhardt, Figulla, and Tripathi (1976) on isolated SA-nodal preparations, and by Akiyama and Fozzard (1979) on isolated AV-nodal tissue, both from rabbits. The results were virtually identical, since it turned out that overshoot and upstroke velocity of the SA- and AV-node action potentials not only depend on the extracellular Ca (Ca_o) concentration but also respond to major changes in the Na content of the surrounding fluid (Na_o).

4.3.3.1. Calcium Dependency.   As to the influence of Ca_o on sinus-node automaticity, a positive chronotropic effect of an elevated Ca_o concentration has been observed by many authors (Reiter and Noé, 1959; Feinberg, Boyd, and Katz, 1962; Paradise, 1963; Seifen, Flacke, and Alper, 1964; Toda and West, 1967; Refsum, 1975). This is because the slope of diastolic depolarization steepens with augmenting Ca_o (Seifen, Schaer, and Marshall, 1964; Lu and Brooks, 1969). Moreover, as shown in Figure 122, upstroke velocity (dV/dt_{max}) and overshoot of the SA-node action potentials rise linearly when the Ca_o concentration is increased from 0.2 to 4.0 mM. Conversely, at a Ca_o concentration lower than 0.2 mM, the sinus pacemaker function ceases. But there is also an impairment of SA-node automaticity if the Ca_o concentration is excessively high, that is to say, above 7mM. An optimum Ca_o concentration seems to exist around 6 to 7 mM. Similar results were also obtained on the AV node. Here too, low Ca_o concentrations (0.8 mM) as well as high Ca_o concentrations (7.2 mM) depressed intranodal conduction (Watanabe, 1978/1980). However, when Ca_o concentrations varied between 0.45 and 3.6 mM, there was in the N cells of the AV node the same linear change in overshoot and upstroke

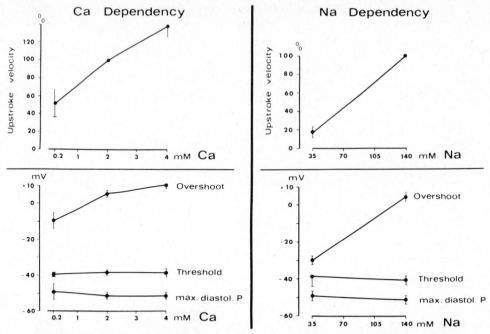

FIGURE 122. Changes in upstroke velocity (dV/dt_{max}) and height of overshoot of spontaneous SA-node action potentials in response to variations of the extracellular Ca or Na concentration. The measurements were made on steadily impaled primary pacemaker cells from isolated rabbit SA nodes. In normal Tyrode solution containing 2.2 mM Ca and 149.2 mM Na, these cells exhibited the following control characteristics: maximal diastolic potential, -53.7 ($\pm$ 7.8) mV; threshold potential, -40.1 ($\pm$ 4.5) mV; overshoot, 8.1 ($\pm$ 4.6) mV; rate of rise of action potential (dV/dt_{max}), 1.7 ($\pm$ 1.1) V/sec. Temperature, 34 ($\pm$ 0.5)°C; pH, 7.3; oxygenation with 95% O_2 and 5% CO_2. In the experiments with low Na_0, sucrose was used for osmotic substitution. From Kohlhardt, Figulla, and Tripathi (1976).

velocity of action potentials as in the sinus node (Matsuda, 1973; Akiyama and Fozzard, 1979). No analogous responses were found in the His conducting system.

4.3.3.2.   Sodium Dependency.   *The involvement of Na* into the electrogenesis of pacemaker action potentials ensues from the fact that the discriminative power of the nodal slow channels against Na ions is high, but still permits a limited transmembrane Na penetration. Thus Akiyama and Fozzard, (1979) calculated that the membrane of the excited AV-nodal cells is about 70 times more permeable to Ca than to Na. This particular preference for Ca is, however, largely compensated by the predominant concentration of Na_o, which exceeds that of Ca_o by a factor of more than 100 in the normal interstitial fluid. Hence the contribution of Na to the slow inward current of nodal cells may finally be equal to or even greater than that of Ca. Consequently, upstroke velocity and overshoot of the SA- and AV-node action potentials are also depressed when the concentration of Na_o is diminished. For instance, in SA-nodal cells, a reduction of the Na_o concentration from 140 to 35 mM affected these bioelectric parameters to the same or even a greater extent than a decrease in the Ca_o concentration from 2 to 0.2 mM did (see Figure 122). The responses of isolated AV-nodal N cells to a reduction of the Na_o concentration from 153 to 38 mM (Akiyama and Fozzard, 1979) did not differ from those observed by Kohlhardt, Figulla, and Tripathi (1976) on Na-deprived SA-nodal tissue. Total removal of Na, like complete withdrawal of Ca, caused nodal inexcitability. This happened without major changes in maximal diastolic potential or threshold potential. Tetrodotoxin (TTX) did not alter the sensitivity of nodal excitation to variations of Na_o or Ca_o. Hence the conclusion is justified that the slow TTX-resistant inward current in SA- and AV-nodal cells essentially consists of two electrogenic cation fluxes, one carried by Ca and the other by Na. The Na ions probably provide a basal current that acts as a nodal-excitation safety factor by keeping the inward transport of positive charges at a sufficiently high level. The Ca inflow, on the other hand, seems to constitute that part of the slow inward current that is more susceptible to regulatory changes such as those produced by β-adrenergic agents.

To elucidate the individual contributions of Ca and Na to the slow inward current in nodal tissues, the use of specific inhibitors again seems very promising. In fact, SA-node automaticity and AV conduction respond to both Ca-antagonistic and Na-antagonistic agents. Thus lidocaine, procaine, procaine amide, and quinidine, which according to our voltage-clamp studies on cat trabeculae predominantly act as Na antagonists (Kohlhardt, Bauer, Krause, and Fleckenstein, 1972), also suppress the nodal functions provided the doses are rather high (Haastert and Fleckenstein, 1975). A typical experiment with lidocaine is shown in Figure 123. The only peculiarity that lidocaine and other Na-antagonistic compounds exhibit in contrast with Ca antagonists (see Figure 115) consists of a spectacular prolongation of QRS. This reflects a large decrease in the rate of fast Na-dependent intraventricular impulse propagation. Similar effects of lidocaine on AV-nodal and ventricular conduction of isolated perfused guinea pig hearts were reported by Carmeliet and Zaman (1979). Even in human subjects, lidocaine may occasionally produce heart block by impairing AV conduction (Gianelly, van der Groeben, Spivack, and Harrison, 1967; Ryden and Korsgren 1969; Lichstein, Chudda, and Gupta 1973). Our results are also consistent with observations of Narimatsu and Taira (1976). These authors applied the inhibitory drugs directly through the nutrient posterior septal artery to blood-perfused canine AV nodes *in situ*. In these experiments too, the Ca antagonists nifedipine, verapamil, and diltiazem as well as the Na antagonists lidocaine, procaine, and quinidine proved to inhibit AV conduction. The relative potencies of these drugs, as indicated by the doses causing an increase in AV conduction time by about 15% of the control values, were as follows: Nifedipine: diltiazem: verapamil: quinidine: lidocaine: procaine $= 1: \frac{1}{2}: \frac{1}{2}: \frac{1}{80}: \frac{1}{200}: \frac{1}{400}$ (on a weight basis). Narimatsu and Taira (1976) suggested that this susceptibility to Na-antagonistic drugs might possibly be due to a partial involvement of the fast Na channel in AV-nodal excitation. But pertinent studies of Akiyama and Fozzard (1979) and Watanabe (1978/1980) indicated that Na ions invariably participate in the slow AV-nodal inward current whether TTX has been added or not. Moreover, Watanabe reported that an augmentation of the Na_o concentration from 145 to 172 mM was even capable of reversing a verapamil-induced block of AV conduction in the

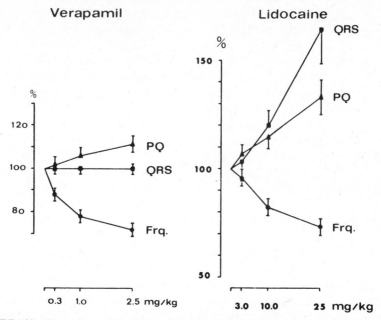

FIGURE 123. Comparison of the effects of the Na-antagonistic compound lidocaine on the guinea pig electrocardiogram with those of the Ca antagonist verapamil. Intermittent intravenous infusion of increasing doses of a Ca antagonist such as verapamil (see also Figure 115) only inhibits Ca-dependent SA-node automaticity and AV conduction, but does not affect NA-dependent intraventricular impulse propagation (QRS). Contrarily, the Na antagonist lidocaine drastically prolongs QRS, but also depresses heart rate and AV conduction velocity by neutralizing the contribution of Na to nodal excitation. Experimental procedure as in Figure 115. From Fleckenstein (1978/1980).

presence of 10 mg/l TTX. Elevation of the Ca_o concentration failed to produce recovery. Thus a promotion of the slow Na current by elevation of the Na_o concentration is obviously a more effective way of relieving a verapamil-induced blockade of AV conduction than is an increase in the Ca_o concentration. Probably in this situation the enhancement of the slow Na current by supplementary Na_o compensates the impairment of the slow electrogenic Ca influx produced by verapamil. In our own experiments on isolated SA and AV nodes of rabbits or guinea pigs, addition of extra Ca was also unable to neutralize the inhibitory effects of Ca antagonists (Haastert, 1973). The assumption is justified that the negative dromotropic action of a high Ca concentration and its failure to relieve a verapamil-induced intranodal block results from an interference of the high Ca_o concentration with the slow transmembrane Na current. Presumably, in AV-nodal cells treated with verapamil, additional Ca is more likely to further impede impulse conduction by reducing the slow inward Na current than to overcome the verapamil-induced inhibition of the slow Ca current.

In conclusion, SA-node automaticity and AV conduction can only be maintained as long as sufficient amounts of extracellular Ca *and* Na are available. Both cations probably serve as indispensable charge carriers of two individual TTX-insensitive electrogenic inward currents that simultaneously pass across the nodal cell membranes. As to the Ca ions, specific Ca antagonists such as verapamil, D 600, nifedipine, or diltiazem suppress the nodal functions by blocking the slow Ca current, whereas β-adrenergic substances (and dibutyryl cyclic AMP) act in the opposite direction by promoting the Ca influx. On the other hand, Na antagonists such as lidocaine, procaine, procaine amide, or quinidine seem to exert their negative chronotropic and dromotropic effects by inhibiting the slow influx of Na. There is no indication that the specific Ca antagonists additionally entangle the slow Na influx or, conversely, that the Na antagonists also interfere with the slow Ca current to a major extent. With respect to these rather particular drug actions, the general term "slow-channel blocker," occasionally used instead of *Ca antagonists,* is incorrect and therefore should be avoided. As a tentative hypothesis of the mechanism of action, we suggest that the organic Ca and Na antagonists specifically displace Ca or Na ions from their individual binding sites at the outer layers of the nodal cell membranes, thus reducing the availability of Ca or Na to the respective channels. Interestingly enough, the Na antagonists of the lidocaine-quinidine type probably restrict the fast as well as the slow inward Na currents. Similarly, a high Ca_o concentration seems to exert Na-antagonistic effects on both Na-transport systems.

CHAPTER FIVE

Suppression by
Calcium Antagonists of
Ectopic Cardiac Autorhythmicity

5.1. ONTOGENIC ROOTS OF CALCIUM-DEPENDENT ECTOPIC PACEMAKER ACTIVITY

There is no doubt that every ordinary myocardial fiber possesses the latent capability of adopting, under certain conditions, the abnormal role of an ectopic pacemaker. This functional change consists of an alteration in the bioelectric membrane properties in that the regular nonundulatory resting potential declines from its high level until, after partial depolarization, spontaneous subthreshold oscillations and lastly overt automaticity are elicited. However, the essence of this transformation of a myocardial fiber is that the excitatory process, with the development of ectopic automaticity, progressively changes from the fast-channel-mediated Na-dependent type into the predominantly Ca-dependent slow form. The occurrence of focal pacemaker activity in previously intact myocardial fibers has to be considered a relapse from a high evolutionary stage, characterized by the presence of an operative fast Na channel, to a lower level of functional perfection, which resembles that of embryonic heart muscle cells.

In fact, an adult fiber that develops ectopic automaticity passes through the same typical forms of excitation, however in the reverse direction, as the embryonic myocardial fibers do during the course of their ontogenesis. For instance, as depicted by Bernard (1975), 10-day-old rat embryonic heart muscle cells exhibit a rather low diastolic membrane potential (-50 mV) with regular spontaneous diastolic depolarizations. In this early stage, the action potentials are sensitive to $MnCl_2$, refractory to TTX, and characterized by a remarkably slow rate of upstroke (dV/dt_{max} : 5 to 8 V/sec). The overshoot too proved to be relatively small and responded much more to changes in Ca_o concentration than to those in Na_o concentration. However the spontaneous diastolic depolarizations disappeared with the thirteenth day of embryonic life, whereas the resting potential rose to approximately -75 mV until at 21 days a final value of around -82 mV was reached. Simultaneously, the action potentials converted more and more from the slow Ca to the fast Na pattern. Thus the 21-day-old embryonic heart muscle cells showed a high upstroke velocity (dV/dt_{max} : 45 to 55 V/sec), a pronounced sensitivity to changes in Na_o concentration and to TTX, but no impairment by $MnCl_2$. Hence there is little doubt that ectopic automaticity means a decay of the adult form of myocardial specialization and a regression to a primitive order of cardiac function in which the excitatory processes are dominated by Ca. Since in embryonic heart muscle cells with a low membrane potential, spontaneous excitation as well as contraction are equally dependent on Ca, the Ca-antagonist D 600 suppresses both functions strictly in parallel (Koidl and Tritthart, 1980, 1982).

Only Purkinje fibers exposed to normal Tyrode solution with a slightly reduced K content (2.7 mM) are able to exhibit a rhythmic activity at a high level of membrane potential (see Figure 127). Here spontaneous Na-dependent activity may occur because of the appearance of diastolic depolarizations in the range between the resting potential (-90 to -95 mV) and the threshold potential (-65 to -70 mV). However, if the membrane is depolarized beyond -55 mV, there is even in Purkinje fibers a transition to the other type of spontaneous activity that is mediated by the slow Ca current, enhanced by adrenaline, unaffected by Na withdrawal or TTX, and depressed by $MnCl_2$ (Imanishi, 1971; Aronson and Cranefield, 1974). Thus pacemaker activity of Purkinje fibers is (1) strongly dependent on Na_o concentration at membrane potentials greater than -55 mV, (2) partially dependent on Na_o concentration at an intermediate potential of -55 to -50 mV, and (3) virtually independent of Na_o concentration at a potential lower than -50 mV.

As a logical consequence, it appears reasonable that ectopic automaticity, occurring at a high level of resting potential, is most responsive to the antiarrhythmic action of Na antagonists such as lidocaine, procaine, procaine amide, or quinidine, whereas, conversely, the Ca antagonists gain in antiarrhythmic potency as the maximal diastolic potential of spontaneously active fibers falls off. This rule seems to apply not only to the His-Purkinje system, but also to fibers from the adult atrial or ventricular myocardium when they develop ectopic automaticity.

5.2.   FUNCTIONAL DIFFERENTIATION BETWEEN SODIUM-ANTAGONISTIC AND CALCIUM-ANTAGONISTIC DRUG ACTIONS ON ECTOPIC PACEMAKERS

5.2.1.   Possible Involvement of Sodium Ions in Cardiac Dysrhythmias at a High Membrane Potential—Role of Purkinje Fibers

According to clinical experiences, atrial fibrillation and flutter as well as ventricular extrasystolic beats and arrhythmias respond favorably, in many cases, to treatment with Na antagonists such as quinidine, lidocaine, or procaine amide. In the light of our present knowledge, it is reasonable to assume that those dysrhythmias that are especially sensitive to Na antagonists originate from ectopic foci that operate at a rather high membrane potential. For this reason, the Purkinje fibers deserve particular interest as a possible source of predominantly Na-dependent ectopic beats and ventricular tachycardias. In fact, Purkinje fibers are prone to sustained rhythmic activity in response to a variety of experimental interventions that may not necessarily induce considerable slow-channel activity.

In this context, particular attention should be paid to the effect of stretch that unstabilizes the Purkinje fiber membrane and thereby evokes or accelerates automaticity without causing a major decay of membrane potential. Since cardiac contractile incompetence frequently leads in humans to a considerable extension of the ventricular wall, stretch-induced ectopic ventricular automaticity certainly deserves more than purely academic interest. A typical experiment carried out in our laboratory by Kaufmann and Theophile (1967) is shown in Figure 124. Here the frequency of spontaneous discharges of an isolated Purkinje fiber of a rhesus monkey was increased from 30/min to 85/min by a stretch that elongated the preparation by 50% above resting length in the unloaded stage (= 100%). In this case even during stretch, automaticity arose from a maximal diastolic potential of about -75 mV, at which the Na current is by no means inactivated. In 10 experiments of this type, the maximal diastolic potential before stretch was -69.9 ($\pm$ 1.4) mV and diminished during stretch by an average of 4.8 mV. There were no changes in threshold potential. However, by stimulating Ca influx, β-adrenergic catecholamines can further enhance the impulse discharge from Purkinje fibers even at such high levels of membrane potential. Interestingly enough, the sensitivity to stretch

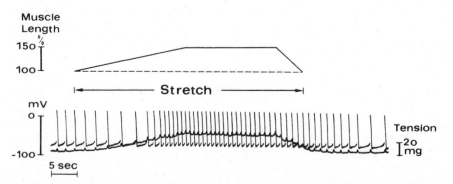

FIGURE 124.   Stretch-induced enhancement of automaticity of an isolated Purkinje fiber from a rhesus monkey heart. Starting from an initial length of the unloaded fiber (L_0 = 3 mm, $\emptyset$ = 0.25 mm) the preparation is stretched to the length of 4.5 mm (= 150% of L_0) within 20 sec. This prolongation produces a rise in basal tension and reversibly increases the rate of spontaneous impulse discharge from 30/min to 85/min. While the diastolic depolarizations become steeper during stretch, the maximal diastolic potential virtually persists at a high level of about 75 mV. Continuous registration of bioelectric activity and mechanical tension with intracellular microelectrode and mechanoelectric transducer (RCA 5734). Control of muscle length with an ocular micrometer. Normal Tyrode solution with 2.68 mM K and 1.8 mM Ca, 30°C, gassed with 95% O_2 and 5% CO_2. From Kaufmann and Theophile (1967).

is distinctly greater in Purkinje fibers than in the ordinary ventricular or atrial myocardium (Kaufmann and Theophile, 1967). Hence ventricular dilation of incompetent hearts is more likely to cause ectopic pacemaker activity by affecting Purkinje fibers than by acting on the ordinary myocardium. On the other hand, in human atria, dilation may reach such high degrees that in this case the common nonspecialized myocardial fibers can also develop stretch-induced automaticity. As generally known, the resulting atrial flutter or fibrillation responds to the traditional treatment with quinidine, in many cases quite satisfactorily. Accordingly, isolated trabeculae from the atria of rhesus monkeys develop stretch-induced automaticity at membrane potentials as high as -65 mV (Kaufmann and Theophile, 1967).

Sodium antagonists such as quinidine, procaine amide, and lidocaine increase the threshold of excitability, reduce the maximal rate of upstroke of action potential, and prolong the effective refractory period. All these alterations occur at a high level of membrane potential and may effectively contribute to the prevention or termination of ectopic automaticity and arrhythmias, provided an exaggerated transmembrane Na influx plays a predominant role in these cases. The aconitine-induced dysrhythmias may serve as an example. They appear in many cases in the -90 to -70 mV range and are suppressed, at least temporarily, by reduction of the Na_o concentration (Schmidt, 1960), by quinidine (Heistracher and Pillat, 1962), by procaine amide (Raschack, 1976b), or by a high Ca_o concentration (Matsuda, Hoshi, and Kameyama, 1959). Verapamil was inefficient (Raschack, 1976b). As reported by Peper and Trautwein (1966), aconitine increases the transmembrane permeability to Na_o so that even during repolarization a TTX-sensitive inward Na current continues to flow. This explains both the efficacy of Na antagonists in inhibiting aconitine-induced dysrhythmias and the failure of verapamil to do so. However, the antiarrhythmic efficacy of Na antagonists declines if the Ca ions take the lead in a lower range of membrane potential.

5.2.2. Effects of Calcium Antagonists on Calcium-Dependent Dysrhythmias in a Low Range of Membrane Potential

The antiarrhythmic potency of Ca antagonists was first recognized by Melville, Shister, and Huq (1964) using verapamil. They found that verapamil can protect the cat heart *in situ* against chloroform-adrenaline-induced ventricular fibrillation and also antagonizes ventricular dysrhythmias caused by continuous intravenous infusion of toxic doses of ouabain. In most cases the onset of T-wave changes was strikingly delayed, and the development of multifocal ectopic automaticity of the ventricles prevented. Essentially similar experimental observations with verapamil, particularly in glycoside-poisoned atrial and ventricular myocardium of different species, were subsequently reported by Schmid and Hanna (1967), Fratz, Greeff, and Wagner (1967), Haas and Busch (1968), Rodriguez-Pereira and Viana (1968), Hanna and Schmid (1970), and Foster, King, Nicoll, and Zipes (1976). Verapamil was also shown to suppress the ouabain-induced increase in automaticity in canine Purkinje fibers (Tse and Han, 1975) and to prevent ventricular fibrillation of dog hearts *in situ* following coronary artery ligation (Kaumann and Aramendia, 1968) or temporary coronary occlusion (Fondacaro, Han, and Yoon, 1978). Other Ca antagonists such as D 600 (Haas and Busch, 1968) or prenylamine (Lindner and Kaiser, 1975) also provided cardioprotection against ventricular arrhythmias. Clinical reports rapidly substantiated the observations on animal hearts. Hence after successful therapeutical tests, intravenous verapamil was introduced in 1966 by Bender, Kojima, Reploh, and Oelmann for the treatment of tachyarrhythmias even before the mechanism of its regularizing action had been fully understood. Special attention should also be paid in this context to the pioneer work of Schamroth (1971) and Krikler (1974a), who also decisively contributed to the further elucidation and propagation of the new therapy (for more details see Section 7.5.2.).

As to the theoretical concept, the antidysrhythmic properties of verapamil were first attributed, erroneously, to a putative β-receptor blocking effect of the drug. But after we had demonstrated that verapamil is, in reality, a Ca antagonist, the true nature of its action on nomotopic and ectopic cardiac pacemakers was soon recognized. Hence Singh and Vaughan Williams (1972) considered verapamil the prototype of a novel fourth class of antidysrhythmic drugs that act by interference with Ca conductance [see also Vaughan Williams (1975)]. In fact, the necessity of putting the different antidysrhythmic drugs in a certain order according to their fundamental mechanisms of action could not longer be disregarded. Besides a differentiation between agents that specifically interfere with the sympathetic drive (group II), and those that merely prolong the refractory period by extending the plateau phase of action potential (group III), the most important classification to be done was certainly that of distinguishing the Na antagonists (group I) from the Ca antagonists (group IV).

The criteria are easily discernible. The *Na antagonists* such as quinidine, procaine amide, or lidocaine aim at the excitatory process in its regular, Na-dependent form. Here they induce changes in threshold, upstroke velocity, overshoot, propagation rate, and so forth. The Na antagonists can also prevent abnormal increases in atrial or ventricular rate in that they slow the recovery of the fast Na-conducting system between the beats. Another rate-limiting influence may result from the fact that some Na antagonists, for instance lidocaine, are capable of reducing the upstroke velocity of the ventricular action potentials much more effectively at high than at normal stimulation frequencies (Tritthart, B. Fleckenstein, and A. Fleckenstein, 1970/1971). This effect too makes the occurrence of ventricular tachycardias and fibrillation less likely. The *Ca antagonists*, on the other hand, let all these Na-dependent parameters, which are reflecting changes in the normal course of atrial or ventricular excitation, unaffected. The Ca antagonists rather aim at a different category of excitation in that they only block the abortive Ca-dependent "slow-response activity" that arises from the altered myocardium. By this action, Ca antagonists can selectively extinguish the uncontrolled firing of Ca-dependent ectopic pacemakers without simultaneous inhibition of the normal excitatory events in the atrial or ventricular musculature. In other words, Ca antagonists, compared with Na antagonists, hit different functional targets when they are successfully used as weapons against arrhythmias.

5.3. ELECTROPHYSIOLOGICAL ASSESSMENT OF THE CARDINAL FACTORS CAUSING ECTOPIC AUTOMATICITY AND THEIR RESPONSIVENESS TO CALCIUM ANTAGONISTS AND CALCIUM PROMOTERS

The electrophysiological features of ectopic automaticity closely resemble the well-known pattern of spontaneous impulse discharge in the SA or AV nodes, although in many cases the dependence on Ca may be yet more pronounced in ectopic than in ordinary pacemaker cells. As discussed in Section 4.3.1, the most typical sign of automaticity consists of an instability of resting potential during diastole. There are two possible manifestations of this peculiarity, namely (1) spontaneous rhythmic oscillations of membrane potential in the subthreshold range or (2) spontaneous diastolic depolarizations that reach the threshold and thereby elicit conducted pacemaker action potentials. Such oscillations as well as overt ectopic automaticity are brought about by a multitude of factors that can, however, be condensed in a simplified concept to only three main determinants, namely:

1. Promotion of transmembrane Ca influx.
2. Augmentation of transmembrane K efflux.
3. Decrease of membrane potential by inhibition of active transport of Na and K. Thereby the passive transmembrane fluxes of Ca and K, and consequently the onset of ectopic automaticity are greatly facilitated.

There is overwhelming evidence that each of these factors can prime ectopic automaticity although they are closely interdependent.

5.3.1. The Significance of Excessive Transmembrane Calcium Influx in Producing Ectopic Automaticity

It has been known for a long time that suitable doses of $CaCl_2$ alone (Rothberger and Winterberg, 1911; van Egmond, 1913; Kolm and Pick, 1920) or in combination with adrenaline or histamine (Kruta, 1934) can resuscitate automaticity in quiescent ventricular and atrial myocardium. This effect is undoubtedly due to an enhancement of the transmembrane inward Ca current. As Bozler reported in 1943, oscillatory changes of membrane potential can be observed in tortoise hearts following an increase in the extracellular Ca concentration. As we have shown in studies on atrial and ventricular myocardium of guinea pigs, such oscillations regularly occur in the form of vacillating afterpotentials if a Tyrode solution with a high Ca content (14 mM) is cooled below 30°C (Kaufmann, Fleckenstein, and Antoni, 1963). The augmentation of Ca_o proved to be most efficient in our experiments if the Na content was simultaneously reduced to 25% of normal. The rhythmic changes of membrane potential always elicit mechanical waves of tension that strictly correspond in time and amplitude to the depolarizing phase of the electric oscillations (See Figure 125).

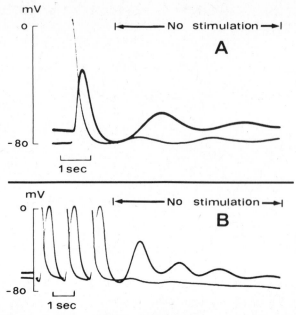

FIGURE 125. Typical occurrence of oscillatory afterpotentials and consecutive aftercontractions in two isolated atrial trabeculae (guinea pig) exposed to a Ca-rich (14.4 m*M*) Tyrode solution at 14°C. After cessation of electric stimulation, a number of damped undulatory changes of membrane potential coupled with mechanical tension waves subsist up to 10 sec. The time lag between the electric and the mechanical peaks is approximately 380 msec. From Kaufmann, Fleckenstein, and Antoni (1963).

This parallelism clearly indicated that both the rhythmic depolarizations and the oscillatory rises in tension have to be considered closely coupled Ca-dependent phenomena that ensue from pulsatory increases in transmembrane Ca inflow. Accordingly the electric and mechanical oscillations immediately disappeared upon extracellular Ca withdrawal.

In the light of these results, it is not surprising that all substances tested so far that increase myocardial contractile tension by promoting the slow Ca current (see Figure 60 in Section 2.8.5) are also capable of enhancing or inducing ectopic automaticity. Thus oscillations of membrane potential or propagated idioventricular impulses can be evoked or at least facilitated (1) by adrenaline, noradrenaline, and other β-adrenergic agents, (2) by histamine (Senges, Randolf, and Katus 1977), or (3) by dibutyryl cyclic AMP (see Figure 134). In all these cases, the oscillations begin at a relatively high membrane potential in the range of about −80 to −70 mV and continuously increase in height and frequency as the diastolic potential declines to the level of −50 to −40 mV, at which excitation is distinctly Ca-dependent. Conversely, as was expected, ectopic automaticity was always suppressed by Ca antagonists, provided the pacemakers operated in this low range of membrane potential.

5.3.2. Ectopic Automaticity Induced by an Increase in Transmembrane Potassium Efflux

We consider an enhancement of the transmembrane efflux of K ions the second cardinal factor that is responsible for the induction of ectopic automaticity (Fleckenstein, 1961b,1963b). As was first shown in experiments of Kehar and Hooker (1935), ventricular myocardium brought to fibrillation by electric shocks loses K. Later reports confirmed these findings on auricular tissue. A particularly careful study with ^{42}K was carried out by Holland and Briggs (1959) and by Briggs and Holland (1960) on isolated rabbit atria. These researchers caused increasing losses of K from the tissue stepwise (1) by exposure to a Tyrode solution with a low K concentration, (2) by adding acetylcholine, which promotes the transmembrane K conductivity of the atrial fibers, and (3) by frequent electric stimulation until sustained fibrillation started. The fibrillation threshold coincided with a 10-fold increase in K efflux relative to the K influx.

Voltage-clamp studies on the transmembrane outward currents in ventricular fibers indicate that there are two outward K currents that are probably involved in the development of ectopic automaticity, namely (1) the time-independent, background K current (I_{bg}), and (2) the time-dependent K current (I_k) according to the terminology of McDonald and Trautwein (1978a,b). The current I_k seems to be virtually identical with the outward current $i_{x(1)}$ in Purkinje fibers (Noble and Tsien, 1969; McAllister, Noble, and Tsien, 1975). *The background K current* does not necessarily increase in a K-deficient solution because a low K_o concentration reduces the K conductance of the myocardial fiber membrane. This permeability change is thought to be responsible, at least in part, for the depolarization in a K-deficient medium as a prerequisite of slow-channel-mediated ectopic automaticity. *The time-dependent K current (I_k),* on the other hand, grows if the extracellular K concentration is lowered. This current is activated by depolarizing pulses and represents the decisive ionic process that subsequently drives the membrane potential back to the diastolic values (see Figure 131). A low K_o concentration increases the steepness of the transmembrane K gradient and thereby potentiates the driving force of I_k. However, the intensification of I_k seems also to enhance the slow-channel-mediated Ca influx, thus facilitating ectopic automaticity. This occurs because both the slow inward Ca current and I_k probably reflect an equivalent transmembrane Ca–K exchange in the potential range below -50 mV. In other words, a low extracellular K concentration has rather peculiar effects on the passive transmembrane K movement in that it exerts an inhibitory influence on the background K current simultaneously with a potentiation of I_k. However, both effects are eventually cooperative in that they favor the onset of ectopic automaticity.

Electrophysiological evidence of the development of ectopic automaticity in a low-K environment is most readily obtainable in Purkinje fibers that are particularly sensitive to K withdrawal. Pertinent observations of Antoni (1961) and of Antoni, Herkel, and Fleckenstein (see Fleckenstein, 1964b) on Purkinje fibers of rhesus monkeys are represented in the Figures 126 and 127. Both experiments demonstrate that there is a rapid decay of membrane potential within 5 min following exposure

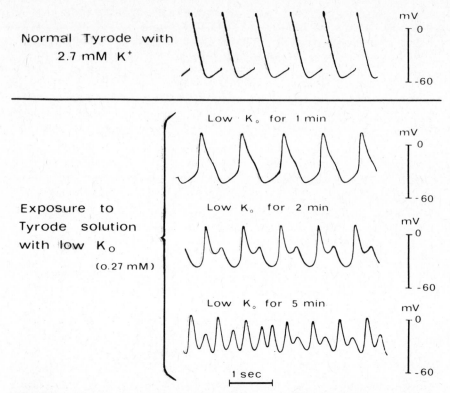

Normal Tyrode with 2.7 mM K⁺

Exposure to Tyrode solution with low K_o (0.27 mM)

Low K_o for 1 min

Low K_o for 2 min

Low K_o for 5 min

1 sec

FIGURE 126. Precipitous decay of membrane potential and onset of irregular flutter in a spontaneously active isolated Purkinje fiber from a rhesus monkey heart upon exposure to a K-deficient Tyrode solution. Decrease of K_o from 2.7 to 0.27 mM. Temperature, 36°C. From Antoni (1961).

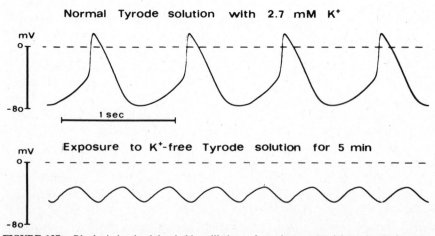

Normal Tyrode solution with 2.7 mM K⁺

1 sec

Exposure to K⁺-free Tyrode solution for 5 min

FIGURE 127. Rhythmic local subthreshold oscillations of membrane potential at a level of approximately −40 mV following exposure of an isolated rhesus monkey Purkinje fiber to K-free Tyrode solution for 5 min. Temperature, 36°C. From Antoni, Herkel, and Fleckenstein; see Fleckenstein (1964b).

to the K-deficient media. Then at a level of -40 mV (Figure 126), irregular flutter developed, whereas in the other experiment (Figure 127) rhythmic subthreshold oscillations appeared. A similar loss of resting potential after immersion into a K-deficient solution was also observed by other authors in dog Purkinje fibers (Weidmann 1956; Hoffman and Cranefield, 1960).

Ordinary ventricular myocardium is less responsive to K_o withdrawal. However, our studies on isolated papillary muscles of guinea pigs have shown that even here sustained automaticity may occur at a low extracellular K concentration if the preparations are continuously stimulated for about 20 to 30 min. An experiment of Antoni (1961) is represented in Figure 128. In this case, an isolated guinea pig papillary muscle had been electrically driven in a K-free Tyrode solution for 35 min until the preparation developed distinct pacemaker activity accompanied by mechanical flutter waves. The spontaneous electric discharges were characterized by rhythmic diastolic depolarizations that elicited plateauless abbreviated action potentials at a level of about -75 to -70 mV. Then 2 min later, there was suddenly a further fall in membrane potential, and the preparation began to fibrillate. The final stage of spontaneous activity of K-deprived guinea pig papillary muscles can be seen from Figure 129. Here only rhythmic oscillatory subthreshold depolarizations, associated with corresponding contraction waves, were left. The depolarizations started from a membrane potential of less than -40 mV, at which only the slow channel is in operation. Thus the oscillatory depolarizations and the concomitant contractions at a low K_o concentration basically correspond to those observed at a high Ca_o concentration since under both circumstances, pulsatory increases in Ca influx seem to be responsible for these phenomena. In keeping with

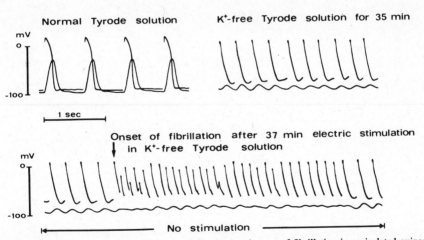

FIGURE 128. Appearance of diastolic depolarizations and onset of fibrillation in an isolated guinea pig papillary muscle following prolonged electric stimulation in K-free Tyrode solution. Apart from automaticity, the muscle also exhibits plateauless abbreviated action potentials. The latter phenomenon is also attributable to the enhancement of K-efflux (I_k) at low K_o because under these circumstances precipitous repolarization takes place. Temperature, 36°C. From Antoni (1961).

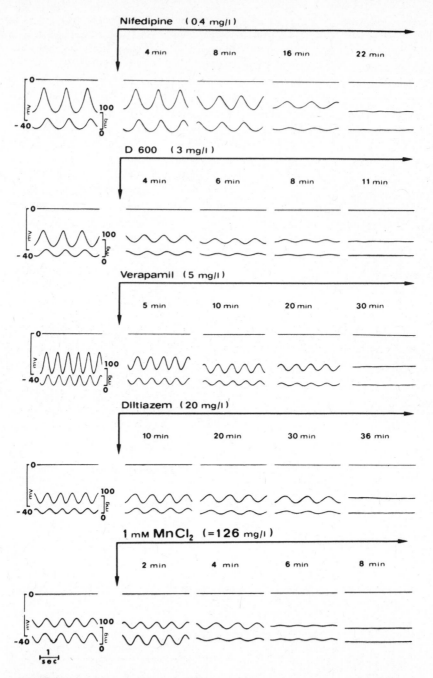

FIGURE 129. Spontaneous rhythmic subthreshold oscillations of isolated guinea pig papillary muscles following prolonged electric stimulation with 30 shocks/min for 20 to 25 min in a Tyrode solution with low K_o (0.4 mM) at a slightly reduced temperature (30°C). Each wave of membrane potential induces an oscillatory contractile response correlated with the depolarizing phase of the electric oscillations. The organic Ca antagonists nifedipine, D 600, verapamil, and diltiazem as well as $MnCl_2$ suppress the bioelectric and mechanical oscillations in parallel. The upstroke velocity (dV/dt_{max}) of the rhythmic depolarizations is extremely slow (approximately 0.2 to 0.5 V/sec). From Fleckenstein and Späh, unpublished.

196

this, we were able to show that the Ca antagonists nifedipine, D 600, verapamil, and diltiazem as well as $MnCl_2$ simultaneously suppress the bioelectric and the mechanical vacillations (see Figure 129 from Fleckenstein and Späh, unpublished observations). Furthermore, it has been established in our studies with ^{45}Ca that a reduction of the K_o concentration enhances myocardial Ca uptake enormously, as depicted in Section 3.5.3 (see Figure 101 in particular). Verapamil, on the other hand, fully neutralized the promoter effect that K deficiency exerts on the ^{45}Ca incorporation (see Figure 102). Hence it is by no means surprising that verapamil and the other specific Ca antagonists can also suppress the electrophysiological manifestations of this abundant inward Ca flux into the K-deprived myocardium.

5.3.3. Induction of Ectopic Automaticity in Partially Depolarized Myocardium after Inhibition of Active Transport of Sodium and Potassium

Apparently a third decisive factor that can enhance ectopic automaticity in ordinary myocardial fibers consists of a labilization of membrane potential in consequence of disturbances of active transport of Na and K and possibly also of Ca extrusion. In fact, every incompetence of the cation pumps in maintaining the normal heights of the transmembrane concentration gradients for Na, K, or Ca necessarily destabilizes the resting state of the myocardial fibers. For instance, spontaneous impulse discharge as a consequence of impairment of active cation transport can be elicited, or at least facilitated, by the following experimental procedures:

1. Cooling of the myocardium to a temperature of 30 to 14°C.
2. Intoxication with cardiac glycosides.
3. Application of anoxia or ischemia.

In all these cases, there is a significant drop in membrane potential that conditions the fibers for the entry of Ca ions as the decisive charge carriers in the electrogenesis of ventricular ectopic automaticity.

As generally known, toxic doses of cardiac glycosides directly block active Na-K transport in atrial and ventricular myocardium (Conn 1956; Schreiber, 1956; Rayner and Weatherall, 1957). In consequence, as early observed in glycoside-poisoned dog and rabbit hearts, the intracellular K content is considerably lowered (Calhoun and Harrison, 1931; Wood and Moe, 1938; Hagen, 1939). Hence with a decrease in the ratio K_i:K_o, the high resting potential of ordinary myocardial fibers progressively declines until finally Na-dependent excitation is replaced by Ca-dependent slow-channel-mediated activity. This transition seems to occur gradually. As we have shown, electric stimuli may elicit the first oscillatory afterpotentials of strophanthin-poisoned guinea pig papillary muscles in normal Tyrode solution (36°C) at a resting potential of about -80 mV, but never induce sustained automaticity under these conditions (Kaufmann, Fleckenstein, and Antoni, 1963). If the membrane potential further decreased or extra Ca was added, the afterpotentials occasionally reached the threshold. However, multifocal Ca-dependent autorhythmicity of the strophanthin-poisoned myocardium generally did not develop except at a membrane potential below -50 mV. Ferrier ad Moe (1973) made similar observations on canine Purkinje fibers poisoned with acetylstrophanthidin. In these experiments too, the afterpotentials increased in amplitude with a rise in the Ca_o concentration and were depressed by Ca-antagonistic Mn ions. The scheme of Figure 130 illustrates summarily the fundamental influence of membrane potential on the electrogenic cation fluxes in nomotopic and ectopic cardiac pacemaker excitation.

The onset of fibrillation in ischemic dog hearts after coronary artery occlusion or ligation (Kaumann and Aramendia, 1968; Fondacaro, Han, and Yoon, 1978) is also attributable to an excessive Ca inflow at a low membrane potential. Indeed, ectopic ventricular autorhythmicity after interruption of coronary blood supply seems to be nothing but an electrophysiological equivalent to the dramatic intrusion of Ca

Cation exchange in nomotopic and ectopic pacemaker excitation

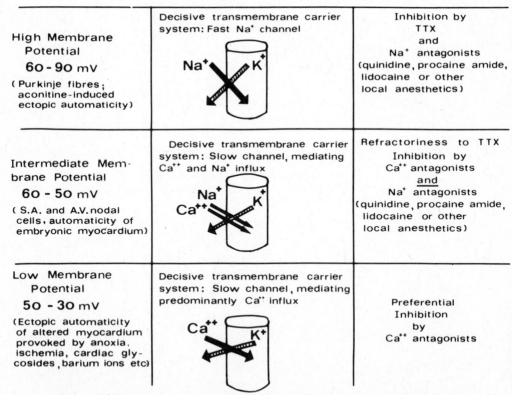

FIGURE 130. Scheme of cation currents that underlie spontaneous cardiac impulse discharge. Transition from fast-channel-mediated Na–K exchange at a high membrane potential to slow-channel-mediated Ca–K exchange in a low range of membrane potential.

that takes place in anoxic or ischemic myocardium (as depicted in Section 3.5.4). The ability of verapamil and other Ca antagonists such as nifedipine or diltiazem to prevent this Ca engulfment is also a well-known fact. Therefore, it is easily understood that Ca antagonists also suppress, together with the excessive Ca uptake into the ischemic myocardium, the bioelectric symptoms of this ion movement. However, we stress that in all probability, not only the electrogenic transmembrane Ca influx but also the resulting intracellular Ca overload are decisively involved in the excitatory disorders of the ischemic myocardium. This applies particularly to the oscillations in a low range of membrane potential. Such oscillations always coincide, according to our observations, with a considerable increase in the intracellular Ca concentration, leading to an exhaustive breakdown of the ATP and CP stores. In consequence, active extrusion of Ca is greatly cut off from the energy supply. Hence a vicious circle may be established in that a low membrane potential initially favours Ca entry and intracellular Ca accumulation, while, in turn, the consecutive high-energy-phosphate deficiency of the Ca-overloaded fibers further promotes Ca overload and membrane-potential decay by restricting active Ca (and Na) transport. The Ca antagonists that inhibit Ca influx, intracellular Ca accumulation, and consequently high-energy-phosphate breakdown, seem to interrupt this positive feedback.

5.3.4. Enhancement of Passive Transmembrane Ca–K Exchange as the Causative Principle of Ectopic Automaticity

Evidence is presented in the preceding sections that ectopic pacemaker activity, at least in a lower range of membrane potential, is necessarily connected with a transmembrane influx of Ca, while K leaks out. Both cation fluxes are closely interdependent, and it seems reasonable to suppose that they merely reflect a variant of the well-known cation exchange occurring in normal excitation. In accordance with the classic notion of Hodgkin, Huxley, and Katz, the ordinary action potentials of intact atrial and ventricular fibers are certainly brought about by an exchange of Na with K (Hodgkin and Huxley, 1947, 1952a, b, c, 1953; Hodgkin, Huxley, and Katz, 1952; Draper and Weidmann, 1951; Weidmann, 1956). Instead, in spontaneous slow-channel-mediated ectopic excitation, the essential exchange partners are, in all probability, represented by Ca and K. *Hence we propose that the crucial reaction in ectopic pacemaker activity consists of an exaggerated passive transmembrane exchange of Ca with an equivalent amount of K down the respective concentration gradients.* According to the scheme of Figure 131A, this exchange process is *disphasic* in that the pulsatory increases in Ca influx that produce the rhythmic depolarizations in oscillating fibers are each time compensated by the subsequent efflux (I_k) of an equivalent amount of K that drives the membrane potential back to the higher diastolic values. Moreover, even propagated ectopic pacemaker action potentials exhibit a distinct disphasic character. Apparently each Ca-mediated spike potential is balanced by an overshooting repolarization that largely exceeds the maximal height of the diastolic potential of preceeding or following subthreshold oscillations (see Figure 131B). This phenomenon naturally

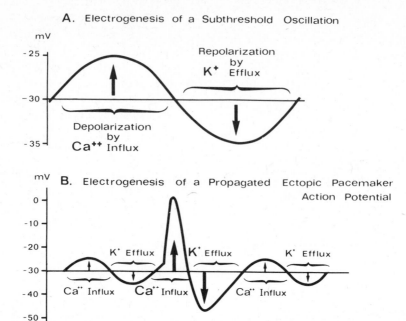

FIGURE 131. Scheme of the coupled Ca–K exchange that underlies the electrogenesis of ectopic subthreshold oscillations (*A*) and propagated ectopic pacemaker action potentials (*B*) in a low range of membrane potential (below -50 mV). In both cases A and B, the depolarizing slow-channel-mediated inward current is carried by Ca ions, while the subsequent repolarization is brought about by the efflux of an equivalent amount of K (I_k), which drives the membrane potential back to the diastolic values. The greater influx of Ca in case of a propagated ectopic pacemaker action potential is apparently compensated by an enhancement of I_k so that an overshooting repolarization is produced. From Fleckenstein (1980/1981).

points to a considerable enhancement of K efflux (I_k) in response to the previous intrusion of a larger amount of Ca during the depolarizing phase of a propagated pacemaker action potential.

Regarding the host of scattered data and opinions on the origin of ectopic automaticity, there is certainly a need for a comprehensive synopsis. The theoretical concept outlined above meets these requirements since it amalgamates many old findings with the new results obtained by means of Ca antagonists. First it explains the close connection that exists, according to our isotope studies, between the changes in the extracellular K concentration (K_o) and the transmembrane Ca uptake. As ensues from the proposed concept, the total driving force F that energizes the coupled transmembrane Ca–K exchange represents the sum of the particular driving forces F_{Ca} and F_K. Hence F varies with the height of both the transmembrane concentration ratio of Ca_o:Ca_i and the ratio of K_i:K_o. In consequence, transmembrane Ca influx (I_{si}) *and* K efflux (I_k), linked together in this exchange cycle, can be equally potentiated by either an augmentation of Ca_o or by a reduction of K_o (see Figure 130).

In fact, high Ca_o concentrations and low K_o concentrations enormously favor transmembrane ^{45}Ca uptake and ectopic pacemaker activity under virtually all circumstances. Conversely, as we have also shown in our studies with ^{45}Ca, the transmembrane uptake of Ca is greatly diminished if the steepness of the K gradient is reduced by increasing the K_o concentration. Thus a high K_o concentration diminishes the uptake of labeled Ca as effectively as a low Ca_o concentration. Simultaneously, a high K_o concentration blocks ectopic pacemakers, an effect that is rather unique among depolarizing agents. For instance, Hering reported as early as in 1904 that "every kind of fibrillation" of isolated ventricles of rabbits, cats, dogs, or monkeys can be immediately abolished and normal contractility eventually restored if additional KCl is given in the perfusion fluid. He even emphasized that this effect might be of therapeutic significance in man. Ventricular fibrillation of isolated dog hearts produced by electric shocks is similarly stopped by intracoronary application of a K-rich solution (Kehar and Hooker, 1935). Glycoside-induced cardiac dysrhythmias also respond favourably to an elevation of the K_o concentration, not only in animal experiments, but also under clinical conditions. Thus oral or intravenous administration of K salts is a widely used therapeutic measure to suppress, in cases of cardiac glycoside intoxication, ventricular ectopic beats, bigeminal rhythm, or ventricular tachyarrhythmias (Sampson and Anderson, 1932; Sampson, Alberton, and Kondo, 1943; Enselberg, Simmons, and Mintz, 1950; Lown, Salzberg, Enselberg, and Weston, 1951). Interestingly enough, also in man, reduction of the Ca_o concentration following injection of the chelating agent EDTA neutralizes glycoside-induced cardiac dysrhythmias in a quite similar manner as elevation of the K_o concentration does. Conversely, low K_o or high Ca_o concentrations greatly potentiate the cardiotoxic glycoside effects. Even in hypoxic hearts, a low K_o concentration seems to promote the occurrence of fibrillation. For instance, Coffman and Gregg (1960) reported that anoxic dog hearts exhibited a higher incidence of fibrillation if the venous K concentration, measured in the right atrial blood, was relatively low.

Apart from the steepness of the respective cation gradients, the intensity of the Ca–K exchange naturally depends on the *gating processes* that regulate the cation permeabilities of the cardiac fiber membranes. The opposite effects of Ca antagonists and Ca promoters (β-adrenergic substances, histamine, dibutyryl cyclic AMP) on ectopic automaticity are due to their contrary actions on transmembrane Ca conductance. Moreover, it is reasonable to assume that antiarrhythmic agents that are able to induce changes in the outward K current (I_k) influence the Ca–K exchange cycle in a low range of membrane potential as effectively as if they acted on the Ca channel. In this context, some antiarrhythmic drugs that belong to group III, according to the classification of Singh and Vaughan Williams (1972), deserve particular interest. Substances of this type produce a "pure" prolongation of the action potential duration and supposedly suppress ectopic tachyarrhythmias merely by increasing the refractory period. Hauswirth and Singh (1979) considered the antiarrhythmic compound amiodarone to be typical of substances that act in this way. Little is hitherto known about the fundamental effects of such drugs on the repolarizing ion shifts. However, there is reason to suppose that this "pure" prolongation of action potential might reflect a retardation or reduction of the repolarizing outward K current (I_k) or, more precisely, that amiodarone and related drugs inhibit the coupled Ca–K exchange in ectopic pacemakers by acting preferentially on the K side. It is up to further studies to shed more light on this problem.

5.3.5. Induction of Typically Calcium-Dependent Ectopic Pacemaker Activity by Barium Ions

One of the most suitable possibilities of inducing ectopic pacemaker activity in animal hearts consists of the application of soluble Ba salts. It has for a long time been recognized that Ba ions are able to start autorhythmicity in isolated quiescent myocardium or in ventricles *in situ* after previous blockade of AV conduction (Rothberger and Winterberg, 1911; van Egmond, 1913; Abderhalden and Gellhorn, 1920; Kolm and Pick, 1920; Kruta, 1934; Boulet and Boulet, 1945). Accordingly, even in man, attacks of Adams-Stokes syncope could be overcome with the help of $BaCl_2$ (Cohn and Levine, 1925). To clarify the mechanism of action, in our laboratory Antoni and Oberdisse (1965) first made use of intracellular registration techniques. The studies were carried out on isolated papillary muscles of rabbits, guinea pigs, cats, and rhesus monkeys. Surprisingly, $BaCl_2$ at a concentration of 1 to 4 mM converted the bioelectric behavior of the total mass of ordinary ventricular fibers into that of synchronously beating pacemaker cells (see Figure 132). In electrically stimulated preparations, this transformation usually took place within a few minutes *pari passu* with a progressive decrease in membrane potential. Two stages of automaticity were discernible. In the range of membrane potential of -70 to -50 mV, diastolic depolarizations of growing steepness appeared. If stimulation was discontinued, such muscles exhibited oscillations that occasionally reached the threshold, but mostly faded away (see Figure 133). But as soon as the membrane potential of the Ba-treated fibers fell below -50 mV, sustained automaticity developed that persisted under appropriate experimental conditions for several hours. Thus Ba-induced ventricular ectopic automaticity is a particularly useful model on which the validity of the proposed Ca–K-exchange concept could be subjected to crucial tests.

In fact, all available data indicate that every measure that promotes transmembrane Ca influx or K efflux potentiates Ba-induced ectopic pacemaker activity. This is evident from the following observations:

1. The steepness of the Ba-induced slow diastolic depolarizations as well as maximal upstroke velocity and overshoot of the propagated ectopic pacemaker action potentials increase considerably if the extracellular Ca (Ca_o) concentration is raised above normal. Contractile tension grows roughly in parallel with the bioelectric parameters (Figure 134).

2. Neural sympathetic stimulation or direct application of adrenaline greatly facilitates the onset of Ba-induced automaticity. This is true of both ven-

A. Isolated rabbit papillary muscle

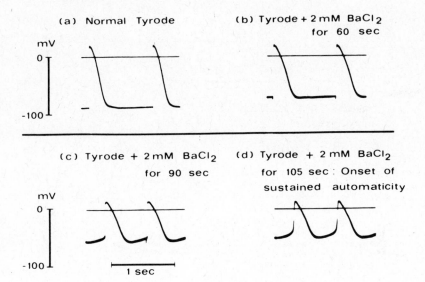

(a) Normal Tyrode

(b) Tyrode + 2 mM BaCl$_2$
for 60 sec

(c) Tyrode + 2 mM BaCl$_2$
for 90 sec

(d) Tyrode + 2 mM BaCl$_2$
for 105 sec : Onset of
sustained automaticity

1 sec

B. Isolated rabbit atrial trabecula

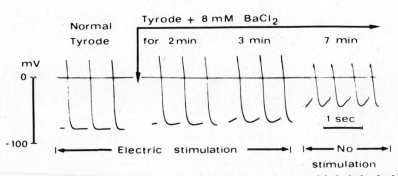

Normal
Tyrode

Tyrode + 8 mM BaCl$_2$

for 2 min   3 min   7 min

1 sec

|◄——— Electric stimulation ———►| |◄—— No ——►|
stimulation

FIGURE 132. Electrogenesis of Ba-induced ectopic pacemaker action potentials in isolated rabbit myocardium. (A) Addition of BaCl$_2$ (2 mM) to ordinary Tyrode solution produces diastolic depolarizations in electrically stimulated ventricular myocardium (b) to (c). Then within 2 min, synchronous electric and mechanical automaticity of all papillary muscle fibers develops (d). (B) Atrial myocardium, in comparison with ventricular fibers, is less sensitive to BaCl$_2$. However, with 8 mM BaCl$_2$, even in atrial preparations, automaticity is elicited. The intracellular records originate in each experiment from one and the same fiber. Experiments from Antoni and Oberdisse (1965).

203

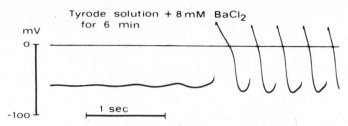

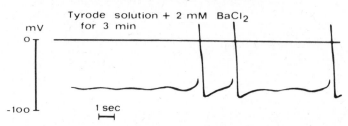

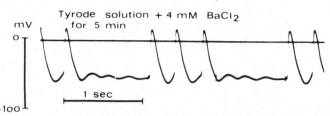

FIGURE 133. Barium-induced oscillatory prepotentials (*A*), (*B*) and afterpotentials (*C*) in isolated papillary muscles from guinea pig and rabbit hearts. As long as the diastolic potentials were more negative than -50 mV, no sustained automaticity appeared. From Antoni and Oberdisse (1965).

tricular myocardium (Rothberger and Winterberg, 1911; van Egmond, 1913) and isolated atria (Kruta, 1934). Figure 134 shows pertinent microelectrode records with noradrenaline. Nicotine, which has to be considered a noradrenaline releaser (see Section 2.8), also potentiates the Ba action (Rothberger and Winterberg, 1911).

3. Stimulation of H_2-receptors with histamine enhances impulse discharge from Ba-induced ventricular pacemakers just like adrenergic β-receptor stimulation does (Späh and Fleckenstein unpublished).

4. A striking promotion of Ba-induced ectopic automaticity also occurs if dibutyryl cyclic AMP is administered (see Figure 134).

5. Moreover, a low K_o concentration favors spontaneous Ba-induced impulse discharge.

Calcium

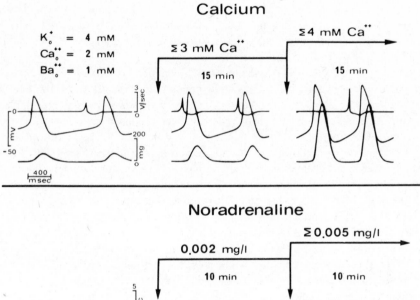

Noradrenaline

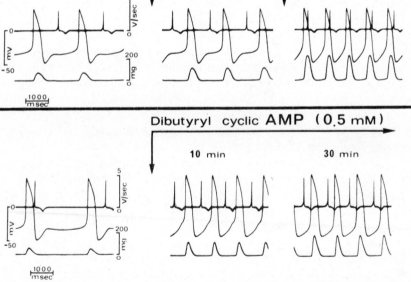

FIGURE 134. Enhancement of Ba-induced ectopic pacemaker activity of guinea pig papillary muscles by promotion of transsarcolemmal Ca entry with additional Ca, noradrenaline, or dibutyryl cyclic AMP. As can be argued from the changes in dV/dt_{max}, the augmentation of contractile tension after addition of extra Ca seems to be due primarily to a greater Ca influx per beat. However, the positive inotropic effect following the addition of noradrenaline or dibutyryl cyclic AMP seems rather to represent a positive-staircase phenomenon in which intracellular Ca accumulation is brought about by the closer succession of the Ca-carried action potentials (see Section 2.6). The intracellular records were taken from one and the same myocardial fiber in each experiment. From Späh and Fleckenstein, unpublished.

All the experimental interventions 1 to 5 are known to strengthen the slow inward Ca current (see Sections 2.8 and 3.5.3). Obviously, Ba-induced automaticity is intensified by any agent or experimental procedure that augments Ca inflow, as illustrated in Figure 60.

Conversely, a decrease in transmembrane Ca conductivity will inhibit Ba-induced ectopic pacemaker activity. Interestingly enough, the sensitivity of Ba-induced ventricular pacemakers to the inhibitory action of Ca antagonists is greater than that of SA- or AV-nodal cells. Thus minute concentrations of nifedipine (0.02 mg/l), D 600 (0.05 mg/l), verapamil (0.1 mg/l), or diltiazem (1.0 mg/l) proved to be highly effective in extinguishing Ba-induced ventricular rhythms (see Figure 135). On the other hand, even strong concentrations of Na antagonists such as lidocaine (50 to 100 mg/l) or procaine amide (50 to 100 mg/l) as well as tetrodotoxin (10 mg/l) failed to abolish Ba-induced ectopic automaticity in our experiments (see Figure 136). This refractoriness against Na antagonists indicates that in contrast with nomotopic SA- or AV-nodal pacemaker activity, there is probably no major involvement of Na ions in ectopic Ba-induced impulse discharge.

In fact, Ba-induced automaticity seems to be based primarily on Ca inflow without an appreciable contribution of Na ions as additional transmembrane electric-charge carriers. Conversely, automatic SA- and AV-nodal action potentials are characterized by an obligatory participation of Ca *and* Na (see Section 4.3.3). It is probably for this reason that the two pacemaker types also respond quite differently to high Ca_o concentrations since elevation of the Ca_o concentration up to 14 mM excessively stimulates Ba-induced automaticity, whereas normal SA-node activity is totally abolished by this treatment (Kohlhardt and Kaufmann, 1970). A high Ca_o concentration presumably suppresses the obligatory inward Na current in nodal cells so that automaticity ceases. In Ba-induced ectopic pacemakers, on the other hand, a high Ca_o concentration merely promotes Ca inflow so that automaticity is enhanced. Moreover, for the same reason, a high Ca_o concentration can overcome the inhibition by Ca antagonists of Ba-induced ectopic automaticity within certain limits. Conversely, the suppression of SA-node automaticity or AV conduction by Ca antagonists is refractory to additional Ca as discussed in Section 4.3.3. In this case, a high Ca_o concentration is more likely to further impede nodal excitation by reducing the obligatory inward Na current than to overcome the blockade of transmembrane Ca conductivity.

In summarizing our observations on Ba-induced pacemakers, we stress that this type of ectopic automaticity represents a model in which the underlying *Ca–K exchange cycle* appears in a rather pure form. Accordingly, Ba-induced ectopic pacemaker activity is more readily extinguished by Ca antagonists than is nomotopic impulse discharge from the SA node or impulse conduction through the AV node. Moreover, the Ca–K exchange cycle is also easily blocked by elevation of the extracellular K (K_o) concentration. Thus it was reported long ago by Kolm and Pick (1920) and by Boulet and Boulet (1945) that Ba-induced ectopic pacemaker activity of ventricular myocardium is even more susceptible to the inhibitory influence of a high K_o concentration than nomotopic SA-node automaticity is. More recent studies with the intracellular registration technique have confirmed these

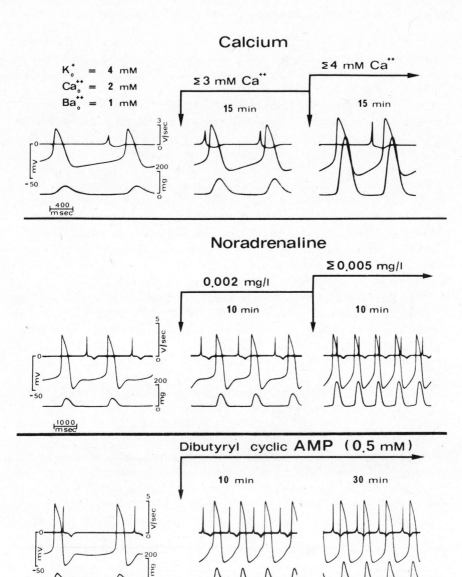

FIGURE 134. Enhancement of Ba-induced ectopic pacemaker activity of guinea pig papillary muscles by promotion of transsarcolemmal Ca entry with additional Ca, noradrenaline, or dibutyryl cyclic AMP. As can be argued from the changes in dV/dt_{max}, the augmentation of contractile tension after addition of extra Ca seems to be due primarily to a greater Ca influx per beat. However, the positive inotropic effect following the addition of noradrenaline or dibutyryl cyclic AMP seems rather to represent a positive-staircase phenomenon in which intracellular Ca accumulation is brought about by the closer succession of the Ca-carried action potentials (see Section 2.6). The intracellular records were taken from one and the same myocardial fiber in each experiment. From Späh and Fleckenstein, unpublished.

All the experimental interventions 1 to 5 are known to strengthen the slow inward Ca current (see Sections 2.8 and 3.5.3). Obviously, Ba-induced automaticity is intensified by any agent or experimental procedure that augments Ca inflow, as illustrated in Figure 60.

Conversely, a decrease in transmembrane Ca conductivity will inhibit Ba-induced ectopic pacemaker activity. Interestingly enough, the sensitivity of Ba-induced ventricular pacemakers to the inhibitory action of Ca antagonists is greater than that of SA- or AV-nodal cells. Thus minute concentrations of nifedipine (0.02 mg/l), D 600 (0.05 mg/l), verapamil (0.1 mg/l), or diltiazem (1.0 mg/l) proved to be highly effective in extinguishing Ba-induced ventricular rhythms (see Figure 135). On the other hand, even strong concentrations of Na antagonists such as lidocaine (50 to 100 mg/l) or procaine amide (50 to 100 mg/l) as well as tetrodotoxin (10 mg/l) failed to abolish Ba-induced ectopic automaticity in our experiments (see Figure 136). This refractoriness against Na antagonists indicates that in contrast with nomotopic SA- or AV-nodal pacemaker activity, there is probably no major involvement of Na ions in ectopic Ba-induced impulse discharge.

In fact, Ba-induced automaticity seems to be based primarily on Ca inflow without an appreciable contribution of Na ions as additional transmembrane electric-charge carriers. Conversely, automatic SA- and AV-nodal action potentials are characterized by an obligatory participation of Ca *and* Na (see Section 4.3.3). It is probably for this reason that the two pacemaker types also respond quite differently to high Ca_o concentrations since elevation of the Ca_o concentration up to 14 mM excessively stimulates Ba-induced automaticity, whereas normal SA-node activity is totally abolished by this treatment (Kohlhardt and Kaufmann, 1970). A high Ca_o concentration presumably suppresses the obligatory inward Na current in nodal cells so that automaticity ceases. In Ba-induced ectopic pacemakers, on the other hand, a high Ca_o concentration merely promotes Ca inflow so that automaticity is enhanced. Moreover, for the same reason, a high Ca_o concentration can overcome the inhibition by Ca antagonists of Ba-induced ectopic automaticity within certain limits. Conversely, the suppression of SA-node automaticity or AV conduction by Ca antagonists is refractory to additional Ca as discussed in Section 4.3.3. In this case, a high Ca_o concentration is more likely to further impede nodal excitation by reducing the obligatory inward Na current than to overcome the blockade of transmembrane Ca conductivity.

In summarizing our observations on Ba-induced pacemakers, we stress that this type of ectopic automaticity represents a model in which the underlying *Ca–K exchange cycle* appears in a rather pure form. Accordingly, Ba-induced ectopic pacemaker activity is more readily extinguished by Ca antagonists than is nomotopic impulse discharge from the SA node or impulse conduction through the AV node. Moreover, the Ca–K exchange cycle is also easily blocked by elevation of the extracellular K (K_o) concentration. Thus it was reported long ago by Kolm and Pick (1920) and by Boulet and Boulet (1945) that Ba-induced ectopic pacemaker activity of ventricular myocardium is even more susceptible to the inhibitory influence of a high K_o concentration than nomotopic SA-node automaticity is. More recent studies with the intracellular registration technique have confirmed these

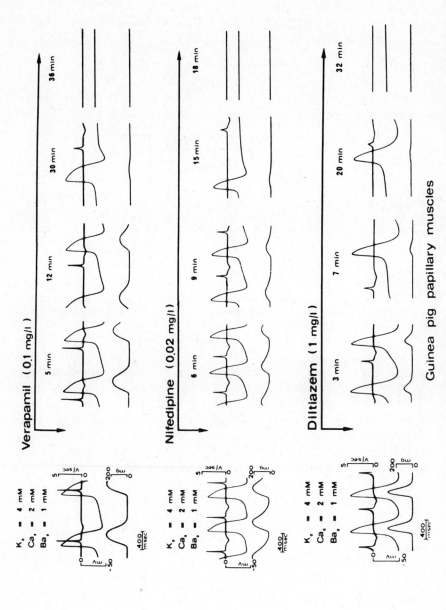

FIGURE 135. Suppression of Ba-induced ectopic pacemaker activity by minute amounts of the specific Ca antagonists verapamil (0.1 mg/l), nifedipine (0.02 mg/l), and diltiazem (1.0 mg/l). Experiments on isolated guinea pig papillary muscles immersed in Tyrode solution with 1 mM Ba, 2 mM Ca, and 4 mM K for 30 min at 30°C until sustained rhythmic automaticity had developed. Then the Ca antagonists were added. The intracellular records originated in each experiment from one and the same myocardial fiber. From Fleckenstein and Späh, unpublished.

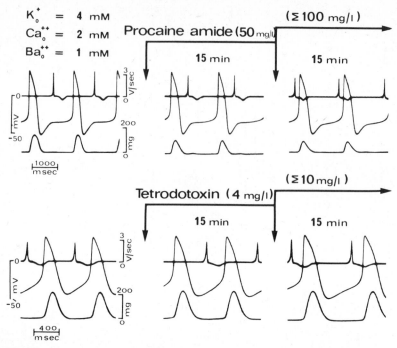

FIGURE 136. Refractoriness of Ba-induced ectopic pacemaker activity to high concentrations of Na antagonists such as procaine amide or tetrodotoxin. The experimental procedure was analogous to that in Figure 135. From Fleckenstein and Späh, unpublished.

findings (Antoni and Oberdisse, 1965). Needless to say, numerous problems related to the origin or suppression of Ba-induced ectopic automaticity still have to be clarified by further investigations. This applies particularly to the specific mechanism of action by which the Ba ions produce such dramatic deviations from the normal cation permeabilities of the intact myocardium. Promising approaches to this goal were made by Hermsmeyer and Sperelakis (1970) and by Hiraoka, Ikeda, and Sano (1980). The use of Ca antagonists certainly represents a landmark in this field of research. Nevertheless, it seems advisable to study not only the action of Ba on the passive cation fluxes, but also the possible interference of Ba ions with active cation transport. For instance, it is by no means ruled out that the Ba ions coming into contact with the sarcolemma membrane impair active Na–K transport by precipitating ATP as the necessary enzyme substrate for this process. There are, in fact, many similarities between ectopic ventricular automaticity produced by Ba and that elicited by high doses of ouabain, which are well known to block the Na-K pump.

CHAPTER SIX

Calcium Antagonism,
A Basic Principle of
Drug-Induced Smooth Muscle
Relaxation

Although smooth and striated muscle exhibit large differences regarding ultrastructure, magnitude of contractile force, or rate of tension rise and decay, the fundamental processes of energy transformation in the contractile system (e.g., Ca-dependent splitting of ATP, sliding-filament displacement, generation of force by actin–myosin interactions) seemed to be quite similar (Rüegg, 1971). Nevertheless, it has turned out in more recent investigations that in smooth muscle this interaction deviates remarkably from the usual pattern found in skeletal and heart muscle since actin–myosin interaction in smooth muscle probably involves phosphorylation of certain of the protein chains of the myosin molecule. The enzyme that catalyzes this phosphorylation has been designated a myosin-light-chain kinase that requires Ca for activation. But Ca is only effective in the presence of "calmodulin," a newly discovered Ca-binding regulatory protein (see Cheung, 1980). It closely resembles troponin C, the well-known Ca-receptor protein of skeletal muscle (Table 2). Both calmodulin and troponin C have molecular weights of about 17,000 to 18,000 and represent the Ca-sensitive components of the contractile systems in smooth and striated muscle (Dabrowska, Sherry, Aromatorio, and Hartshorne, 1978; Sherry, Gorecha, Aksoy, Dabrowska, and Hartshorne, 1978). According to this new concept, smooth muscle contraction is believed to occur if the myosin-light-chain kinase phosphorylates myosin in the presence of Ca. Conversely, when Ca is removed, the kinase is inactivated, and a second enzyme, a myosin-light-chain phosphatase, splits the phosphate groups off, thereby causing relaxation (for more details see Hartshorne 1980; Hartshorne and Gorecka, 1980; Stull and Sanford 1981).

Irrespective of several unsettled points of controversy (see Ebashi, 1980), there is no doubt that the trigger function of Ca ions in initiating contraction of smooth muscle corresponds in principle with that found in striated muscle. Consequently, also in smooth muscle cells, the contractile responses are always lost more or less rapidly in the absence of Ca whatever the special stimulus may be (see the pertinent review articles of Bozler, 1962; Bohr, 1964; Schatzmann, 1964; Somlyo and Somlyo, 1968, 1970; Rüegg, 1971; and Weiss, 1977). Therefore, it was not surprising that the specific Ca antagonists too proved to be able to produce a general inhibition of contractile smooth muscle activation that is basically similar to that resulting from extracellular Ca withdrawal. But again, as in cardiac muscle, the Ca antagonists do not interfere directly with actin-myosin interaction. Accordingly in our experiments, when shortening was caused by immediate administration of Ca and ATP to isolated contractile structures obtained by glycerol extraction or to skinned smooth muscles fibers without cell membranes, the Ca antagonists were totally unable to suppress tension development. In fact, the Ca antagonists only interrupt the supply of Ca to the contractile apparatus without blocking the Ca-dependent activation of the internal contractile machinery itself. Again, in smooth muscle as in heart muscle, the decisive action of Ca antagonists seems to consist of a displacement of Ca ions from specific Ca-binding sites at the cell membrane and the transmembrane Ca carrier systems. This basic action manifests itself in two particular ways, namely:

1. As *inhibition of the electrogenic transmembrane Ca influx,* thereby impeding automatic Ca-mediated impulse generation as well as Ca-mediated spike discharge upon stimulation.
2. As *interference with Ca-dependent excitation–contraction coupling,* thereby interrupting the linkage between membrane excitation (local depolarization, conducted impulses) and the mechanical responses.

Interestingly enough, the effects 1 and 2 do not develop strictly in parallel, so they can be studied separately in certain types of smooth muscle and with special experimental arrangements. On the contrary, the Ca antagonists do not seriously impair the "membrane-stabilizing" function of Ca ions, which consists of maintaining a high level of membrane potential when the smooth muscle cells are at rest. Or in other words, *the Ca antagonists only counteract the inward movements of Ca ions connected with activity but spare the "static" functions of Ca in quiescent fibers.*

6.1. FUNDAMENTAL ACTIONS OF CALCIUM ANTAGONISTS ON VISCERAL SMOOTH MUSCLE

6.1.1. Inhibition by Calcium Antagonists of Electrogenic Calcium Influx

Spontaneous or evoked action potentials occur in a wide variety of smooth muscle cells. For instance, as established by the pioneering work of Bozler and of Bülbring, spike discharge represents the dominant form of bioelectric activity in visceral smooth muscle. Observations were made with microelectrodes on the taenia coli of guinea pigs (Bülbring, 1955, 1957, 1962; Bülbring, Burnstock, and Holman, 1958; Bülbring and Kuriyama, 1963) and on cat small intestine (see Prosser, 1962). Further confirmatory results were obtained on tbe longitudinal and circular muscle of guinea pig duodenum, jejunum, ileum, caecum, and rectum (Kuriyama, Osa, and Toida, 1967a). The occurrence and electrogenesis of action potentials in ureteric smooth muscle was first investigated with extracellular electrodes by Bozler (1942) and by Kobayashi (1965) and subsequently studied with intracellular techniques by Bennett and Burnstock (1966), and Kuriyama, Osa, and Toida (1967b). Natural spike activity is also present in the estrogen-dominated myometrium (Bozler, 1941; Marshall, 1962; Casteels and Kuriyama, 1965; Anderson, Ramon, and Snyder 1971), in the guinea pig vas deferens (Hashimoto, Holman, and Tille, 1966), in gastric smooth muscle, and in the wall of portal veins (for further references see Table 14). Tracheal and arterial smooth muscle preparations, on the other hand, are electrically silent, as usual, but even here action potentials could be evoked by various stimuli after pretreatment with tetraethylammonium (Kroeger and Stephens, 1975; Casteels and Droogmans, 1976; Kitamura, Kuriyama, and Suzuki, 1976).

In the course of these extensive studies, it soon became evident that the bioelectric behavior of the spontaneously discharging smooth muscle fibers closely resembles that of cardiac pacemaker cells. The following observations reflect this conformity:

1. The resting potential of smooth muscle fibers, as that of cardiac nodal cells, is relatively small and mostly ranges between -50 and -60 mV.

2. In smooth muscle there is a typical occurrence of slow oscillatory prepotentials that trigger a spike discharge when their depolarizing amplitudes reach the firing level.

3. The maximum rate of rise of smooth muscle action potentials is always low. In guinea pig taenia coli dV/dt_{max} amounts to 7 to 8 V/sec (Bülbring and Kuriyama, 1963). This value corresponds to the upstroke velocity of AV-nodal action potentials (see Table 11).

4. As shown by Anderson, Ramon, and Snyder (1971) in voltage-clamp studies on uterine smooth muscle, spike activity requires the presence of extracellular Na and Ca. But as found by Bülbring and Kuriyama (1963), both the rate of rise and the amplitude of the spike of the taenia action potentials are a function of the external Ca (Ca_o) concentration, whereas changes in the Na_o concentration between 0 and 137 mM did not influence the height of overshoot.

5. One of the most characteristic properties of smooth muscle excitation is that the fast-Na-influx inhibitor tetrodotoxin (TTX), in analogy to its inefficacy on SA- or AV-nodal cells, has also no effect on spontaneous or evoked spike discharge. This is true of all types of smooth muscle studied so far: taenia coli (Nonomura, Hotta, and Ohashi, 1966; Bülbring and Tomita, 1967; Kuriyama, Osa, and Toida, 1967a), ureter (Washizu, 1966; Kuriyama, Osa, and Toida, 1967b), vas deferens (Bennett, 1967), uterus (Anderson, Ramon, and Snyder, 1971), and arterial smooth muscle (Keatinge, 1968a).

6.   To the contrary, Mn ions block smooth muscle excitation. This applies to taenia coli (Nonomura, Hotta, and Ohashi, 1966; Brading, Bülbring, and Tomita, 1969), ureter (Kuriyama, Osa, and Toida, 1967b), and myometrium (Anderson, Ramon, and Snyder, 1971). Other Ca-antagonistic cations such as Co^{2+} and La^{3+} acted similarly.

All these findings indicate that (1) visceral smooth muscle exhibits functional membrane peculiarities that are similar to those of the cardiac SA and AV-nodal cells (see Chapter 4, Figure 114), (2) the generation of smooth muscle spike potentials depends on the availability of Ca ions as electric-charge carriers, and (3) the smooth muscle cell membranes, in contrast with myocardial fibers, are not provided with a TTX-sensitive Na-carrier system.

Nevertheless, it remained for some time rather uncertain whether Ca-mediated action potentials really do represent the regular form of smooth muscle excitation under physiological conditions. Still in 1962 Bülbring stated that the ability to produce Ca-mediated action potentials might be a mechanism available for the smooth muscle of taenia coli when it is *deprived of Na*. She wrote: *"For the explanation of spike activity in normal solution, there is at present no need for abandoning the sodium-dependent mechanism."* However, during the following years, with a deeper analysis of the excitatory processes of smooth muscle, the new Ca concept steadily gained ground (see Bülbring and Kuriyama, 1963; Kobayashi, 1965; Bennett, 1967; Bülbring and Tomita, 1970). In this situation, definite proof came from the use of Ca antagonists. In fact, the observations made after addition of these drugs to Ringer or Tyrode solution with normal Na and Ca contents were more informative than most of the earlier experiments in which the external cation concentrations had been unphysiologically altered. For instance, Ca withdrawal unstabilizes and thereby depolarizes the visceral smooth muscle cell membranes in addition to affecting the Ca-dependent excitatory and contractile processes. The inhibitory effects of Ca antagonists, on the other hand, are clearly restricted to those smooth muscle functions that depend on the *transmembrane* Ca influx, that is, spike discharge and excitation–contraction coupling. Moreover, the organic Ca antagonists proved to represent the most powerful and specific inhibitors of these processes yet discovered, since they possess, in comparison with Mn salts for instance, an up to 10,000 times higher potency without causing tissue damage.

The long series of studies with organic Ca antagonists on smooth muscle was initiated in 1969, when we reported that verapamil, D 600, and prenylamine, previously identified by us as specific inhibitors of excitation–contraction coupling of mammalian myocardium, are also capable of blocking excitability and contractility of the rat uterus by virtue of the same Ca-antagonistic action (Fleckenstein and Grün, 1969; Grün, Fleckenstein, and Tritthart, 1969). The electrogenesis of spontaneous uterine spike potentials was even more sensitive to the Ca-antagonistic drugs than excitation–contraction coupling (Grün, Byon, Tritthart, and Fleckenstein, 1970; Tritthart, Grün, Byon, and Fleckenstein, 1970; Grün, Fleckenstein, and Byon, 1971a; Fleckenstein, Grün, Tritthart, and Byon (1971). Thus, in a Tyrode solution containing 1 mM Ca, automaticity was totally abolished with 0.1 mg D

600/1 ($\approx 2 \times 10^{-7}M$), whereas in the same experiments, the suppression of excitation–contraction coupling always required a nearly 10-fold dose. Apart from D 600, the 1,4-dihydropyridine derivatives such as nifedipine and niludipine exerted the strongest depression of uterine automaticity (Grün and Fleckenstein, 1972; Fleckenstein, Fleckenstein-Grün, Byon, Haastert, and Späh, 1979). Reduction of the extracellular Ca concentration to less than 1 mM always potentiated the Ca-antagonistic drug actions, whereas in the presence of the Ca antagonists, automaticity fully recovered from standstill when the Ca content was elevated from 1 to 3 or 5 mM. Our findings were soon confirmed and extended by Golenhofen and Lammel (1972) in a careful study on guinea pig smooth muscle preparations. These researchers established that verapamil, in analogy with the effect of Ca-deprivation, also suppresses spike discharge in taenia coli, portal vein, ureter and stomach (antrum). Another brilliant study, by Riemer, Dörfler, Mayer, and Ulbrecht, (1974), concentrated upon the guinea pig taenia coli. They also found that verapamil primarily affects the Ca-dependent mechanisms that underlie the formation of spontaneous or evoked spike potentials. Thus the slow pacemaker potentials preceding automatic spike discharges, as well as the rates of rise and the amplitudes of the spikes themselves, were strongly inhibited (see Figure 137). The reduction in contractile force resulted primarily from the decreased number and height of spike potentials, but an impairment of excitation–contraction coupling was also discernible. Dose–response curves obtained at different Ca concentrations revealed a competitive type of antagonism between Ca and verapamil. One molecule of verapamil was able to counteract about 8000 Ca ions in this study. The effective concentration of verapamil that blocked spontaneous spike discharge of the guinea pig taenia coli was in the range of 10^{-6} M, compared with 10^{-3} M MnCl$_2$ (Brading, Bülbring, and Tomita, 1969).

The outstanding potency of the Ca antagonists verapamil, D 600, and nifedipine has been further documented by a multitude of investigations on visceral smooth muscle in which these drugs were used to suppress *evoked* bioelectric activity. This applies, for instance, to spike discharge elicited by electric and mechanical stimuli (quick stretch) or by depolarization with high K$_o$ concentrations. Moreover, the Ca antagonists abolished spike discharge brought about by application of pharmacological agents such as oxytocin and prostaglandin F$_{2\alpha}$ on the uterus, acetylcholine and prostaglandin E$_2$ on the taenia coli, or noradrenaline on the portal vein. Action potentials of tetraethylammonium-pretreated tracheal or arterial smooth muscle cells were also extinguished by Ca antagonists in the usual concentration range between 10^{-7} and 10^{-5} M. More details are available in Table 14. Needless to say, the Ca antagonists always suppressed both the bursts of action potentials and the resulting phasic (tetanic) contractions simultaneously, often before excitation–contraction coupling itself had been directly impaired. However, apart from producing spike potentials, an electrogenic influx of Ca may also lead to slow depolarization waves or protracted depolarization. This slow type of Ca-dependent excitation is accompanied by sustained shortening. The Ca antagonists are also highly effective against such sustained contractions (contractures) partially because of interference with Ca-dependent depolarization and partially because of a blockade of excita-

TABLE 14. Blockade by Ca Antagonists of the Generation of Ca^{++}-Carried Spike Potentials and of the Resulting Phasic Contractions in Smooth Muscle of Different Origin

Type of Smooth Muscle	Ca Antagonist Used	Registration Technique	Effects of Ca Antagonists	Authors
Virginal Myometrium (rat)	Verapamil (2 to 5 × 10^{-6} M) D 600 (10^{-7} M) Prenylamine (5 × 10^{-6} M) Nifedipine (10^{-7} M)	Sucrose-gap method	Spike potentials elicited by high K_o or oxytocin are extinguished	Tritthart, Grün, Byon, and Fleckenstein (1970) Fleckenstein, Grün, Tritthart and Byon (1971) Grün and Fleckenstein (1972)
Myometrium (guinea pig)	D 600 (10^{-6} to 10^{-5} M)	Intracellular recordings	Spike potentials elicited by oxytocin are extinguished	Golenhofen and Neuser (1974) see Golenhofen (1976)
Myometrium (pregnant rat)	D 600 (10^{-7} to 10^{-5} M) Experiments on ^{45}Ca influx with 5 × 10^{-5} M	Intracellular recordings Measurements of Ca influx and efflux with ^{45}Ca	Spike potentials during spontaneous activity and upon electric or chemical stimulation (with $PGF_{2\alpha}$) are abolished Blockade of ^{45}Ca influx	Reiner and Marshall (1975, 1976) Kroeger, Marshall and Bianchi (1975)

Tissue	Drug (concentration)	Method	Effect	Reference
Taenia coli (guinea pig)	Verapamil (10^{-6} to 10^{-5} M)	Intracellular recordings	Upstroke velocity, height, and frequency of spontaneous and K-induced spike potentials are depressed	Golenhofen and Lammel (1972) Riemer, Dörfler, Mayer, and Ulbrecht (1974) den Hertog and van den Akker (1979)
Taenia coli (guinea pig)	D 600 Blockade with 1.2×10^{-6} M	Sucrose-gap method Flux measurements with ^{45}Ca	Depolarization and spike activity elicited by PGE$_2$ are suppressed, together with tension development	
Taenia coli (human)	Verapamil	Intracellular recordings	Spontaneous and acetylcholine-induced spike activity is abolished; TTX is inefficient	Kirk and Duthie (1977)
Gastric antrum and *Ureter* (guinea pig)	Verapamil (10^{-6} to 10^{-5} M)	Intracellular recordings	Preferential suppression of spike activity	Golenhofen and Lammel (1972)
Canine trachea and *rabbit ear artery*	D 600 Trachea: (10^{-5} M) Ear artery: (5×10^{-7} M)	Intracellular recordings	Tetraethylammonium-induced generation of spike potentials is abolished	Stephens, Kroeger, and Kromer (1975) Kroeger and Stephens (1975) Casteels and Droogmans (1976)
Portal vein (guinea pig, rat)	Verapamil (10^{-6} to 10^{-5} M) D 600 (10^{-6} M) Nifedipine (more than 10^{-7} M)	Extracellular and intracellular recordings	Spike potentials elicited by noradrenaline are abolished	Golenhofen (1976) Jetley and Weston (1980)

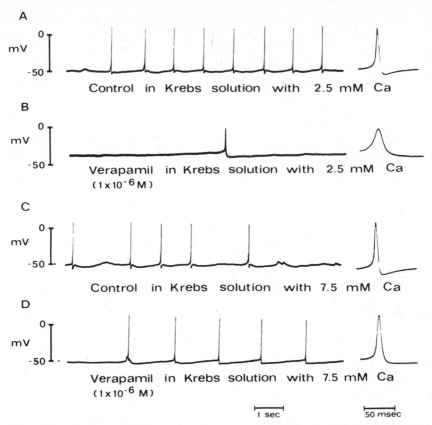

FIGURE 137. Inhibitory influence of verapamil on spontaneous electric activity of the guinea pig taenia coli in Krebs solution with different Ca contents. (*A*), (*B*) At a Ca concentration of 2.5 m*M*, verapamil (1 × 10⁻⁶ *M*) strongly reduces the rate of automatic impulse discharge as well as upstroke velocity and height of overshoot of the individual action potentials. (*C*), (*D*) At an elevated Ca content of 7.5 m*M*, the same concentration of verapamil is nearly ineffective. The tracings were recorded from different cells of the same strip, after 35 and 45 min equilibration with the 2.5- and 7.5-m*M* Ca solution, respectively. The action potentials on the right are shown at an enlarged time scale to illustrate the change in their shape. From Riemer, Dörfler, Mayer and Ulbrecht (1974).

tion–contraction coupling. A clear differentiation between these two possibilities would, however, require an electrophysiological analysis in each particular case.

6.1.2.   Blockade by Calcium Antagonists of Excitation–Contraction Coupling of Visceral Smooth Muscle

Inhibition of excitation–contraction coupling means that the Ca antagonists are also capable of blocking the messenger function of Ca ions between the excited (depolarized) smooth muscle cell membrane and the contractile system. In visceral smooth muscle, the cessation of spike discharge is usually the first response to the administration of Ca antagonists, whereas excitation–contraction uncoupling develops more slowly or requires a somewhat higher concentration of the Ca-antagonistic inhibitors. Excitation-contraction uncoupling by verapamil, D 600, and prenylamine was first demonstrated by us in uterine smooth muscle (Fleckenstein and Grün, 1969; Tritthart, Grün, Byon, and Fleckenstein, 1970). In these studies isolated segments of virginal rat uteri were immersed into an isotonic Tyrode solution with 136.9 mM K, substituted for Na, and the changes in membrane potential and isometric tension continuously recorded. As shown in Figure 138A, the normal

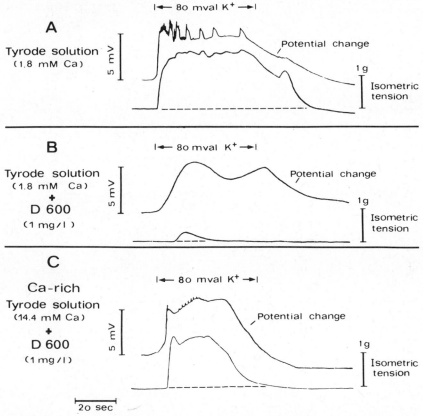

FIGURE 138. Reversible suppression of spike discharge and blockade of excitation–contraction coupling by D 600 in a K-depolarized segment of a rat uterus. The control experiment (A) demonstrates the parallel changes in membrane potential and mechanogram upon depolarization in a K-rich (80 mval) Tyrode solution with normal Ca content. Subsequently (B), under the influence of D 600, the onset of K-induced depolarization was slowed, superimposed spike discharge abolished, and the mechanogram reduced to 5% of normal according to a planimetric evaluation. Finally (C), the inhibitory effects of D 600 on the K-depolarized uterus were almost nullified after the Ca content of the D 600–containing solution had been increased by 8 times up to 14.4 mM. The exposure to the D 600–containing media always took 20 minutes, previous to administration of the solutions with 80 mval K. The potential changes were continuously recorded using the sucrose-gap technique. From Fleckenstein, Grün, Tritthart, and Byon (1971).

reaction of a control preparation to the application of the high-K-concentration solution consists of (1) a rapid onset of depolarization with additive spike discharges, and (2) a large, but uneven, contracture that reflects the irregular bursts of the superimposed action potentials. The characteristic action of D 600, on the other hand, consists of (1) abolishing these superimposed spike potentials so that the K-induced depolarization curve becomes perfectly smooth without, however, being decreased, and (2) simultaneously blocking the mechanical response to the depolarization (see Figure 138*B*). The restorative potency of additional Ca is demonstrated in Figure 138*C*. Here both rapid spike discharge and excitation–contraction coupling recovered to a considerable extent after the external Ca concentration had been raised from 1.8 to 14.4 m*M* in the presence of D 600. Figure 139 represents

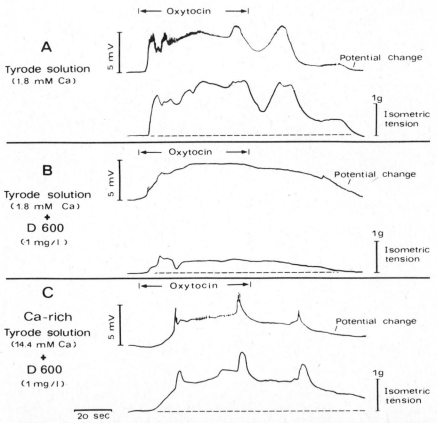

FIGURE 139. Reversible suppression of spike discharge and partial blockade of excitation–contraction coupling by D 600 in an oxytocin-activated rat uterine smooth muscle segment. The degree of inhibition by which D 600 reduced the oxytocin effects at a normal extracellular Ca concentration can be judged from the records in (*B*) compared with those in (*A*). As shown in (*C*), the influence of D 600 could again be overcome by elevation of Ca$_o$ concentration up to 14.4 m*M*. The dose of oxytocin was 3 IU per 100 ml. The experimental arrangements were analogous to those in Figure 138, particularly with respect to the use of the sucrose-gap technique for a continuous registration of the potential changes. From Fleckenstein, Grün, Tritthart, and Byon (1971).

an analogous experiment in which the uterine segment was depolarized with oxytocin. Again D 600 strongly depressed superimposed oxytocin-induced spike activity as well as the mechanical reactions, and once more there was a rapid return nearly to normal upon addition of extra Ca to the D 600-containing Tyrode solution. Lastly, we depolarized isolated rat uterine segments directly with cathodic DC currents to elicit a contractile response. Even under these conditions, D 600 rendered the membrane depolarization mechanically ineffective (see Figure 140). However, there was again *no* blockade of excitation–contraction coupling by D 600 when the drug had been applied in a Ca-rich Tyrode solution.

Abolition of spike discharge and interruption of excitation–contraction coupling by Ca antagonists naturally produce an *additive* decrement of the visceral smooth muscle mechanogram. However, these two factors contribute quite differently to the inhibition of contractile performance depending on the experimental conditions (dose of Ca antagonists, time of exposure, special drugs used for smooth muscle excitation, etc.). As an example, Figure 141 represents three experiments in which suitable doses of verapamil, prenylamine, and D 600 were applied in order to minimize the contractile responses of rat uterine smooth muscle segments to a high K_o concentration, oxytocin, and $BaCl_2$. In the first case, when shortening was induced with a high K concentration, the suppression of the mechanical reactions by verapamil proved to be due primarily to excitation–contraction uncoupling. However, in the second case, when oxytocin was used for stimulation, the inhibitory action of prenylamine was based to a comparably greater extent on the restriction of Ca-dependent electric membrane activity. This applies even more to the third experiment with $BaCl_2$. In this case, enormous bursts of Ca-dependent spike potentials were elicited by $BaCl_2$, so the resulting contraction adopted a predominantly tetanic character. Under these conditions, D 600 operated primarily by decreasing exaggerated spike discharge. Further "agonists" that can also evoke Ca-dependent, TTX-insensitive contractions of visceral smooth muscle and consequently lose their

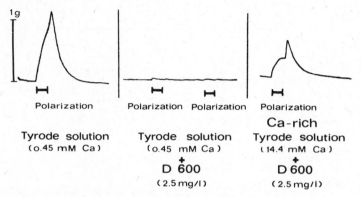

FIGURE 140. Total suppression by D 600 of the contractile responses of an isolated rat uterine segment to direct depolarization with a cathodic DC current in Tyrode solution with 0.45 mM Ca. Partial neutralization of the effect of D 600 by increasing the external Ca concentration up to 14.4 mM. From Fleckenstein, Grün, Tritthart, and Byon (1971).

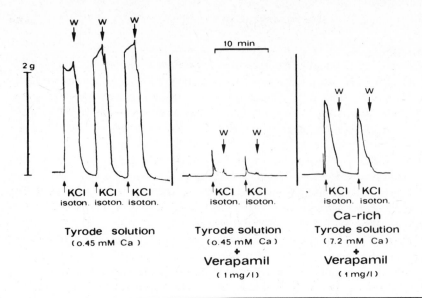

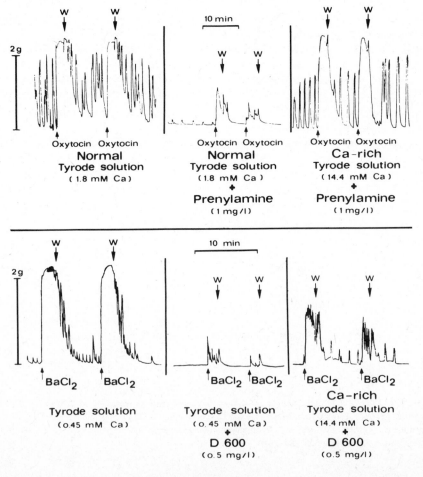

power under the influence of Ca antagonists are listed in Table 15. According to our observations, Ca antagonists also depress those Ca-dependent contractile responses that are additionally producible in completely K-depolarized visceral smooth muscle preparations by administration of acetylcholine, carbachol, serotonin, and so forth (see Evans, Schild, and Thesleff, 1958; Durbin and Jenkinson, 1961; Edman and Schild, 1962, 1963). In this situation supplementary tension is developed without a further fall in membrane potential, thus reflecting a purely receptor-mediated increase in Ca conductance or Ca release. Hence the Ca antagonists seem to interfere also with potential-independent Ca movements.

It is generally accepted that the activation of the contractile machinery by all these various agonists is brought about by voltage- or receptor-dependent facilitation of transmembrane influx of extracellular Ca and/or by liberation of sequestered Ca from certain cellular stores. Although there is still a great deal of speculation about the special location of such mobilizable Ca deposits in the SR or other structures, the plasma membrane of visceral smooth muscle cells with its invaginations and associated vesicles is probably one of the most important storage sites from which activator Ca can be released. Thus in all probability, the plasma membrane not only provides the gates for electrogenic Ca influx but also serves, like the myocardial sarcolemma membrane, as a Ca-accumulating system. Observations on various kinds of visceral smooth muscle indicate that the activation of the contractile machinery by agonists is mostly inhomogenous because there is an obvious overlap of phasic and tonic contractile components that probably reflect different ways or different sources of Ca supply. For instance, in visceral smooth muscle, the phasic contractions are mostly the consequence of an electrogenic influx of Ca associated with spike discharge or rapid depolarization. Such forms of contractile activation that are directly connected with transmembrane inward Ca movement are preferably blocked by Ca antagonists. However, as a rule the Ca antagonists, at least after prolonged incubation, also affect the tonic components of contraction that in visceral smooth muscle are more likely produced by the release of sequestered Ca. This effect can be explained by the assumption that there is no sufficient replenishment of the Ca stores in or underneath the plasma membrane if the Ca conductivity of these structures has been impaired.

The Ca shifts connected with reversible activation and inactivation of the contractile machinery do not manifest themselves by appreciable changes in the total Ca content of visceral smooth muscle. This is also true of the effect of Ca antagonists. Nevertheless, it could be realized with the more sensitive lanthanum method that there is, in fact, a demonstrable gain in labeled intracellular ^{45}Ca when the

---

FIGURE 141.   Three analogous experiments on isolated rat uterine segments in which the contractile responses to (1) K-induced depolarization (Tyrode solution with isotonic KCl substituted for NaCl), (2) oxytocin, and (3) $BaCl_2$ were minimized by addition of suitable amounts of verapamil, prenylamine, or D 600. In all these cases, the Ca antagonists lost most of their power upon elevation of Ca_o concentration to 14.4 mM. The W marks washings of the uterine segments with the different experimental solutions in the absence of the respective stimulatory agents, i.e., isotonic KCl, oxytocin, $BaCl_2$. From Fleckenstein, Grün, Tritthart, and Byon (1971).

TABLE 15. Inhibition of Ca-Dependent, TTX-Insensitive Visceral Smooth Muscle Contractions by Ca Antagonists

Type of Smooth Muscle	Contractile Activation (Agents Used)	Ca Antagonists Used	Effects of Ca Antagonists	Authors
Virginal uterus (rat)	Acetylcholine Carbaminoylcholine	Verapamil (2 to 5 × 10^{-6} M) D 600 (10^{-7} M) Prenylamine (5 × 10^{-6} M) Nifedipine (10^{-7} M)	Complete suppression of contractile responses	Fleckenstein and Grün (1969) Fleckenstein, Grün, Tritthart, and Byon (1971)
Stomach (guinea pig)	Acetylcholine	Verapamil (5 × 10^{-6} to 10^{-5} M)	Phasic contraction more readily suppressed than tonic responses	Golenhofen and Wegner (1975)
	Acetylcholine Prostaglandin E_1	Verapamil (10^{-5} M)	PGE_1-induced contractions are relatively resistant to verapamil	Ishizawa and Miyazaki (1977)
Forestomach (sheep)	Acetylcholine	D 600 (10^{-6} to 10^{-5} M)	Complete suppression of phasic contractility in all parts of forestomach	Vassilev, Stoyanov, Lukanov, and Vassileva (1975)
Ileal longitudinal muscle (guinea pig)	Muscarinic stimulation with cis-2-methyl-4-dimethylaminomethyl-1,3-dioxolone methiodide (CD)	D 600 (10^{-8} to 10^{-7} M) Nifedipine (2 × 10^{-8} to 5 × 10^{-9} M)	Tonic component more effectively inhibited than phasic component of mechanical response	Rosenberger, Ticku, and Trigle (1979)

Tissue	Substance	Drug	Effect	Reference
Taenia coli (guinea pig)	Substance P	Verapamil (4.4×10^{-6} M)	Complete suppression of contractile responses	Szeli, Molina, Zappia, and Bertaccini (1977)
	Acetylcholine and calcium-ionophore A 23187	D 600 (3×10^{-6} M) D 600 (2×10^{-5} M)	Complete suppression of contractile responses	Mandrek and Golenhofen (1977)
Descending colon (rat)	Prostaglandin E$_1$	Verapamil (3.5×10^{-6} M)	Partial inhibition of contractile responses	Torok, Vizi, and Knoll (1974)
	Angiotensin II	SKF 525 A (2.6×10^{-5} M)		Crocker, Mayeka, and Wilson (1979)
	Prostaglandin E$_2$			
Circular duodenal muscle (rabbit)	Acetylcholine	Verapamil (2×10^{-6} M according to personal communication)	Suppression of spike activity and contractile responses	Mayer, Ruppin, Riemer, Kölling, Domschke, Wünsch, and Demling (1977)
	13-Norleucine motilin			
Stomach (antral circular muscle), duodenum, jejunum (rabbit)	13-Norleucine motilin	Verapamil (4.4×10^{-6} M)	Total suppression of contractile responses	Strunz, Domschke, Mitznegg, Domschke, Schubert, Wünsch, Jaeger, and Demling (1975)
Antral part of human stomach	13-Norleucine motilin			
Ureter (pig)	Adrenaline	Nifedipine (3×10^{-7} M)	Complete suppression of phasic contractions and subtotal inhibition of tonic component	Golenhofen and Hannappel (1978)

smooth musculature contracts, and conversely, that the cellular ^{45}Ca uptake is blocked by practically the same concentrations of verapamil, D 600, and nifedipine that abolish these contractile responses (see Mayer, van Breemen, and Casteels, 1972; Kroeger, Marshall, and Bianchi, 1975; Rosenberger, Ticku, and Triggle, 1979). Lanthanum cations displace superficial Ca from the outer layers of the plasma membranes, but sequester the true cellular Ca that has been taken up during activity. This allows a determination of the particularly important intracellular Ca fraction in the La-treated smooth muscle strips. The findings with ^{45}Ca are again fully consistent with the general concept of the mechanism of action of Ca antagonists, that is, competitive displacement of Ca from its transmembrane carrier system. On the other hand, all attempts to correlate the relaxing potency of Ca antagonists to other than ionic effects have failed. This applies first of all to certain biochemical reactions such as papaverinelike inhibition of phosphodiesterase, or interaction with cyclicAMP or cyclicGMP metabolism, since the Ca antagonists proved to be virtually inert in this respect.

In summary of the host of observations on visceral smooth muscle, the Ca antagonists interfere with the Ca-dependent excitatory and contractile processes beyond the receptor level. This means that the Ca antagonists restrict the delivery of Ca ions to the cellular reaction sites in a rather direct way, that is to say, without regard to the multitude of different agonists used as smooth muscle stimulants and irrespective of the variety of receptors at which these stimulants may act. There is in fact no other experimental possibility of inhibiting the reactivity of isolated visceral smooth muscle in a more effective manner. Clinical studies on this matter are hitherto scarce. However, recent reports indicate that nifedipine, for instance, is highly effective in suppressing myometrial hypercontractility in cases of premature labor or dysmenorrhea (Ulmsten, Andersson, and Forman, 1978; Andersson and Ulmsten, 1978; Sandahl, Ulmsten, and Andersson, 1979; Ulmsten, Andersson, and Wingerup, 1980).

6.2. CALCIUM ANTAGONISTS AND VASCULAR SMOOTH MUSCLE

The most sensitive reponses to Ca antagonists are those of the vascular system. Surprisingly, vascular smooth muscle relaxation may still be discernbile under the influence of the Ca antagonists nifedipine, niludipine, nimodipine, or D 600 in a concentration range of 10^{-9} to 10^{-10} M. Hence small doses of Ca antagonists are able to diminish Ca-dependent smooth muscle tone and contractility of the coronary, cerebral, intestinal, or renal arteries, as well as of the peripheral resistance vessels, without causing a concomitant cardiodepression or a parallel inhibition of the visceral smooth muscle functions. It is, however, not only with respect to this outstanding susceptibility to Ca antagonists but also to a number of other peculiarities that the involvement of Ca in contractile activation of vascular smooth muscle deserves special consideration.

6.2.1. Particular Pathways of Calcium Supply in Contractile Activation of Vascular Smooth Muscle

Because of methodological difficulties, bioelectric data on the vascular smooth muscle function are still relatively rare. Nevertheless, there is general agreement about the following points:

1. In contrast with visceral smooth muscle, spike discharge does not occur, or occurs only exceptionally, in the arterial vasculature. Therefore it does not play any role in the regulation of basal arterial tone.

2. Transmembrane Ca uptake, like Ca uptake in visceral smooth muscle, can be regulated by changes in membrane potential ("potential-dependent Ca influx") in that depolarization is again a determinant factor for the initiation of Ca influx and tension rise. The mechanical response to a depolarizing high-K_0 concentration is exemplary of this type of contractile activation. Extracellular Ca withdrawal and particularly chelation of loosely bound membrane Ca with EDTA block this "potential-dependent" pathway of transmembrane Ca supply almost instantaneously.

3. However, there is still an alternative "receptor-dependent" mechanism, stimulated by certain vasoconstrictor agents, which also provides activator Ca to the contractile system but bypasses the "potential-dependent" pathway in that it operates unrelated to bioelectric membrane excitation. Vasoconstrictor agonists such as adrenaline, noradrenaline, histamine, serotonin, or pitressin may enhance Ca entry in this manner, or may even liberate sequestered Ca from a pool within the cell membrane. In this latter case, the inhibitory influence of extracellular Ca withdrawal on contractile activation by such vasoconstrictor agents often manifests itself with a considerable delay.

Most observations indicating the existence of different sources of activator Ca in vascular smooth muscle were made on isolated strips or segments from intestinal canine arteries, rat tail arteries, rabbit or rat aortas, sheep carotid arteries, and on the vascular system of isolated rabbit ears (see Waugh, 1962; Hinke, Wilson, and Burnham, 1964; Shibata and Briggs, 1966; Hudgins and Weiss, 1968; Hiraoka, Yamagishi, and Sano, 1968; Wende and Peiper, 1970). The conclusion that adrenaline, noradrenaline, and histamine preferentially open an alternative pathway for Ca that is not necessarily connected with membrane depolarization relies on particularly solid experimental grounds. For instance, as Waugh pointed out in 1962, vasoconstriction by adrenaline can still be elicited in arterial smooth muscle that has been completely predepolarized by external application of K_2SO_4. Therefore, he concluded that the primary essential process in vasoconstriction by adrenergic neurohormones is a mechanism that stimulates the translocation of Ca *nonelectrically*. This effect was attributed to a release of Ca ions from certain membrane stores (Hinke, Wilson, and Burnham, 1964, Hiraoka, Yamagishi, and Sano, 1968; Hudgins and Weiss, 1969). As reported by Shibata and Briggs (1966) and by Keatinge (1968b), the contractile responses to adrenaline or noradrenaline may even be accompanied by an increase in membrane potential. However, according to observations of Casteels and Droogmans (1976) on rabbit ear arteries, noradrenaline (10^{-9} to $10^{-6}M$) and histamine (10^{-8} to $10^{-7}M$) usually cause a dose-dependent contraction that develops *without* a concomitant change in cellular membrane potential. In the noradrenaline-stimulated (10^{-8} to $10^{-7}M$) vasculature of the rabbit main pulmonary artery, there was also no discernible decrease in membrane potential (Kitamura, Kuriyama, and Suzuki, 1976). But depolarization occurred at concentrations of noradrenaline or histamine higher than 1 to $2 \times 10^{-7}M$. This means that such agonists can also produce mixed effects in that they cause an additional "potential-dependent" Ca-influx by depolarization apart from enhancing Ca supply by stimulating the electroneutral mechanism of "receptor-dependent" Ca supply. For instance, adrenaline or noradrenaline in the high concentration of around $1 \times 10^{-5}M$ usually produce a biphasic contractile response of arterial smooth muscle consisting of a rapid phasic and a slow tonic component. The initial phasic component is considered to reflect a fast receptor-mediated release of activator Ca from cellular storage sites, whereas the subsequent tonic component seems to depend directly on transmembrane Ca influx connected with depolarization. Accordingly, at a low Ca_0 concentration, the tonic responses to adrenaline or noradrenaline more readily disappear than the phasic contractions do (see Bohr, 1963, 1964; Godfraind and Kaba, 1969a, b; Peiper, Griebel, and Wende, 1971; Sitrin and Bohr, 1971; Godfraind, 1976). Thus the biphasic activation of vascular smooth muscle by α-adrenergic stimulants utilizes Ca that originates from at least two sources: Ca entering the cell from outside, and Ca supposed to be delivered from cellular depots.

The most precise characterization of the different sources of Ca utilized for agonist-induced activation of vascular smooth muscle relies on data obtained from Ca-washout experiments. A first differentiation was made in the late 1960s between a depletion-resistant and a readily removable Ca fraction (Hinke, Wilson, and Burnham, 1964; Hinke, 1965; Hudgins and Weiss, 1968, 1969; Hiraoka, Yamagishi, and Sano, 1968). More recently, this research work has been considerably advanced by van Breemen and his group and by Weiss and his associates. They analyzed the ^{45}Ca binding and washout kinetics with rather refined techniques on rabbit aortic smooth muscle (van Breemen and Lesser, 1971; van Breemen, Farinas, Gerba, and McNaughton, 1972; Deth and van Breemen, 1974; Karaki and Weiss, 1979, 1980; Wheeler and Weiss, 1979) and on canine renal arteries (Hester, Weiss, and Fry, 1979). All these studies have definitely established that, at least in these types of vascular smooth muscle, contractile activation by a depolarizing high K_0 concentration or alternatively by vasoconstrictor agonists such as norepinephrine, histamine, or angiotensin takes place through different Ca-operated pathways. Depolarization by a high K_0 concentration initiates an influx of Ca from superficial "low-affinity" binding sites into the La-resistent compartments of the cell. This superficial low-affinity Ca readily equilibrates with the extracellular Ca. Transmembrane entry of low-affinity Ca is strongly blocked by D 600 (Hester, Weiss, and Fry, 1979; Karaki and Weiss, 1980), as it is by extracellular Ca withdrawal. Noradrenaline, histamine or angiotensin, on the other hand, appear to mobilize Ca from more remote "high-affinity" binding sites that can also rapidly provide activator

Ca, although the uptake of labeled extracellar Ca into this fraction is slow. The release of high-affinity Ca, which underlies the phasic component of the noradrenaline response, seems to be rather resistant to D 600. The same is true of resting Ca exchange and Ca efflux into a low-Ca-plus-EDTA solution. The situation may be even more complex, since it has been suggested, considering some ultrastructural findings, that the principal sources of activator Ca might consist of the following:

1. Superficial, loosely membrane bound Ca.
2. Tightly membrane bound Ca,
3. Ca located at the internal surface of the membrane.
4. Ca stored in the SR (see Yamashita, Takagi, and Hotta 1977).

Clearly, definite information about the anatomic location and the particular contribution of these pools to the critical increase in cytoplasmic activator Ca is still lacking. Moreover, any attempt to generalize such findings, obtained on a special type of vascular smooth muscle (mostly rabbit aorta), would be premature with respect to the many individualities that the vasculature of different origin exhibits. Thus the following sections deal with the effects of Ca antagonists on a deliberately broad variety of vessels. Nevertheless, in our report preference will be given to the vasculature of the coronary bed because of its outstanding physiological and pathophysiological importance.

6.2.2. Coronary Smooth Muscle Relaxation by Calcium Antagonists, Particular Significance of the Extramural Coronary Stem Arteries

The ability of Ca antagonists to increase coronary blood flow is one of their most obvious circulatory effects. Thus the coronary vasodilation following administration of *prenylamine* (see Lindner 1960; Böhm, Schlepper, and Witzleb, 1960; Kochsiek, Bretschneider, and Scheler, 1960; Braasch and Fleck, 1961), *verapamil* (Haas and Härtfelder, 1962; Schlepper and Witzleb, 1962; Melville, Shister, and Huq, 1964; Luebs, Cohen, Zaleski, and Bing, 1966), or *D 600* (Haas and Busch, 1967) had already been noticed before the primordial Ca-antagonistic action of these drugs was clarified in our laboratory. Similarly, coronary vasodilation by *perhexiline* (Hudak, Lewis, and Kuhn, 1970) and by *nifedipine* (Bossert and Vater, 1971; Vater, Kroneberg, Hoffmeister, Kaller, Meng, Oberdorf, Puls, Schlossmann, and Stoepel, 1972) was observed in pharmacological screening tests without prior knowledge of the basic mode of action, and even in the case of *diltiazem*, the identification as a specific Ca antagonist by Nakajima, Hoshiyama, Yamashita, and Kiyomoto (1975) lagged 4 years behind the first report on its coronary vasodilator effects (see Sato, Nagao, Yamaguchi, Nakajima, and Kiyomoto, 1971).

However, all these measurements were carried out on hearts *in situ* or on perfused preparations using Langendorff's technique. Needless to say, with these rather indistinctive methods, no differentiation could be made between the older generation of coronary vasodilators such as adenosine, dipyridamole, theophylline, chromonar, and so forth, and the new Ca-antagonistic agents. Moreover, the results obtained by measuring global flow primarily reflected the reactions of the small intramural resistance vessels, particularly arterioles, which quantitatively control coronary perfusion. But these crude techniques could certainly not provide sufficient information about the physiological contractile behavior and the drug susceptibilities of the *great extramural coronary stem arteries,* which are clinically of much greater importance. The reasons are as follows:

1. In patients with occlusive coronary disease, more than 95% of the stenosing processes are located in these big extramural vessels.
2. If the atherosclerotic intima processes develop eccentrically, even in diseased coronary trunk arteries parts of the vascular wall will remain, at least for a while, functionally intact.
3. This residual contractility often manifests itself in the form of spasms, so blood flow in the narrowed extramural arteries dramatically deteriorates (see Section 7.3).
4. Accordingly, only those drugs are satisfactory in coronary therapy that are capable of exerting pronounced vasodilator or spasmolytic effects in this extramural part of the coronary bed (stem arteries, collaterals, anastomoses). As will be shown in the subsequent Sections, the Ca antagonists are particularly suitable for this purpose.

Thus our interst specifically concentrated on the basic physiology and pharmacology of the extramural coronary smooth musculature that had been rather neglected for a considerable time in experimental research. Our approach was direct in that we primarily used isolated coronary smooth muscle strips that mostly originated from the wall of the descending branch of the left coronary artery of pigs and rabbits. The total number of pigs whose freshly dissected coronaries have been studied in this investigation since 1968 is about 2500.

6.2.3. Calcium Dependency of Coronary Vascular Tone and Contractility; Natural Interactions of Calcium with Calcium-Antagonistic Magnesium and Hydrogen Ions

Calcium Requirements.   To illustrate the crucial role of Ca, Figure 142 represents an exemplary experiment in which a pig coronary strip was depolarized by increasing the extracellular K concentration up to 43 mM. As discussed in Section 6.2.1, the K contracture produced by this procedure is mediated by an increased Ca influx through the K-depolarized smooth muscle cell membrane. Therefore, relaxation occurred when (middle part of Figure 142) the coronary strip was transferred into a Ca-free solution, in spite of the fact that the depolarizing K concentration of 43 mM remained unchanged. However, as shown on the right, contractile tone completely recovered after return into the Ca-containing medium. Chelation of Ca by EDTA produced the same type of reversible relaxation even more rapidly.

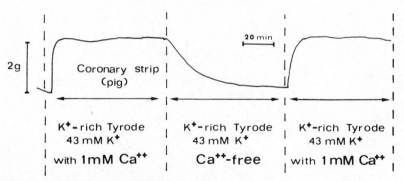

FIGURE 142. Reversible relaxation of a K-depolarized pig coronary strip by Ca withdrawal in a Ca-free Tyrode solution. From Grün and Fleckenstein (1972).

Mutual Antagonism Between Magnesium and Calcium Ions. Interestingly enough, contractile tension development of the K-depolarized coronary preparations was also suppressed by administration of a high dose of $MgCl_2$, exceeding the Ca concentration by a factor of 10 to 20 (Grün and Fleckenstein, 1972). This relaxing effect of Mg is obviously due to competition with Ca. Accordingly, additional Ca restored the mechanical activity of the K-depolarized preparations in the presence of a high Mg concentration. Thus contractile tension development of coronary smooth muscle seems to be more determined by the Ca:Mg ratio than by the absolute Ca content of the medium. Further experiments by Nakayama, Fleckenstein, Byon, and Fleckenstein-Grün (1978) on electrically stimulated pig coronary strips led to identical results (see Figure 143). Here at a constant Ca concentration of 2 mM, contractile tension rose considerably when the Mg concentration was lowered to one half (0.53 mM) of normal (1.05 mM). On the other hand, a stepwise reduction of isometric tension took place when the Mg concentration was increased up to 2.1, 4.2, or 8.4 mM. With 16.8 mM Mg, contractility completely ceased. But the contractile responses were promptly restored by raising the extracellular Ca content up to 6 mM. Figure 144 represents an evaluation of six experiments in which the Mg effects on active tension development of electrically driven pig coronary strips were studied in the concentration range between 0.53 and 16.8 mM. The log dose–response curve obtained in this way clearly shows that regarding contractile force, any aberration from the normal extracellular (1.05 mM) Mg content bears considerable consequences.

Calcium-Antagonistic Influence of Extracellular Hydrogen Ions. As to the natural Ca-antagonistic action of H ions, it has since long been recognized that coronary smooth muscle tone is also highly sensitive to changes in pH (see Iwai, 1924; Anrep, 1926). For instance, in K-depolarized pig coronary strips, there is a gradual loss of contractile tension as the *extracellular* concentration of H ions increases. Accordingly, as shown in Figure 145, the K-depolarized preparations relaxed when the original pH of 7.4 was successively lowered to 7.0, 6.2, and finally to 6.0. At a pH of 6.0, contractile tone was completely abolished as in the

Pig Coronary Artery Strip

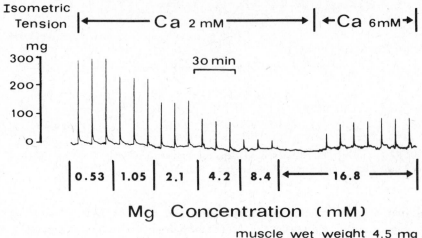

FIGURE 143. Influence of changes in the extracellular Mg concentration on isometric tension development of an electrically stimulated pig coronary strip. The physiological Mg content of a normal Tyrode solution is 1.05 mM. Reducing the Mg concentration below this control level intensifies contractile force, whereas contractility gradually declines at higher Mg concentrations. Additional Ca restores tension development. Intermittent electric-field stimulation in the bath by rectangular alternating pulses (voltage, 10 V/cm; frequency, 10 Hz; duration, each time 16 sec). Isometric tension is measured at optimal muscle length, i.e., elongation to 150% related to the initial length (= 100%) of the unloaded preparation. From Nakayama, Fleckenstein, Byon, and Fleckenstein-Grün (1978).

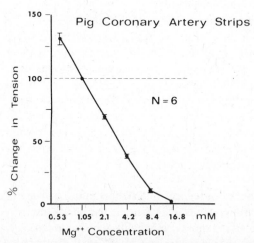

FIGURE 144. Relative changes in active tension development of electrically driven pig coronary strips (N = 6) at varying extracellular Mg concentrations. Isometric tension observed at the different Mg concentrations is expressed as percentage of that developed at the normal control level of 1.05 mM Mg (= 100%). Each point represents the mean ± SE. Experimental conditions as in Figure 143. From Nakayama, Fleckenstein, Byon, and Fleckenstein-Grün (1978).

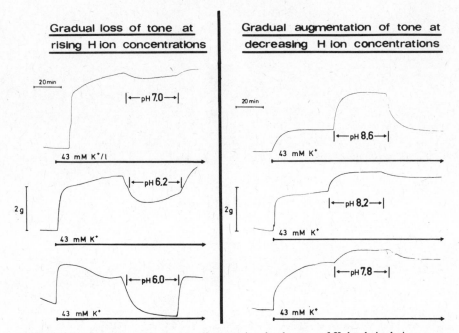

Gradual loss of tone at rising H ion concentrations

Gradual augmentation of tone at decreasing H ion concentrations

FIGURE 145.   Influence of changes in pH on tension development of K-depolarized pig coronary strips starting from an original pH of 7.4. From Fleckenstein, Nakayama, Fleckenstein-Grün, and Byon (1975).

state of full Ca deficiency. Conversely, at a pH of 8.6, contractile tension was usually doubled compared with that at a pH of 7.4. Electrically stimulated coronary strips behaved similarly. A typical experiment of Nakayama, Fleckenstein, Byon, and Fleckenstein-Grün (1978) is shown in Figure 146. Here the pH of the Tyrode solution was systematically altered over a relatively narrow range between 6.8 and 7.8. Consequently, under the influence of acidosis (pH 6.8), the isometric contraction amplitude was reduced to about one half of that observed at the control pH of 7.35. Alkalosis, on the other hand, dramatically potentiated the mechanical reactions. For instance, shifting the pH from 7.35 to 7.6 not only produced bigger phasic contractions but also led to the appearance of a very pronounced contracture. This increase in tone reached a rather excessive degree at a pH of 7.8 in the form of a large and long-lasting spasm.

Excitation–Contraction Uncoupling by Intracellular Hydrogen Accumulation.   Relaxation of K-depolarized coronary strips can also be produced, even at a constant extracellular pH of 7.4, under all conditions that favor acute *intracellular* H-ion accumulation. Thus relaxation regularly occurred in our experiments when the glycolytic activity of the K-depolarized coronary preparations was intensified in anoxia or under the influence of inhibitors of respiration or oxidative phosphorylation such as NaCN or 2,4-dinitrophenol (Grün, Bayer, and Fleckenstein, 1972;

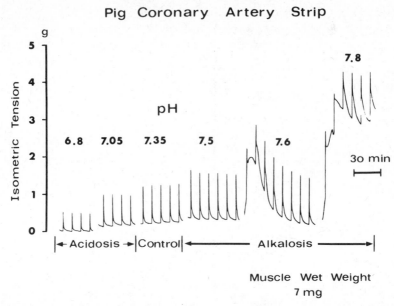

FIGURE 146. Influence of changes in pH on the contractile responses of an electrically stimulated pig coronary strip. Variation of pH over the range from 6.8 to 7.8 in Tris-buffered Tyrode solution. Acidosis by way of accumulation of Ca-antagonistic H ions lowers isometric tension development. Conversely, alkalosis, by diminishing the number of H ions, removes their physiological brake effect on Ca-dependent excitation–contraction coupling so that the mechanical reactions are dramatically potentiated. Experimental conditions as in Figure 143. From Nakayama, Fleckenstein, Byon, and Fleckenstein-Grün (1978).

Grün, Weder, and Fleckenstein, 1972; Fleckenstein, Nakayama, Fleckenstein-Grün, and Byo.. 1975, 1976a). Figure 147 demonstrates the reversible loss of tone brought about by anoxia or 2,4 dinitrophenol in two K-depolarized pig coronary strips at a strictly constant extracellular pH of 7.4. Recovery of tension could readily be achieved with an alkaline Tris buffer solution, whereas a NaHCO$_3$ buffer was practically useless because it fails to exert an appreciable influence on intracellular pH. This means that the relaxation due to anoxia, NaCN, or 2,4-dinitrophenol probably results more from a blockade of Ca-dependent utilization of high-energy phosphates by intracellularly accumulated H ions than from a true high-energy-phosphate deficiency.

All our observations suggest that the metabolic H production interferes with Ca-dependent excitation–contraction coupling of coronary smooth muscle and thereby temporally precludes the fundamental function of Ca, that is, maintenance of vascular tone and contractility. Although in comparison with the small intramural resistance vessels, the great extramural coronary stem arteries *in situ* are less exposed to the influence of acid metabolites of the myocardium, they nevertheless obey the general law that the smooth musculature of the vascular walls relaxes and blood flow increases in response to acidosis. Conversely, alkalosis induces vasoconstric-

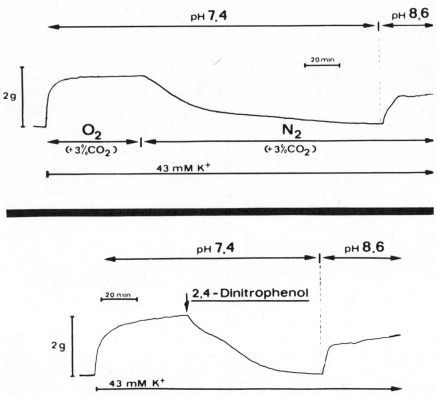

FIGURE 147. Reversible loss of tone produced by anoxia or 2,4-dinitrophenol in two K-depolarized pig coronary strips at a constant extracellular pH of 7.4. Recovery of tone only occurs in an alkaline Tris-buffer solution, whereas a $NaHCO_3$ buffer is inefficient. From Fleckenstein, Nakayama, Fleckenstein-Grün, and Byon (1976a).

tion. This basic regulatory mechanism of blood supply obviously operates without involvement of sympathetic or parasympathetic transmitters, since the pH-induced changes in coronary tension development were not altered in our experiments by atropine or by a blockade of adrenergic α- or β-receptors. In other words, the H ions, by interaction with Ca, are capable of directly influencing coronary tone, irrespective of the presence or absence of an intact autonomic nerve control. The H ions seem to compete with Ca for the same active sites, both at the Ca-transport system of the plasma membrane and at the myofibrillar ATPase. It is well known that (1) tension development of the isolated contractile system of glycerol-extracted muscle fibers is considerably reduced by a shift from pH 7 to pH 6 (Briggs and Portzehl, 1957) and (2) the ATPase of vascular smooth muscle is particularly responsive in this respect (Schädler, 1967). Hence even mild degrees of acidosis, unable to impair Ca-dependent splitting of ATP and tension development in skeletal muscle, may strongly inhibit these functions in vascular smooth muscle so that vasodilation occurs.

In summary, the present results indicate that tone and contractility of the great extramural coronary stem arteries is basically determined by the cation ratio $Ca^{++}/(Mg^{++}, H^+)$. Thus high Ca concentrations, Mg deficiency, and alkalosis enhance contractile activation of the coronary vascular wall, whereas relaxation is produced in a Ca-deficient medium, at a high Mg level, or if the H ions accumulate. These mutual interactions of Ca, Mg, and H ions in excitation–contraction coupling of the coronary vasculature are obviously quite similar to those previously depicted with respect to the myocardium (see Section 3.5.1 to 3.5.4).

6.2.4. Powerful Blockade of Excitation–Contraction Coupling of Coronary Smooth Muscle by Organic Calcium Antagonists; Differentiation Between Calcium Antagonists and Nitrites

Calcium Antagonists.   Certainly the most effective way of interrupting excitation–contraction coupling of the great extramural coronary stem arteries consists of the use of organic Ca antagonists. By suitable doses of these drugs, the extramural coronary bed can be enlarged and the occurrence of coronary vasospasms prevented. As to the fundamental mechanism of action, the Ca antagonists are most powerful inhibitors of "potential dependent" Ca entry through the depolarized coronary smooth muscle cell membranes. For instance, in K-depolarized strips from pig and rabbit stem arteries, one molecule of verapamil, D 600, prenylamine, and particularly nifedipine proved to block the effect of up to several thousand Ca ions in excitation–contraction coupling (Fleckenstein, 1970/1971b; Grün and Fleckenstein, 1971, 1972). Figure 148 represents four experiments on pig coronary strips in which K-induced *in vitro* spasms were completely neutralized by addition of suitable doses (1 to 4 mg/l) of fendiline, prenylamine, verapamil, and diltiazem. Terodiline and perhexiline maleate acted in the same concentration range. By restricting transmembrane Ca supply, all these drugs produce reversible relaxation, similar to that after extracellular Ca withdrawal, whereas depolarization persists (cf. Figure 142).

However, as is to be expected, the Ca-antagonistic depression of contractile tension development also depends on the transmembrane Ca gradient and the actual pH. Thus the reduction in transmembrane Ca conductivity can always be compensated, at least in part, by increasing the extracellular Ca concentration above normal. Thereby Ca influx is intensified and tension restored to a corresponding extent. Another experimental means of partially reversing the contractile depression induced by Ca antagonists is the application of an alkaline Tris buffer solution, a measure that also modifies the intracellular Ca:H ratio in favor of Ca. Figure 149 shows an exemplary experiment with D 600. Here the relaxing power of three concentrations of D 600 (0.01, 0.02, and 1.0 mg/l) was counterbalanced by shifting the reaction from pH 7.4 to pH 8.6. Low concentrations of Ca antagonists are, of course, more readily neutralizable by alkalization than strong ones.

With the exception of D 600, the most powerful Ca-antagonistic coronary vasodilator drugs originate from the 1,4-dihydropyridine group (nifedipine, niludipine,

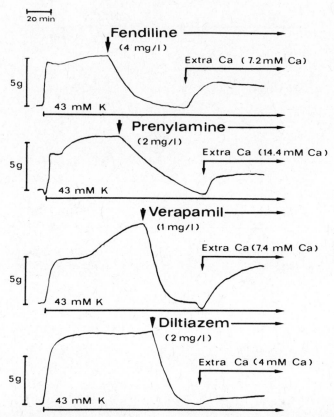

FIGURE 148. Relaxation of K-depolarized pig coronary strips by different Ca antagonists. Partial restitution of contractile tension by additional Ca at the end of the experiments. From Fleckenstein (1970/1971b) and Grün and Fleckenstein (1972).

nimodipine, nisoldipine, ryosidine). For instance, in Figure 150 the tremendous efficacy of nifedipine in blocking Ca-dependent excitation–contraction coupling in a K-depolarized, fully contracted rabbit coronary strip is shown. At the climax of spasm, minute amounts of nifedipine were added to produce relaxation of the coronary muscle preparation: 0.05, 0.1, and 2,8 µg/l. At a concentration of 6 × 10^{-10} M, excitation–contraction coupling was inhibited by about 60%. Full relaxation was obtained with less than 1 × 10^{-8} M nifedipine. No other drugs are known that relax the coronary musculature at such a low concentration. In Figure 151 are shown the results of a comparative study on pig coronary strips with different Ca antagonists. The ordinate indicates the percentages of excitation–contraction uncoupling obtained. The abscissa shows on a logarithmic scale the molar concentrations of the Ca-antagonistic compounds applied. Obviously, all Ca antagonists tested in this series are more potent than papaverine. In comparison with papaverine, nifedipine is approximately 3000 times stronger.

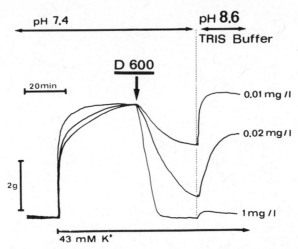

FIGURE 149. Partial neutralization of the relaxing effect of D 600 on a K-depolarized pig coronary strip by shifting the intracellular Ca: H ratio in favor of Ca with an alkaline Tris-buffer solution. From Grün and Fleckenstein, unpublished.

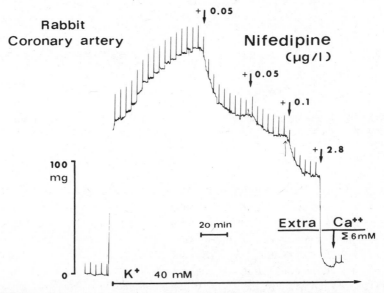

FIGURE 150. Suppression by nifedipine of a spastic *in vitro* contraction of a rabbit coronary strip depolarized with a high K^+ concentration (40 mM) in Tyrode solution. In addition to the high K concentration, alternating electric square-wave stimuli were applied to test excitability. Minute amounts of nifedipine, successively administered to the bath after the climax of shortening had been reached, produced gradual relaxation. With a total dose of 3 μg nifedipine/l (1×10^{-8} M), relaxation was completed and electric excitability abolished. Extra Ca given at the end of the experiment restored excitability. From Nakayama and Fleckenstein (1975); see Fleckenstein-Grün and Fleckenstein (1978/1980).

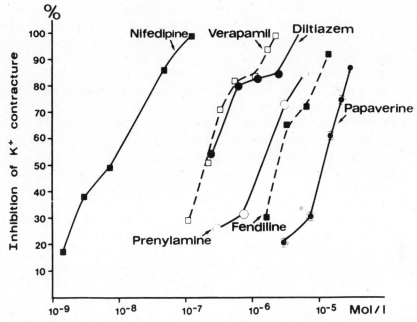

FIGURE 151. Suppression of K-induced contractures of pig coronary strips by Ca-antagonistic inhibitors of excitation–contraction coupling. The strips were depolarized with a K-rich Tyrode solution (43 mM KCl) for 40 min to produce full contractures. Then different concentrations of the Ca-antagonistic compounds were added so that depending on the dose applied, the tension development was more or less inhibited. The degree of relaxation obtained is expressed as percentage of peak tension just before addition of the Ca-antagonistic drugs. Each point represents the average relaxation calculated from at least 15 individual experiments for each concentration, SE not exceeding ± 2%. Before administration of the K-rich Tyrode solution, the coronary strips were kept in a Tyrode solution with a normal K content (concentrations in millimol per liter: NaCl, 155; KCl, 4; NaHCO$_3$, 11.9; CaCl$_2$, 1.0; NaH$_2$PO$_4$, 0.48; glucose, 5.6) for a period of 60 min under a load of 2.0 g. Throughout the experiment a gas mixture of 97% O$_2$ and 3% CO$_2$ was used for oxygenation of the bath at a constant temperature of 35°C and at a pH of 7.4. Isometric tension was continuously recorded with the use of a mechanoelectronic transducer. From Fleckenstein, Nakayama, Fleckenstein-Grün, and Byon (1976b) and Fleckenstein (1977).

Nitroglycerin and Sodium Nitroprusside. Nitroglycerin and related compounds as well as sodium nitroprusside also interfere with the Ca-dependent processes of excitation–contraction coupling of coronary vascular smooth muscle, even though these drugs have no corresponding action on myocardial fibers (Grün and Fleckenstein, 1972; Weder and Grün, 1973; Fleckenstein, Nakayama, Fleckenstein-Grün, and Byon, 1976a). However, the kinetics of vascular relaxation by the nitrocompounds when thoroughly compared on K-depolarized coronary strips with the action of Ca antagonists proved to be rather different. The peculiarities of the nitrocompounds are as follows:

1. The onset of relaxation is rather rapid, particularly when nitroglycerin or amyl nitrite is applied. In fact, nitroglycerin-induced relaxation of coronary smooth muscle reaches its maximum within a few minutes, whereas it takes approximately 1 hour until the climax of the relaxing action of nifedipine, for instance, is attained (see Figure 152).

2. Relaxation produced by organic nitrates or sodium nitroprusside always remains incomplete. Even at high concentrations of these drugs, a residual K contracture of 20 to 40% regularly persists (Figures 153 and 154).

3. Relaxation by organic nitrates is in most cases transient, so coronary tone tends to recover spontaneously in the presence of the drugs (Figure 153). An almost instantaneous neutralization of the nitrocompounds is achieved with increasing Ca_o concentration or with an alkaline Tris buffer solution.

Our experimental findings on isolated coronary smooth muscle show that only the Ca antagonists of the verapamil-nifedipine type can abolish vascular tone completely and permanently. The results also correspond with the old clinical experience that nitroglycerin and amyl nitrite, because of their rapid coronary (and systemic) effects, are most suitable for the interruption of an acute anginal attack. But for the basic long-term treatment of coronary heart diesase, the Ca antagonists seem to be more promising because of their protracted action. This applies particularly to the prevention of spastic coronary troubles classified as "variant angina" according to Prinzmetal's terminology (see the clincial Section 7.3).

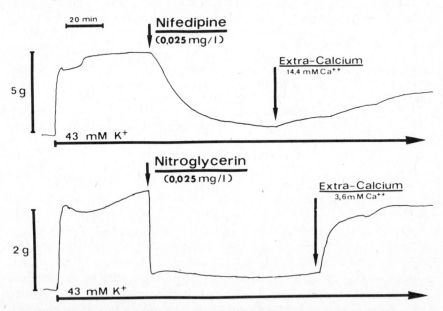

FIGURE 152. Extremely rapid relaxation of a K-depolarized pig coronary strip produced by a small dose of nitroglycerin (0.025 mg/l) within a few minutes. Coronary smooth muscle relaxation following administration of nifedipine (0.025 mg/l) proceeds more slowly. From Grün and Fleckenstein (1972).

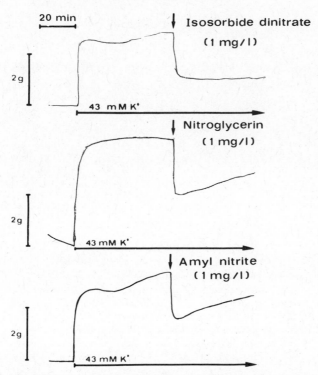

FIGURE 153. Rapid but incomplete relaxation of three K-depolarized pig coronary strips by different organic nitrates. From Fleckenstein, Nakayama, Fleckenstein-Grün, and Byon (1976a).

Nitroglycerin and sodium nitroprusside do not seem to impair potential-dependent Ca influx as the Ca antagonists do (Haeusler and Thorens, 1976; Verhaeghe and Shepherd, 1976; Zsoter, Henein and Wolchinsky, 1977; Thorens and Haeusler, 1979). However, on the basis of comparative measurements of the ^{45}Ca fluxes on canine renal vasculature, Hester, Weiss, and Fry (1979) concluded that sodium nitroprusside, in contrast with D 600, probably acts by increasing the affinity or the number of binding sites for Ca in or on the cell membrane so that activator Ca will be neutralized by sequestration. Thus sodium nitroprusside appears to directly counteract the effects of those vasoconstrictor agonists that release "high-affinity" Ca. In accordance with this concept nitroglycerin and sodium nitroprusside are particularly efficient in antagonizing the phasic components of angiotensin- or epinephrine-induced contractile responses that primarily depend on liberation of bound Ca (Hester, Weiss, and Fry, 1979); Watkins and Davidson, 1980; Karaki, Hester, and Weiss, 1980).

There are several reports suggesting that the relaxation of smooth muscle by nitroglycerin and sodium nitroprusside might be attributable to an increase in the cellular concentration of cyclic 3',5'-GMP (Katsuki, Arnold, and Murad, 1977; Schultz, Schultz, and Schultz, 1977). Particularly in coronary smooth muscle, a

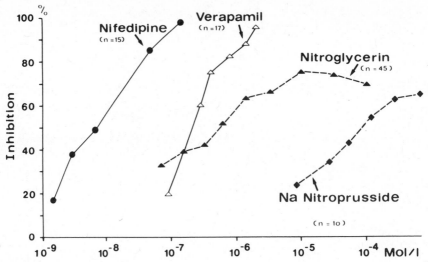

FIGURE 154. Inhibition of K-induced contractures of pig coronary strips by increasing concentrations of Ca antagonists (nifedipine, verapamil), nitroglycerin, and sodium nitroprusside. In contrast with the dose–response curves of nifedipine and verapamil, those of nitroglycerin and sodium nitroprusside become more and more flat as the doses increase. Thus a residual contracture of 20 to 40% always persists even at high nitroglycerin or nitroprusside concentrations. The points represent average values, SE not exceeding ± 3%. From Fleckenstein-Grün, Fleckenstein, Späh, and Assmann (1978/1979).

rapid rise in cyclic GMP, amounting up to a 50-fold increase above the control values, could be observed under the influence of maximum relaxant concentrations of nitroglycerin and sodium nitroprusside (Kukovetz, Holzmann, Wurm, and Pöch, 1979). In the latter study the correlation between the changes in cyclic GMP concentration and the course of relaxation was highly significant both quantitatively and temporally.

Thus the conclusion is justified that Ca antagonists and nitrates (including sodium nitroprusside) restrict the Ca supply to the contractile elements by two fundamentally different mechanisms. The Ca antagonists apparently block Ca entry by competing with Ca at the transmembrane transport system. The nitrates, on the other hand, seem to minimize the availability of free Ca ions by stimulating biochemical mechanisms of cellular Ca sequestration or by enlarging the capacities for Ca storage. However, the possible extension of these capacities seems to be limited, so the nitrate-induced relaxation of K-depolarized coronary smooth muscle always remains incomplete and transient as shown above.

Nevertheless, Ca antagonists and nitrates, although acting on different cellular sites, share the following decisive abilities:

1. They inhibit coronary vascular tone and contractility at the roots, that is, by directly restricting the availability of activator Ca.

2. They exert these drug effects with particularly high efficacy on the great extramural coronary arteries as the clinically most important part of the coronary bed.

By contrast, other coronary vasodilators such as adenosine, dipyridamole (Persantin®), chromonar (carbocromene, Intensain®), theophylline, and caffeine, even in excessive concentrations (30 to 100 mg/l), do not interfere with Ca-dependent excitation–contraction coupling of the extramural coronary vasculature (Fleckenstein-Grün and Fleckenstein, 1975). But these drugs obviously relax the small intramural resistance vessels, that is, the coronary arterioles. However, in coronary patients, arteriolar relaxation is likely to produce a "steal phenomenon" rather than to improve coronary flow through a diseased subepicardial stem artery. Thus it is not surprising that in contrast with Ca antagonists or nitrates, the therapeutic value of coronary vasodilators with a preferentially arteriolar action is widely considered questionable or even nil.

6.2.5. Calcium-Synergistic Potentiation of Coronary Smooth Muscle Contractility and Tone by Cardiac Glycosides, Neutralization of the Coronary Vasoconstrictor Effects of Cardiac Glycosides by Calcium Antagonists

Careful measurements of coronary flow on dog hearts *in situ* have revealed that cardiac glycosides can produce, under certain conditions, a significant rise in coronary vascular resistance. For instance, pertinent observations were made using *acetylstrophanthidin* (Waldhausen, Kilman, Herendeen, and Abel, 1965), *lanatoside C* (Gracey and Brandfonbrener, 1962), *ouabain* (Vatner, Higgins, Franklin, and Braunwald, 1971; Vatner, Higgins, McKown, Franklin, and Braunwald, 1970), or *digoxin* (Steiness, Bille-Brahe, Hansen, Lomholdt, and Ring-Larsen, 1978). Moreover, the severity of myocardial ischemic injury following experimental coronary occlusion was increased by ouabain (Maroko, Braunwald, and Covell, 1970; Maroko, 1971). Therefore, all these authors called attention to the significance of coronary vasoconstriction as a rather neglected side effect of cardiac glycosides and simultaneously suggested that rapid digitalization of patients with serious coronary heart disease might possibly be, for this reason, rather hazardous.

However, glycoside-induced coronary vasoconstriction probably does not occur in all parts of the coronary bed with equal strength and with equally serious consequences. For instance, the direct vasoconstrictor influence on the small intramural resistance vessels seems to be greatly counterbalanced by an indirect metabolic vasodilation that the cardiac glycosides produce in consequence of their positive inotropic action on the myocardium. Hence a measurable decrease in global flow may even be missed in digitalized hearts of normal animals. But the situation is necessarily different if vasoconstriction by cardiac glycosides takes place in the great extramural stem arteries or collaterals of a patient with occlusive coronary heart disease. In this case an additional narrowing of the extramural coronary bed may critically jeopardize the residual blood supply to the ischemic myocardium. Unfortunately, the great extramural stem arteries and collaterals are shielded from the ischemic ventricular wall by fat and connective tissue, so they cannot be reached by the natural vasodilator metabolites from the altered myocardium (particularly H ions). However, it turned out in our studies that glycoside-induced coronary vasoconstriction is extremely susceptible to the vasodilator action of Ca antagonists. The reason is that cardiac glycosides and Ca antagonists influence Ca-dependent coronary tone and contractility in an exactly opposite direction. Or more precisely, the essence of the glycoside effects on coronary smooth muscle consists of potentiating the crucial action of Ca in phasic and tonic contractile tension development (Fleckenstein and Byon, 1974; Grün, Fleckenstein, and Weder, 1974; Fleckenstein and Fleckenstein-Grün, 1975; Fleckenstein, Nakayama, Fleckenstein-Grün, and Byon, 1975, 1976a, b), whereas the Ca antagonists minimize all Ca-dependent mechanical parameters.

Typical experiments are shown in Figures 155 and 156: As can be seen from Figure 155, a coronary strip, like smooth musculature of other origin, responds to appropriate electric stimuli with absolutely regular phasic contractions. When the original Ca content (2 mM) of the medium is doubled, the isometric-contraction amplitude increases. The Ca-antagonistic compounds such as verapamil, on the

Pig Coronary Artery Strips

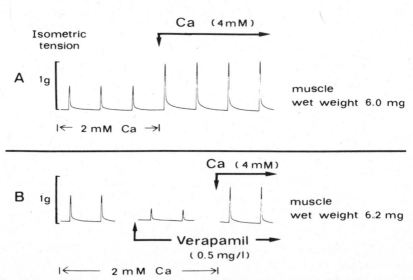

FIGURE 155. Changes in contractile tension development of 2 electrically stimulated pig coronary strips (*A*) upon elevation of Ca concentration of normal Tyrode solution from 2 to 4 mM and (*B*) upon addition of verapamil to normal Tyrode solution with 2 mM Ca. Neutralization of the Ca-antagonist action by raising extracellular Ca concentration from 2 to 4 mM. Alternating square-wave stimulation, 10 Hz; strength of stimulation, 10 V/cm; duration of stimulation, 16 sec each time with 10 min interval; temperature, 35°C. From Fleckenstein, Nakayama, Fleckenstein-Grün, and Byon (1975).

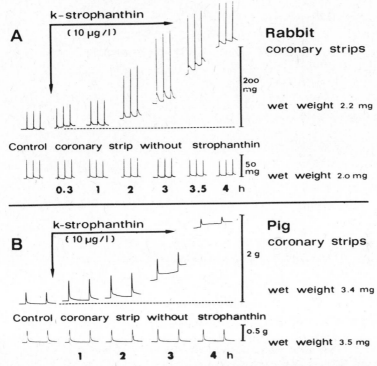

FIGURE 156. Rabbit and pig coronary strips; augmentation of phasic mechanical responses to electric stimuli, and increase in basal tone under the influence of 10 μg k-strophanthin/l during an observation period of 4 hours. By contrast, the control strips without strophanthin (dissected from the same coronary arteries as the test preparations) did not show any change in their contractile behavior. Tyrode solution with 2 mM Ca and 1.05 mM Mg; mode of stimulation as in Figures 143 and 155, however, with only a 5-min interval; temperature, 35°C. From Fleckenstein, Nakayama, Fleckenstein-Grün, and Byon (1975, 1976a).

other hand, lower or suppress the contractions. Conversely, cardiac glycosides are capable of potentiating the Ca-dependent coronary smooth muscle reactions to a striking extent. In fact, all cardiac glycosides, even in concentrations as low as 3 to 10 μg/l, considerably increase the contractile responses of coronary smooth muscle to electric stimuli. Simultaneously, the coronary smooth muscle tone is augmented and even long-lasting contractures develop. For instance, in Figure 156A, two strips dissected from the same rabbit coronary artery were electrically stimulated during an observation period of 4 hours, the upper strip with k-strophanthin, the lower strip without k-strophanthin. It can be easily seen that there is a striking augmentation of the phasic mechanical responses and a strong increase in basic tone under the influence of 10 μg k-strophanthin/l, whereas the control strip without k-strophanthin does not show any change in its contractile behavior. An identical experiment on two pig coronary strips is shown in Figure 156B. As found in a comparative study, the glycoside-induced potentiation of isometric tension in elec-

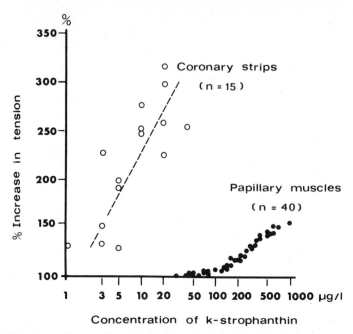

FIGURE 157. Glycoside-induced potentiation of isometric tension (1) in electrically stimulated rabbit coronary strips and (2) in electrically stimulated rabbit papillary muscles. The maximal increases in peak tension attained within a 4-hour observation period are expressed as percentages related to the initial tension before glycoside administration (= 100%). All preparations were stretched to optimal length. Stimulation rate of the papillary muscles was 60/min. Stimulation of coronary strips was carried out as in Figure 156. Tyrode solution containing 2 mM Ca and 1.05 mM Mg; temperature, 35°C. From Fleckenstein, Nakayama, Fleckenstein-Grün, and Byon (1975).

trically stimulated rabbit coronary strips is even greater than in electrically stimulated papillary muscles of the same animals. The graphs in Figure 157 demonstrate the glycoside-induced potentiation of isometric tension on both electrically stimulated rabbit coronary strips and electrically stimulated papillary muscles following the administration of k-strophanthin. Obviously, with a k-strophanthin dose as small as 5 μg/l, contractile tension of the coronary strips is already doubled, whereas more than 100 μg k-strophanthin/l are required to produce a significant positive-inotropic effect on the papillary muscles.

However, with the help of Ca-antagonistic compounds, the glycoside effects on electrically stimulated coronary strips can easily be neutralized. Figure 158 shows again the typical increase in basal coronary smooth muscle tone and the augmentation of the mechanical responses to electric stimuli under the influence of 3 μg k-strophanthin/l. But as soon as 0.5 mg verapamil/l was added to the solution, an immediate relaxation took place. An analogous experiment with nifedipine is shown in Figure 159. Here, a nifedipine concentration of 10 μg/l completely suppressed the strophanthin effects.

Further studies were carried out by us on *nonstimulated* coronary smooth muscle

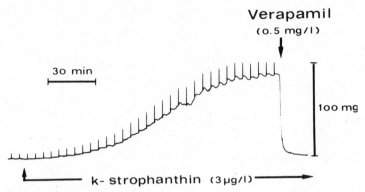

FIGURE 158. Rabbit coronary strip; increase in basal coronary smooth muscle tone and augmentation of mechanical responses to electric stimuli under the influence of 3 μg k-strophanthin/l. Immediate relaxation produced by verapamil. Tyrode solution containing 2 mM Ca and 1.05 mM Mg; wet tissue weight of coronary strip, 1.3 mg; stimulation as in Figure 156; temperature, 35°C. From Fleckenstein, Nakayama, Fleckenstein-Grün, and Byon (1975, 1976a).

preparations that were made to contract by exposure to large glycoside concentrations. In fact, all cardiac glycosides of practical interest such as ouabain, digoxin, β-methyldigoxin, lanatoside C, proscillaridin A, digitoxin, or k-strophanthin are able to evoke sustained contractile responses of resting pig or rabbit coronary strips if a standard dose of 0.5 mg/l is added to the bath. This glycoside concentration certainly exceeds by far the clinically interesting range, but such studies proved to be useful for a rapid pharmacological assessment of the relative coronary vasodilator potencies of the different Ca antagonists. As an example, two sets of experiments are represented in Figures 160 and 161. Here a verapamil concentration of 0.5 mg/l or a nifedipine concentration of 0.01 mg/l totally abolished the contractile responses to all cardiac glycosides included in these series. Full relaxation could also be obtained in analogous experiments with other Ca antagonists such as diltiazem (1

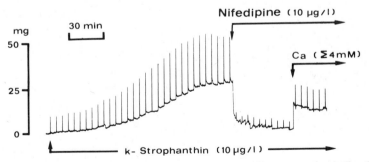

FIGURE 159. Instantaneous neutralization of the strophanthin effects on an electrically stimulated rabbit coronary strip (wet weight, 0.9 mg) with a small dose of nifedipine. Experimental procedure as in Figure 158. From Nakayama, Byon, and Fleckenstein (1976); see Fleckenstein and Fleckenstein-Grün (1977).

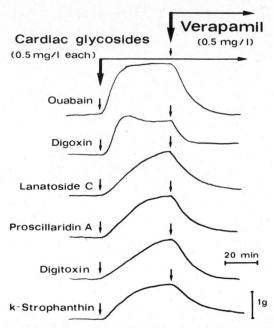

FIGURE 160. Contractures of pig coronary strips following administration of relatively high concentrations of different cardiac glycosides (0.5 mg/l in each experiment) without electric stimulation or addition of other vasoconstrictor agonists. Complete relaxation of the glycoside-contractured vasculature by verapamil. The strips were kept in Tyrode solution containing 1 mM Ca at a temperature of 35°C. From Fleckenstein, Nakayama, Fleckenstein-Grün, and Byon (1975, 1976a).

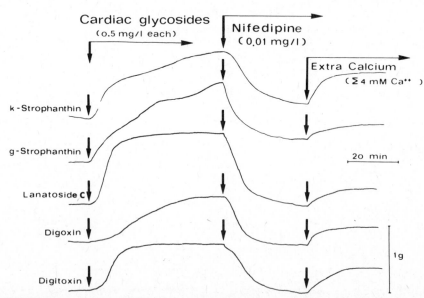

FIGURE 161. Neutralization of various glycoside-induced contractures of pig coronary strips with nifedipine. The standard concentrations of cardiac glycosides (0.5 mg/l) and of nifedipine (10 μg/l) were administered in Tyrode solution containing 1 mM Ca; Temperature, 35°C. From Fleckenstein, Fleckenstein-Grün, Byon, Haastert, and Späh (1979).

mg/l), prenylamine (2 mg/l), perhexiline (2 mg/l), or fendiline (2 to 4 mg/l). Moreover, the coronary glycoside action is antagonized by nitroglycerin and related nitrates (Figure 162). But again, as in K-depolarized strips, the relaxing effects of the nitrocompounds are incomplete and in most cases spontaneously reversible. Figure 163 demonstrates the inability of amyl nitrite (1 mg/l) to abolish a glycoside contraction of a pig coronary strip produced by k-strophanthin. In contrast, an immediate relaxation is obtained with D 600 (1 mg/l). Other coronary vasodilators, which do not significantly interfere with excitation–contraction coupling, are practically unable to prevent or abolish the glycoside-induced coronary smooth muscle contractions. This applies to adenosine, dipyridamole, chromonar, theophylline, and caffeine.

A fundamental property of cardiac glycosides is to "sensitize" the coronary vasculature to the tonic influence of an elevated extracellular Ca level. Figure 164 shows an experiment in which two strips of the same coronary artery were initially kept in a Tyrode solution with 1 mM Ca. Then the Ca content was gradually increased up to 4; 8 and 16 mM. The control strip, without k-strophanthin, responded

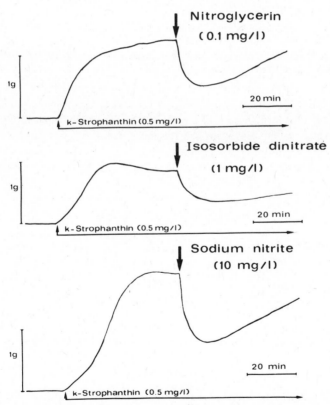

FIGURE 162.   Attenuation of k-strophanthin-induced coronary contractures by means of nitroglycerin, isosorbide dinitrate, or sodium nitrite. As in K-depolarized coronary strips, relaxation by nitrocompounds is incomplete and transient. From Fleckenstein, Nakayama, Fleckenstein-Grün, and Byon (1976a).

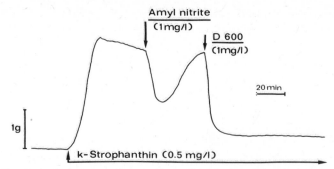

FIGURE 163. Typically fugitive relaxation of a strophanthin-contractured pig coronary strip under the influence of amyl nitrite. Full and permanent relaxation produced by the Ca-antagonistic compound D 600. From Fleckenstein, Nakayama, Fleckenstein-Grün, and Byon (1976a).

with only a moderate increase in tone. Pretreatment with 50 μg k-strophanthin/l, on the other hand, produced an enormous potentiation of the Ca effects so that a strong coronary smooth muscle contracture developed. These results demonstrated that the mutual potentiation of cardiac glycosides and Ca ions found by 0. Loewi as early as 1917 not only affects the myocardium but also, to an equal or even greater extent, the smooth musculature of the great extramural coronary arteries. Obviously cardiac glycosides facilitate the access of extracellular Ca to the interior of the smooth muscle cells. Interestingly enough, coronary strips contractured either by elevation of the K_0 concentration or by cardiac glycosides practically do not differ with respect to their sensitivities to Ca antagonists. Accordingly, the log dose–response curves of Figure 151, obtained on K-depolarized coronary preparations, are also rather representative for the efficacy of Ca antagonists against glycoside-induced coronary contractures. Moreover, the characteristic features of nitrate-induced relaxation (rapid onset, incompleteness, spontaneous reversibility)

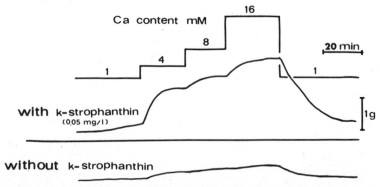

FIGURE 164. Pig coronary strips; potentiation by pretreatment with k-strophanthin of the contractile responses to a stepwise increase in the extracellular Ca concentration from 1 to 4.8 and 16 mM; temperature, 35°C. From Fleckenstein, Nakayama, Fleckenstein-Grün, and Byon (1975).

are equally pronounced in K-depolarized and glycoside-treated coronary strips. In the rat portal vein and the rabbit ear artery, ouabain was found to depolarize the cell membranes (Kuriyama, Ohshima, and Sakamoto, 1971; Hendrickx and Casteels, 1974). Also in dog coronary arteries, significant depolarization developed 15 to 20 min after addition of 1×10^{-7} M ouabain (Berne, Belardinelli, Harder, Sperelakis, and Rubio, 1978/1980). Hence the contractile responses to depolarizing cardiac glycoside concentrations can simply be related to a "potential-dependent" enhancement of transmembrane Ca supply, a pathway that is characterized by a particularly high responsiveness to the inhibitory influence of Ca antagonists. However, even before the cardiac glycosides produce any significant depolarization, they may already elicit an "electrogenic" transmembrane Ca influx that manifests itself in the form of spontaneous spike potentials, provided the coronary preparations have been pretreated with tetraethylammonium. In these muscles, elevation of the Ca_o concentration caused a marked increase in amplitude, rate of rise, and frequency of the spike potentials (Belardinelli, Harder, Sperelakis, Rubio, and Berne, 1979). Conversely, verapamil (5×10^{-6} M) completely abolished automatic impulse discharge as well as the action potentials evoked by additional electric stimulation. Thus all data obtained on coronary smooth muscle indicate that the increases in phasic contractility and basal tone, as well as the facilitation of spontaneous spike discharge, arise from the same promoter action of cardiac glycosides on the transmembrane inward Ca movements.

As to the therapeutic significance of these findings, it is important to note that the dose range in which the Ca-antagonistic drugs protect the coronary smooth musculature against glycoside-induced vasoconstriction is considerably lower than that which diminishes the inotropic glycoside action on the myocardium. Or in other words, in a suitable drug combination of a cardiac glycoside and a Ca-antagonistic compound, the beneficial positive-inotropic glycoside effect on the myocardium can retain its full potency, whereas the undesired coronary vasoconstriction is abolished.

6.2.6. Suppression by Calcium Antagonists of Experimental Coronary Vasospasms Produced with Serotonin, Histamine and Acetylcholine or with Noradrenaline after β-Receptor Blockade

The Ca antagonists, by interrupting transmembrane Ca influx into vascular smooth muscle cells, generally block two processes:

1. The "potential-dependent" transmembrane Ca supply, thus inhibiting contractile activation *directly*, as in K-depolarized or glycoside-treated preparations.

2. The transmembrane refilling of cellular Ca pools from which activator Ca is released "nonelectrically" by vasoconstrictor agonists such as noradrenaline, histamine, or serotonin. Therefore, with a certain delay, an *indirect* depression of agonist-induced (phasic) contractile activity is also to be expected.

Nevertheless, the capacities of these cellular Ca stores (and consequently the rate of exhaustion following a blockade of transmembrane Ca influx) seem to vary in different vascular smooth muscle types. For instance, many observations on smooth muscle preparations from systemic arteries have established that Ca withdrawal, EDTA, or Ca antagonists inhibit the contractions evoked by vasoconstrictor agonists more slowly or to a lesser extent than those produced by a high K_0 concentration. This phenomenon is believed to indicate the existence of well-developed cellular Ca depots. However, in coronary smooth muscle the situation is somewhat different. This appears from our observation that the efficacy of Ca antagonists in neutralizing the contractile responses to vasoconstrictor agonists is nearly as great as their ability to suppress K-induced contractures. Presumably, the Ca stores in coronary smooth muscle cells are less capacious and thus require a more rapid transmembrane replenishment than those in the vasculature of peripheral arteries. Thus the Ca antagonists, besides of blocking "potential-dependent" contractile activation of coronary smooth muscle, also inhibit the Ca supply for "agonist-induced" phasic contractions rather effectively. Conversely, the contractile responses to vasoconstrictor agonists are strongly potentiated by cardiac glycosides.

An evaluation of a great number of experiments on pig coronary strips with increasing concentrations of *serotonin* and *histamine* is given in Figures 165 and 166. Here, beginning with a small dose of 25 μg/l, the drug concentrations were increased stepwise every 40 min until at 1000 μg/l the contractures (calculated as tension times time) attained a maximum. However, in the presence of diltiazem (0.2 mg/l) or nifedipine (0.01 mg/l), the serotonin and histamine effects were minimized, whereas a highly significant potentiation resulted from the addition of 10 μg k-strophanthin/l.

As to the particular influence of sympathetic or parasympathetic neurotransmitters on coronary tone and contractility, Langendorff in 1907 was the first to clearly demonstrate that smooth muscle preparations from large bovine stem arteries exhibited a peculiar behavior in that they relaxed under the influence of adrenaline, in contrast with the typical contractile responses of systemic arteries. Although there are probably certain species differences, the isolated coronary arteries of most animals react to adrenaline by dilation. Conversely, vagal stimulation or acetylcholine produces coronary vasoconstriction. The classic literature on the parasympathetic rise in coronary resistance has been extensively reviewed by Anrep (1926). From these and more recent data (Rein, 1931; Gollwitzer-Meier and Krüger, 1935), it appears that coronary smooth muscle, whether *in situ* or isolated, generally tends to relax when the sympathetic drive is high, as during physical exercise, whereas coronary constriction is likely to occur when the parasympathetic impulses predominate, as during sleep. The latter effect is also of clinical importance since in patients with Prinzmetal's spastic variant angina, the coronary attacks preferably occur at rest and can be provoked even experimentally by injection of parasympathetic agents such as methacholine.

Accordingly, as illustrated by Figure 167, acetylcholine also produces powerful contractures in pig coronary strips. In comparison with serotonin and histamine, the coronary constrictor effects of acetylcholine are considerably stronger. They

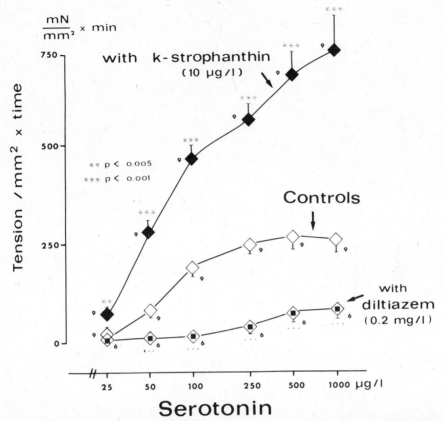

$$\frac{mN}{mm^2} \times min$$

with k-strophanthin
(10 µg/l)

** p < 0.005
*** p < 0.001

Controls

with
diltiazem
(0.2 mg/l)

Tension / mm² × time

25   50   100   250   500   1000 µg/l

Serotonin

FIGURE 165. Potentiation by k-strophanthin and suppression by diltiazem of the contractile responses of pig coronary strips to serotonin. The coronary strips were exposed to stepwise increased concentrations of serotonin, each time for 40 min, in normal Tyrode solution (controls) or in Tyrode solution containing k-strophanthin (10 µg/l) or diltiazem (0.2 mg/l). In all experiments with k-strophanthin or diltiazem, these drugs were administered 30 min before the lowest concentration of serotonin (25 µg/l) was tested. To quantify size and duration of the contractile responses, the records were planimetrically evaluated. Each point plotted in the diagrams represents the product of isometric tension (mN), produced per square millimeter cross section of cylindric coronary smooth muscle strip, multiplied by the time of tension sustained (min) during the observation period (40 min). The mean values ($\pm$ SE) and the number of coronary strips included in the series are indicated for each point. The Ca content of the Tyrode solution was 1 mM. Temperature, 35°C. From Fleckenstein-Grün and Fleckenstein, unpublished.

always consist of a transient phasic and a more protracted tonic component. Verapamil and other Ca antagonists greatly depress both components, although the tonic part seems to be slightly more sensitive. An evaluation of a series of experiments with increasing concentrations of acetylcholine from 10 to 500 µg/l, is shown in Figure 168. The size of contracture is again expressed as the product of tension multiplied by the time of tension development always during an observation period of 40 min. As is clear from these graphs, the inhibitory influence of 0.1 mg

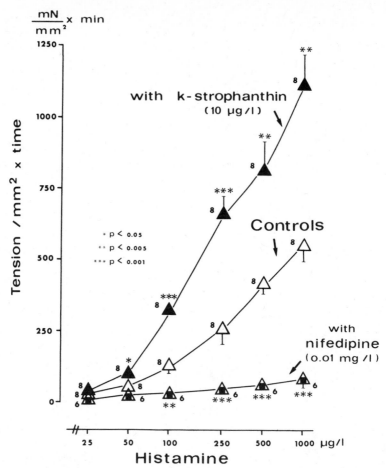

FIGURE 166.   Potentiation by k-strophanthin and suppression by nifedipine of the contractile responses of pig coronary strips to histamine. Experimental procedure as in Figure 165. From Fleckenstein-Grün and Fleckenstein, unpublished.

verapamil/l and, conversely, the potentiation of the acetylcholine effects by strophanthin are again highly significant. Strophanthin and other cardiac glycosides intensify and prolong especially the tonic phases of the acetylcholine-induced contractions.

The behavior of the coronary stem arteries is, in fact, similar to that of the bronchi. This means that the smooth musculature of the coronary stem arteries and the bronchi share the peculiarity of contracting in response to acetylcholine, whereas the sympathetic neurotransmitters normally induce relaxation. The reason is that in both coronary vasculature and bronchi, the number of available adrenergic β-receptors is usually greater than the number of available α-receptors. In consequence, adrenaline and noradrenaline, by stimulating more β-receptors than α-receptors, normally produce coronary relaxation and bronchodilation. However, as

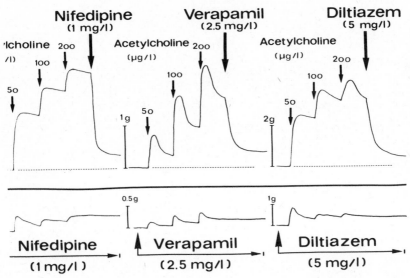

FIGURE 167. Suppression of acetylcholine-induced spasms of pig coronary smooth muscle strips by different Ca antagonists, irrespective of whether they are added before or after acetylcholine. Fleckenstein-Grün and Fleckenstein (1978/1980).

soon as a β-blocker is administered, the α-receptors prevail, so the sympathetic transmitter substances then act as coronary constrictors and bronchoconstrictors. A typical experiment on two strips excised from the same pig coronary artery is shown in Figure 169. The normal control preparation (lower curve) exhibited a small additional relaxation each time it was exposed to noradrenaline (5 mg/l) for 4 min (followed by a washout period of 16 min). Pretreatment with the selective β-blocker pindolol, on the other hand (see upper curve), converted the ordinary noradrenaline-induced relaxations into huge contractions. However, with nifedipine (0.1 mg/l), this special type of coronary smooth muscle activation could also be effectively antagonized.

In summary of our results, the Ca antagonists are the most powerful coronary relaxants hitherto discovered that can protect the heart against all kinds of experimental coronary spasms, whatever the special reasons for the coronary smooth muscle activation may be. The outstanding efficacy of Ca antagonists also is reflected in a growing number of clinical reports that emphasize the therapeutic achievements resulting from the introduction of Ca antagonists, especially for the treatment of spastic forms of coronary disease (for more details see Section 7.3).

6.2.7. Inhibitory Effects of Calcium Antagonists on Potential-Dependent and Receptor-Mediated Activation of Smooth Muscle from Pulmonal and Systemic Arteries

Two principal types of vascular smooth muscle relaxation by Ca antagonists are distinguishable according to the mode of contractile activation:

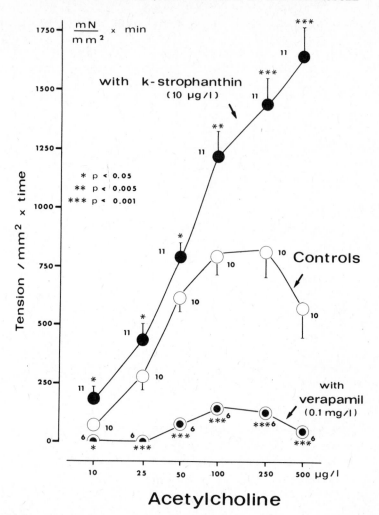

FIGURE 168.   Potentiation by k-strophanthin and suppression by verapamil of the contractile responses of pig coronary strips to acetylcholine. Experimental procedure as in Figure 165. From Fleckenstein-Grün and Fleckenstein, unpublished.

1. Direct relaxation produced by interruption of Ca influx through "potential-dependent," "voltage-sensitive" membrane channels or through certain "receptor-operated" Ca channels.
2. Indirect relaxation produced by depletion of cellular Ca pools in cases of contractile activation by Ca-releasing vasoconstrictor agonists.

The strongest arguments in favor of this dualistic concept came from observations on smooth muscle from pulmonal and systemic arteries. Haeusler (1972) was the first to show in a brilliant study that verapamil in a concentration range of 2 ×

R. descendens (Pig Coronary Artery)

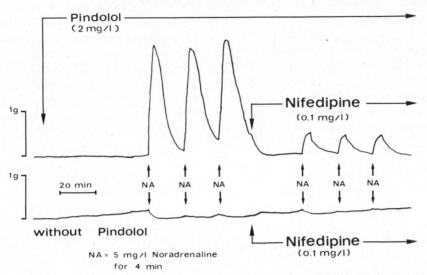

FIGURE 169. Noradrenaline-induced spasms of a pig coronary strip pretreated with the β-receptor blocking agent pindolol (upper experiment). Adrenergic β-receptor blockade unmasks the coronary vasoconstrictor potency of α-receptor stimulation. Nifedipine and all other Ca antagonists minimize even this kind of coronary vasoconstriction. However, as long as under normal physiological conditions the β-receptors prevail numerically in extramural coronary smooth muscle (lower experiment), noradrenaline produces relaxation. From Fleckenstein-Grün and Fleckenstein (1978/1980), and from Fleckenstein and Fleckenstein-Grün (1980).

10^{-8} to 2×10^{-7} M competitively antagonized Ca-induced contractions of depolarized strips of the *rabbit main pulmonary artery*, whereas the inhibition of the contractile response to noradrenaline failed to exhibit a competitive pattern and also required higher doses of the Ca antagonist. Verapamil did not interfere with membrane depolarization, but apparently acted in this study by blocking two different pathways of Ca-dependent contractile activation, distinguishable by their particular drug susceptibilities and kinetics. In accordance with our own concept, Haeusler concluded that "verapamil prevents the increase in calcium permeability of the cell membrane due to depolarization," but "is less effective in antagonizing the liberation of Ca from binding sites by norepinephrine."

Many subsequent observations on the smooth musculature from different systemic arteries confirmed and extended the essence of these statements, not only with respect to the action of sympathetic amines but also regarding other vasoconstrictor agonists. Thus verapamil and D 600, also in *rat aortic strips* or ring preparations, inhibited the contractile responses to K-induced membrane depolarization much faster and more effectively than those to noradrenaline (Bilek and Peiper, 1973; Bilek, Laven, Peiper, and Regnat, 1974; Massingham, 1973). In the latter study, Ca-induced contractions of K-depolarized preparations could be blocked by 50% with 1×10^{-8} M D 600, whereas a 10 times higher concentration was needed to produce a similar inhibition of the responses to noradrenaline. Interestingly enough, Schümann, Görlitz, and Wagner (1975), using spiral strips from *rabbit aortae* and *mesenteric arteries,* noticed an even 1000 times higher relaxing potency of D 600 and nifedipine in the case of Ca-induced spasms of depolarized preparations than in the case of noradrenaline-evoked contractions. Papaverine, on the other hand, did not exhibit specific Ca-antagonistic properties since it blocked both Ca-induced and noradrenaline-evoked contractile responses with equal strength.

One should, however, remember that adrenaline, noradrenaline, and other vasoconstrictor agonists, particularly in a higher concentration range, mostly produce a biphasic contractile response, consisting of a rapid initial peak and a slower tonic component. As already discussed in Section 6.2.1, the initial component is considered to reflect the fast receptor-mediated release of activator Ca from cellular storage sites (usually called phase A), whereas the subsequent tonic component seems to depend directly on transmembrane Ca influx connected with depolarization (phase B). Therefore, it is not surprising that phases A and B differ with respect not only to their susceptibilities to extracellular Ca withdrawal (or Ca chelation with EDTA), but also to Ca antagonists. Thus in general, the tonic phase B is more readily neutralizable by Ca antagonists than is phase A. Using verapamil on the musculature from *rabbit ear arteries,* Bevan, Garstka, Su, and Su (1973) showed that the preferential suppression of phase B was equally discernible, irrespective of whether noradrenaline, histamine, or serotonin were applied as vasoconstrictor agonists. Nevertheless, the initial peak A also decreases considerably if the time of exposure to the Ca antagonists is sufficiently prolonged and the vasoconstrictor agents repeatedly applied in order to empty the cellular Ca depots. A typical experiment of this type on isolated smooth musculature from a *rabbit femoral artery* is shown in Figure 170. Here a series of successive standard doses of noradrenaline (0.1 mg/l) were administered each time for 4 min, followed by a washout period of 8 min. If the Ca antagonists verapamil or diltiazem were present from the beginning (lower lines), phase B was totally abolished so that only sharp transient peak contractions, corresponding to phase A, were left. However, the height of these contractions diminished more and more under the influence of the Ca antagonists until within 2 to 3 hours, all mechanical activity disappeared. Thus a considerable time lag exists until the Ca antagonists, after instantaneous abolition of the tonic phase B, are also able to suppress, probably via exhaustion of mobilizable cellular Ca stores, the peak contractions of phase A. An unexpected result that deserves further investigations is that nifedipine is rather weak in inhibiting the vasoconstrictor effects of noradrenaline (own observations) or of phenylephrine and serotonin (Allen and Banghart, 1979) on the femoral vasculature.

The *cerebral arteries,* on the other hand, are extremely sensitive to Ca antagonists, particularly to those of the 1,4-dihydropyridine group, irrespective of the type of contraction. As an example, Figure 171A demonstrates full relaxation of a K-depolarized strip from a *rabbit basilar artery* after administration of a total of 3 μg nifedipine/l ($1 \times 10^{-8}M$). Similarly in Figure 171B, a low dose of nifedipine abolished a strophanthin-induced contracture of an electrically stimulated rabbit basilar strip. The contractures of K-depolarized or glycoside-treated *rabbit basilar*

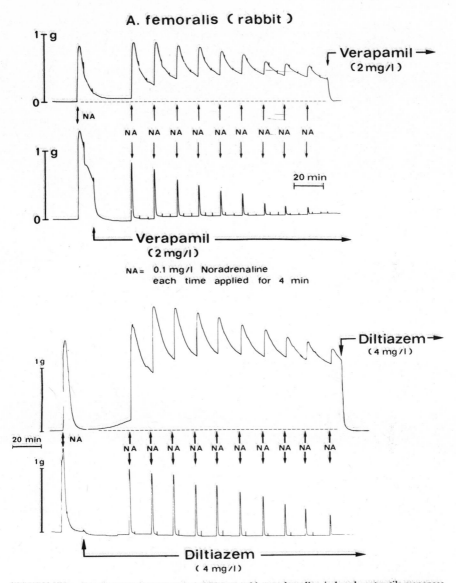

FIGURE 170. Interference of verapamil or diltiazem with noradrenaline-induced contractile responses of 4 smooth muscle strips dissected from a rabbit femoral artery. Obviously verapamil or diltiazem instantaneously suppresses the slow tonic components of the noradrenaline action, whereas it takes 2 to 3 hours until the sharp phasic peak contractions in the corresponding lower experiments are abolished as well. From Fleckenstein-Grün and Fleckenstein (1978/1980; 1980/1981).

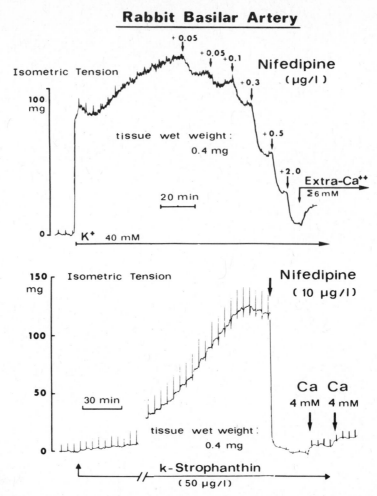

FIGURE 171. Complete relaxation by minute concentrations of nifedipine of two contractured rabbit basilar artery strips. (*A*) The contractile response of a K-depolarized basilar strip is abolished by a total of 3 µg/l nifedipine. (*B*) Instantaneous suppression of strophanthin-induced spasm of an electrically stimulated basilar strip with 10 µg/l nifedipine. Experiments of Nakayama, Byon, and Fleckenstein-Grün (1976), see also Fleckenstein-Grün and Fleckenstein (1978/1980).

strips are nearly as susceptible to relaxation by nifedipine or other Ca antagonists as those of *coronary strips* dissected from the same animals (Nakayama, Byon, and Fleckenstein-Grün, 1976). In another comparative study, both nifedipine and nimodipine inhibited K-induced rabbit coronary and basilar contractures by 50 to 60% at a concentration of $1 \times 10^{-9}\ M$, whereas a total suppression regularly took place under the influence of the same compounds at $1 \times 10^{-8}\ M$ (Nakayama and Fleckenstein, 1977, unpublished). Verapamil abolished these contractures at a concentration of $10^{-6}\ M$. The particularly high sensitivity of ouabain-induced contractions of *dog and monkey cerebral arteries* to verapamil and nifedipine has also recently been emphasized by Toda (1980).

Two other examples of vasoconstriction that were found to be responsive to Ca antagonists probably result from metabolic disorders of vascular Ca metabolism, namely (1) a rise in *pulmonal vascular resistance* following alveolar hypoxia, and (2) an increase in cerebrovascular flow *resistance* produced by previous cerebral ischemia. As to hypoxic pulmonal vasoconstriction, McMurtry, Davidson, Reeves, and Grover (1976) observed a sensitivity to verapamil that was so great that they attributed this kind of spasm to a direct depolarizing effect of hypoxia leading to an increased Ca uptake into the pulmonal vasculature. Also the postischemic reduction of cerebral blood perfusion seems to ensue from a basically similar mechanism. For instance in cats, cerebral flow resistance considerably increases with a time lag of about 30 min following total interruption of brain circulation for 7 min. Most animals will die within 24 hours. However, Kazda, Hoffmeister, Garthoff, and Towart (1979), using nimodipine (1 mg/kg orally), were able to prevent this delayed impairment of cerebral blood supply. Accordingly, the mortality of the cats decreased from 90 to 10%. Since the researchers observed a postischemic rise in the interstitial K concentration, they suggested that the cerebral vasoconstriction might be due to local spasms produced by an augmentation of Ca influx upon K-induced depolarization of the cerebral vasculature. In fact, as shown in our studies, nimodipine, besides nifedipine and niludipine, is the most powerful antidote against this kind of contractile activation. Other vasodilators that increase cerebral blood flow in normal cats such as papaverine, moxaverine, cinnarizine, isoxsuprine, and vincamine did not influence the postischemic vasospasm and survival (Kazda and Hoffmeister, 1979).

Obviously Ca antagonists counteract, also on systemic arteries, rather different types of vasoconstriction with remarkable strength. Among the arterial spasms neutralizable with Ca antagonists, those produced by Ca-synergistic cardiac glycosides are clinically most interesting. This is because such spasms may superimpose themselves on organic stenosing processes in overdigitalized elderly patients with generalized atherosclerosis. The best documented vascular complication of digitalization consists of a *spastic constriction of the superior mesenteric artery*. Even in healthy dogs and monkeys, cardiac glycosides narrow this vessel (Harrison, Blaschke, Phillips, Price, de Cotten, and Jacobson, 1969; Shanbour, Jacobson, Brobmann, and Hinshaw, 1971; Treat, Ulano, Jacobson, 1971; Brobmann, Barth, Strecker, Schmidt-Hieber, and Schmidt, 1975). Mesenteric blood flow decreases in response to even low glycoside concentrations that fail to significantly alter systemic arterial and portal venous pressures or heart rate and rhythm. The extent of mesenteric vasoconstriction proved to be dose related and rose steadily with the amounts of drug injected or infused.

Clearly, these findings on dogs and monkeys are also relevant to clinical pathology because there is ample evidence that strong doses of cardiac glycosides can also severely impair intestinal blood supply in humans (Ferrer, Bradley, Wheeler, Enson, Preisig, and Harvey, 1965). As a possible consequence, infarctlike ischemic necrosis of the gut may develop (Gazes, Holmes, Moseley, and Pratt-Thomas,

1961; Polansky, Berger, and Byrne, 1964; Muggia, 1967; Hess and Stucki, 1975). However, it is to be expected that these intestinal complications of overdigitalization, which are often lethal, can also be overcome with the help of Ca antagonists as antidotes. As an example, Figure 172 shows angiograms, taken by Brobmann, Barth, Strecker, Schmidt-Hieber, and Schmidt (1975), of the main branches of the mesenteric arterial tree of a dog before and 30 min after intravenous injection of k-strophanthin (0.05 mg/kg body weight). Under the influence of the glycoside, the width of these branches was decreased, due partially to even vasoconstriction, partially to severe local vasospasms. Thus in a series of experiments, mesenteric blood flow was lowered in strophanthin-treated dogs by 50% on the average. How-

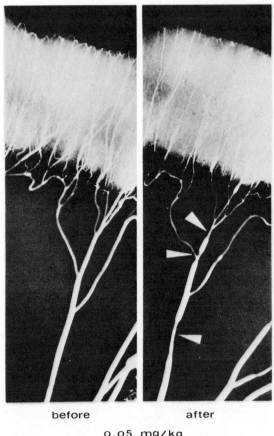

before   after

o.o5 mg/kg
k- strophanthin

FIGURE 172.   Angiogram of canine mesenteric artery. Occurrence within 30 min of spastic contractions of branches of upper mesenteric artery following intravenous injection of k-strophanthin (0.05 mg/kg) in an anesthetized dog. Complete suppression of strophanthin-induced spasms could be achieved within 3 min by intravenous injection of verapamil. From Brobmann, Barth, Strecker, Schmidt-Hieber, and Schmidt (1975).

ever, with the help of verapamil, the glycoside-induced spasms were not only abolished within 3 min, but mesenteric blood flow even increased by 50% above the initial values measured prior to glycoside administration (Brobmann, Mayer, Grimm, and Safer, 1978/1980). Traditionally, clinical practice has focussed upon the cardiac actions of the glycosides but has not sufficiently taken account of the vasoconstrictor effects that can, under certain conditions, seriously jeopardize the therapeutic success. A simultaneous prophylactic treatment with Ca antagonists would certainly improve the safety of glycoside administration.

6.2.8. Inhibition by Calcium Antagonists of Stretch-Induced Autoregulatory Vasoconstriction

When the distending pressure within a blood vessel increases, it is one of the most fundamental properties of the vascular wall to respond by constriction. This reaction reflects the well-known tendency of the vascular system to maintain constant blood flow through an organ, despite changes in arterial perfusion pressure. As postulated first by Biedl and Reiner (1900) and by Bayliss (1902), the phenomenon of vasoconstrictive "autoregulation" of blood supply is of "myogenic" nature in that pressure-induced stretch of the vascular wall acts as a mechanical stimulus for vascular smooth muscle contraction. Thus the mechanical strain on the vascular wall is an important factor that can, in addition to various tissue metabolites, hormones, and neurotransmitters, actively change the arterial caliber. This is true of the small resistance vessels as well as of the large arteries. For instance, vasoconstriction produced by intravascular pressure elevation has been described in kidney, skeletal muscle, brain, intestine, myocardium, and liver (see Johnson, 1964). Since naturally these contractile responses require Ca, they are also susceptible to Ca antagonists.

Pressure-Flow Studies on Intact Vessels. Evidence for the existence of autoregulation has usually been obtained from pressure-flow studies. When in such experiments the perfusion pressure is suddenly elevated to a higher level, flow initially increases to a peak value following passive expansion of vessels. But as soon as autoregulation commences flow tends to return toward the control level because of an active increase in vascular resistance. The significant Ca dependency of autoregulatory vasoconstriction can easily be seen from Figure 173. Here the vascular responses of an isolated rabbit ear to a stepwise increase of perfusion pressure were examined by measurement of the flow rates at elevated, normal, and minute Ca concentrations. The left part of the figure represents the behavior of a rabbit ear when the Ca concentration of the perfusion fluid was doubled. Here the graded increase in perfusion pressure evoked reactive vasoconstriction. By this well-known autoregulatory mechanism, the high initial outflow rates were partially reduced at each pressure step. The middle part of the figure represents the same rabbit ear perfused with Tyrode solution of normal Ca content. Now the same stepwise increases of perfusion pressure produced only small reactive vasoconstrictions. On the right, the perfusion fluid was Ca-free. This led to a complete loss of

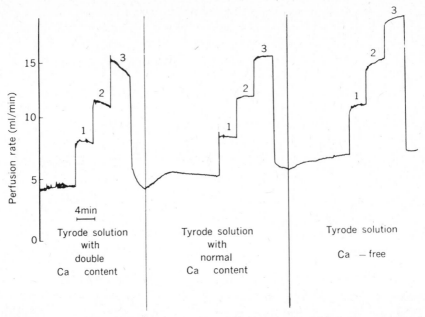

FIGURE 173. Perfusion of an isolated rabbit ear with Tyrode solutions of different Ca concentrations. Decrease in vascular tone and loss of reactive vasoconstrictor responses to stepwise augmentation of hydrostatic pressure as a result of perfusion with a Ca-free fluid. Increase in tone and reactive vasoconstriction produced by doubling the normal Ca concentration of 1.8 mM (pH 8.3; temperature, 18°C). Basal perfusion pressure, 40 cm H_2O; step 1, 50 cm H_2O; step 2, 60 cm H_2O; step 3, 70 cm H_2O. Reproduced from Grün and Fleckenstein (1972).

vascular tone and of stretch-activated vasoconstriction so that passive extensibility of the vascular bed became the only limiting factor for the perfusion rate.

As expected, the Ca antagonists prenylamine, verapamil, D 600, nifedipine, and other 1,4-dihydropyridines also exactly imitate the effects of Ca deficiency on rabbit ears (Grün, Fleckenstein, and Byon, 1971/1972; Grün and Fleckenstein, 1972; Fleckenstein, Fleckenstein-Grün, Byon, Haastert, and Späh, 1979). Figure 174, for instance, shows the action of 1 mg D 600/l in the perfusion fluid. On the left, without D 600, vascular tone and reactive vasoconstriction were marked. Under the influence of D 600, in the middle part of the figure, tone and vascular reactivity disappeared. But as soon as an extra dose of Ca was administered, on the right, the effect of D 600 was rapidly overcome and vascular tone and reactive vasoconstriction were even potentiated. The same type of experiment with the use of nifedipine is shown in Figure 175. Here addition of a dose as low as 0.2 mg/l led to an immediate vasodilation and produced contractile irresponsiveness to increases in perfusion pressure. But even in this case the vascular reactivity could be restored in the presence of nifedipine by an eightfold augmentation of the Ca concentration of the perfusion fluid (up to 14.4 mM).

In comparison with phasic vasoconstriction by noradrenaline, the pressure-induced contractions of the rabbit ear vessels are characterized by a higher sensitivity

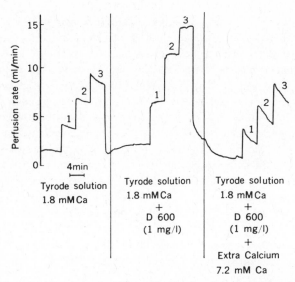

FIGURE 174. Perfusion of an isolated rabbit ear with Tyrode solution containing the Ca-antagonistic compound D 600 (1 mg/l). This produces a decrease in vascular tone and a loss of reactive vasoconstriction as if the ear were perfused with a Ca-free fluid. Subsequent neutralization of drug effects by addition of extra Ca (pH 8.3; temperature, 18°C). Basal perfusion pressure, 15 cm H_2O; step 1, 25 cm H_2O; step 2, 35 cm H_2O; step 3, 45 cm H_2O. Reproduced from Grün and Fleckenstein (1972).

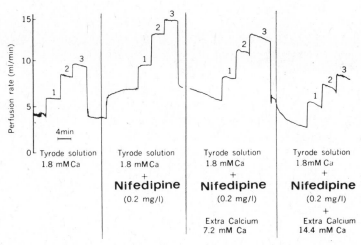

FIGURE 175. Perfusion of an isolated rabbit ear with Tyrode solution containing nifedipine in a concentration as low as 0.2 mg/l. Upon addition of the drug, the extensibility of the ear vessels immediately increases so that the outflow volume grows even at the baseline pressure of 35 cm H_2O. Stepwise augmentation of perfusion pressure (step 1, 45 cm H_2O, step 2, 55 cm H_2O; step 3, 65 cm H_2O) finally produces an almost maximal outflow volume without any sign of autoregulatory vasoconstriction. Elevation of the Ca concentration in the nifedipine-containing Tyrode solution from 1.8 to 7.2 and eventually 14.4 mM even overcompensates the Ca-antagonistic nifedipine effects. Principal experimental conditions as in Figures 173 and 174. From Grün and Fleckenstein (1972).

to Ca withdrawal and Ca antagonists (Grün and Fleckenstein, 1972). Similarly, in the absence of Ca, the contractile responses of human umbilical arteries to increases in transmural pressure ceased much faster than the responses to bradykinin, 5-hydroxytryptamine, or angiotensin did (Davignon, Lorenz, and Shepherd, 1965). These observations suggest that stretch-induced autoregulatory vasoconstriction is obligatorily dependent on transmembrane Ca supply rather than caused by receptor-mediated Ca release from cellular storage sites. Although direct evidence is hitherto lacking, it seems reasonable to suppose that Ca entry into stretched vascular smooth muscle cells is as "potential-dependent" (or in other words caused by membrane depolarization) as in visceral smooth muscle where the first reaction to stretch consists of local or conducted electric membrane discharges (Bozler, 1947; Bülbring, 1955; Burnstock and Prosser, 1960). Accordingly, there are obvious analogies between (1) vascular smooth muscle activation by an elevated extracellular K concentration, representing the prototype of potential-dependent vasoconstriction, and (2) the contractile responses to a rise in intravascular pressure. The common features found in our perfusion experiments are as follows:

1. Instantaneous cessation of contractile activity upon Ca withdrawal, administration of organic Ca antagonists, or acidification of the extracellular fluid.
2. Enormous potentiation of tension development in a Ca-rich alkaline medium.
3. No suppression of the mechanical responses by adrenergic α- or β-receptor blockade, atropine, histaminergic H_1 or H_2 blockade, or pretreatment with reserpine.

Our results, obtained on perfused vessels of rabbit ears, fit well with observations on other organs. Thus changing the pH to lower values or increasing the pCO_2 is a well-known measure to abolish vascular tone and autoregulatory constriction in brain arteries (Rapela and Green, 1964). Conversely, an alkalotic shift of cerebral blood pH is a constrictive stimulus (see the review on brain circulation of Betz, 1975). Next to brain, most investigations into the mechanism of autoregulation have been performed on perfused kidneys, where the maintenance of a stable level of blood flow in spite of fluctuation in arterial blood pressure seems to be of primary physiological importance. Using the smooth muscle relaxant papaverine, Thurau and Kramer (1959) first abolished "myogenic" renal autoregulation with pharmacological means. However, in the light of our present knowledge, the inhibitory action of papaverine on autoregulatory renal vasoconstriction is rather modest in comparison with the outstanding efficacy of specific Ca antagonists (see Ono, Kokubun, and Hashimoto, 1974). For instance, in a more recent study by Hashimoto, Ono, and O'Hara (1978/1980), renal autoregulation was completely abolished in anesthetized dogs of 10 to 20 kg body weight by intraarterial infusion of the following drugs: papaverine, 5 mg/min; perhexiline, 0.5 mg/min; verapamil, 0.1 mg/min; diltiazem, 0.03 mg/min; and nifedipine, 0.01 mg/in. This would indicate an order of potency of 1 (papaverine): 10 (perhexiline): 50 (verapamil): 150 (diltiazem); 500 (nifedipine). Furthermore, as a unique characterization of "specific"

Ca antagonists, it turned out that renal autoregulation could be protected by simultaneous infusion of extra Ca (30 mg CaCl₂/min). On the other hand, "common" smooth muscle relaxants such as papaverine or aminophylline were not neutralized by this treatment (Hashimoto, Ono, and O'Hara (1978/1980). In principle, the above order of potency is consistent with our own observations, although in our experience the strength of diltiazem does not exceed that of verapamil.

Stretch Experiments on Isolated Vascular Smooth Muscle. Since stretch appears to be the determinant factor in autoregulatory vasoconstriction, it seems feasible to study the nature of this phenomenon in a direct way also, that is to say, by stretch experiments on isolated smooth muscle strips from the vascular wall. This procedure offers the possibility of exact measurements on the quantitative relationship between passive distension and active constriction under rigidly controlled experimental conditions. Studies of this type were first carried out by Sparks and Bohr (1962) and by Sparks (1964) on helical strips of canine superior mesenteric and cerebral as well as human umbilical arteries. In analogous investigations of our laboratory, Nakayama and Fleckenstein used spiral strips of rabbit coronary and cerebral arteries. Figure 176 represents an experiment in which a series of quick stretches of increasing amplitude (elongation by 10 to 40%, related to the "resting length") were applied to a rabbit basilar artery strip, whereas the rate of stretch (10 cm/sec) was kept constant. The total tension that developed in response to these stretches was measured with a mechanoelectric transducer. The records consist of two components, that is, a passive viscoelastic force (A), and an actively generated tension (B) that is superimposed on the passive force (A). However, there is no difficulty in discriminating between these two components, since it turned out in

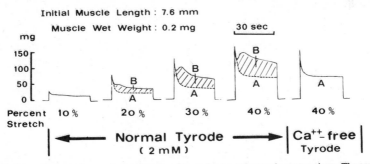

FIGURE 176. Ca dependency of stretch-induced vascular smooth muscle contractions. The generation of active tension (represented by the hatched area, (B) is superimposed on the passive viscoelastic force, (A), during a series of quick stretches of a steady rate (10 cm/sec) but of increasing amplitude (10 to 40% of the control resting length). *Resting length* is defined as the muscle length 20% above the "initial length" of the unloaded preparation. With a quick stretch of 40% above resting length, optimal contractile activation is obtained. However, in the absence of free Ca, the active contractile responses to stretch, (B), totally disappear. General experimental procedure: ultrathin isolated strips excised from the wall of rabbit cerebral arteries (A. basilaris) in Tyrode solution, gassed with 97% O₂ and 3% CO₂ at a temperature of 35°C and a pH of 7.35. From Nakayama and Fleckenstein, unpublished.

our studies that the generation of active tension (hatched areas in Figure 176) completely ceases in a Ca-free medium or in the presence of Ca antagonists such as verapamil (1 mg/l), diltiazem (1 mg/l), or nifedipine (100 μg/l). Thus following Ca withdrawal or addition of Ca antagonists, only the passive viscoelastic force A is left. Figure 177 shows that the contractile responses to a 40% stretch were fairly reproducible, with an interval of 20 min, for more than 2 hours until, at the end of the experiment, verapamil suppressed the active component. Divalent Mg, Mn, Co, and Ni ions, which also compete with Ca in excitation–contraction coupling of vascular smooth muscle, acted alike.

However, it is to be remembered that the first reaction that precedes excitation–contraction coupling in the sequence of events probably consists of a stretch-induced decrease in membrane potential. The theory that depolarization of the membrane triggers the active responses to stretch has been strongly supported in studies on spiral strips of human umbilical arteries by Sparks (1964). He found that predepolarization with a Tyrode solution of elevated K content increased the sensitivity to stretch considerably. On the other hand, stabilization of the membrane at a high Ca content of the medium caused desensitization to stretch. Our own observations on rabbit coronary and basilar artery strips have fully confirmed these findings. Certainly under resting conditions, the extracellular Ca ions, even at the physiologically low interstitial concentration of around 1 mM, predominantly act as a brake on stretch-induced active vasoconstriction by virtue of an elevation of threshold. With higher extracellular Ca concentrations, this effect further increases. Conversely, also in our experiments, predepolarization with a K-rich Tyrode solution (10 to 20 mM K), strongly potentiated height and duration of stretch-induced active tension development (Figure 178). When, however, verapamil (1 mg/l) was added in the presence of 20 mM K, the overshooting active responses were again totally blocked. A similar potentiation of the active responses to stretch as with high K could be produced in our studies on rabbit basilar artery strips, also with

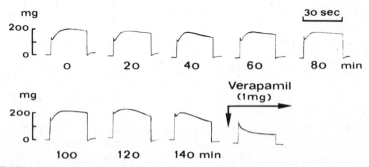

FIGURE 177.   Perfect reproducibility of the contractile responses to repetitive stretches (40% above resting length) of an isolated rabbit basilar artery strip (wet weight 0.5 mg) during an observation period of 140 min. Following addition of verapamil (time of incubation in Figures 177 to 181 always 20 min), contractile reactivity to stretch completely ceases. General experimental procedure as in Figure 176. From Nakayama and Fleckenstein, unpublished.

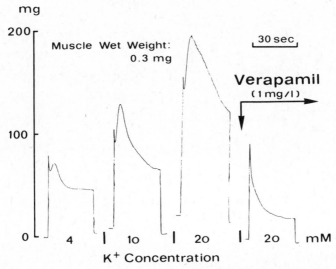

FIGURE 178. Partial predepolarization by elevation of K_o of the Tyrode solution (from 4 to 10 and finally 20 mM) strongly sensitizes the isolated vasculature (rabbit basilar artery strip) to active tension development upon repetitive quick stretches (40% above resting length). The dramatic increase of responsiveness to stretch as well as every contractile vascular reaction is totally abolished by a small dose of verapamil (1 mg/l). General experimental procedure as in Figure 176. Unpublished observations of Nakayama and Fleckenstein.

noradrenaline, histamine, serotonin, tetraethylammonium, and *cardiac glycosides.* These substances obviously lower the threshold of stretch-induced activation. The doses that facilitate in this way the switching from membrane quiescence to action proved to be identical with those necessary for a slight increase in potential-dependent basal tone. Thus also in these cases, the sensitization to stretch-induced active tension development is in all probability due to predepolarization. Needless to say, again a standard dose (1 mg/l) of verapamil regularly abolished every kind of reactive vascular motility (see Figures 179 to 181). But with suitable doses of additional Ca, not exceeding a final concentration of 6 to 8 mM, the active responses to stretch could mostly be resuscitated in the verapamil-treated vasculature (Figure 180). However, the simultaneous stabilization of membrane potential by an elevated level of extracellular Ca may sometimes limit the extent of recovery of stretch-induced vascular constriction.

6.2.9. Vasodilator Actions of Calcium Antagonists on Peripheral Resistance Vessels in Hypertension

With respect to hypertension, it is an open question whether autoregulatory vasoconstriction, apart from its physiological role, might also be a phenomenon of pathophysiological significance. In fact, autoregulatory vasoconstriction represents

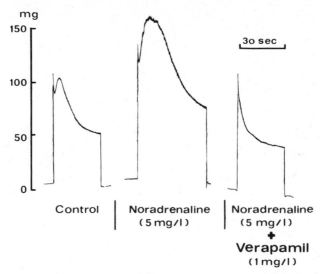

FIGURE 179. Noradrenaline, like predepolarization with an elevated extracellular K-concentration in Figure 178, also provokes potentiated contractile responses of a rabbit basilar artery strip (wet weight, 0.3 mg) to repetitive quick stretches (40% above resting length). This sensitization occurs in connection with a moderate increase in potential-dependent basal tone. Again verapamil (1 mg/l) completely suppresses the large active component of the stretch-induced tension curves. General experimental procedures as in Figure 176. From Nakayama and Fleckenstein, unpublished.

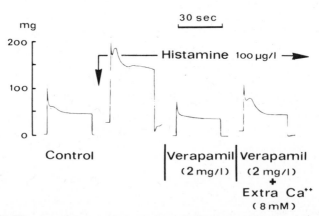

FIGURE 180. Sensitization by histamine of a rabbit basilar artery strip (wet weight, 0.3 mg) to repetitive stretches (40% above resting length). After the active response has disappeared under the influence of 2 mg verapamil/l, addition of extra Ca to the Tyrode solution (elevation of Ca_o from 2 to 8 mM) restores the reactivity to stretch in the presence of verapamil. From Nakayama and Fleckenstein, unpublished.

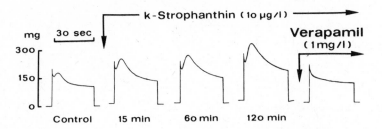

Muscle Wet Weight : 0.4 mg

FIGURE 181. Strophanthin, by potentiating Ca-dependent mechanical vascular smooth muscle activity, also enhances the contractile responses to a series of quick stretches (40% above resting length) of a rabbit basilar strip. Conversely, verapamil abolishes not only the sensitization by strophanthin, but also the total contractile responsiveness to stretch. From Nakayama and Fleckenstein, unpublished.

a positive feedback mechanism in that an initial rise in intravascular pressure evokes a contractile response that in turn further increases pressure in the vascular bed. Moreover, vasoconstrictor agonists strongly potentiate the efficacy of the stretch impulses. Without effective brakes, a mechanism of this kind would easily escape control. Thus an exaggerated autoregulatory vasoconstriction could possibly bear on the origin of hypertension. Folkow (1964) has insinuated this idea with the following statement: "There arises here a matter of potential interest in some types of hypertension. Perhaps these brake mechanisms can be overpowered, leading to increased flow resistance if a primary transmembrane ionic shift has facilitated the myogenic activity and enhanced the Bayliss mechanism in the small resistance vessels. In dealing with a multifaceted pathophysiological disturbance such as hypertension, I think one must be open to *all* possibilities."

Indeed, the main effort in the treatment of hypertension has for a long time aimed primarily at lowering sympathetic vascular tone of the resistance vessels in systemic circulation. For this purpose nearly all practicable measures have been tried, such as the following:

1. Damping central sympathetic activity with tranquilizers.
2. Ganglionic blockade.
3. Depletion of catecholamine stores with reserpine.
4. Inhibition of sympathetic transmitter release with guanethidine.
5. Use of α-methyldopa to cause biosynthesis of unnatural, less-effective, sympathetic transmitters.
6. Adrenergic α-receptor blockade.

But now, with the help of Ca antagonists, a more direct intervention is possible. These drugs, by interference with Ca, counteract the common final link in the chain

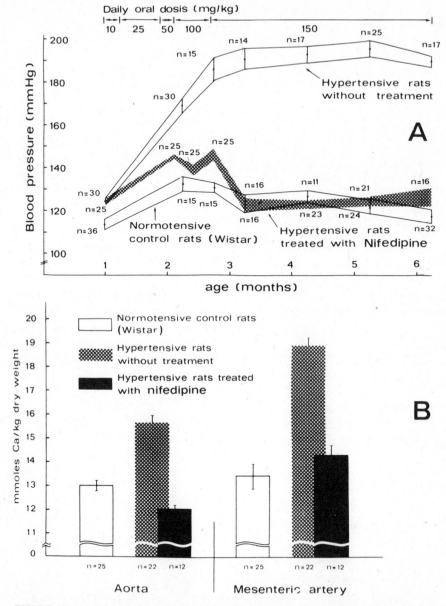

FIGURE 182. (*A*) Normalization of mean arterial blood pressure of rats suffering from spontaneous hypertension by chronic oral administration of nifedipine during 5 months. Treatment with nifedipine lasted from the end of the first to the end of the sixth month of age. However, there was a rapid rise in tension to the level of untreated hypertensive rats as soon as therapy was discontinued. Data from v. Witzleben, Frey, Keidel, and Fleckenstein (1980); see Fleckenstein and Fleckenstein-Grün (1980). (*B*) Restriction of Ca overload of the arterial walls of spontaneously hypertensive rats by the treatment with oral nifedipine over 5 months [same rats as in (*A*)].

of vasoconstrictive reactions irrespective of the special circumstances, that is, regardless of whether hypertension results from an excessive concentration of pressor agents or from excessive vascular reactivity.

To visualize the antihypertensive effect of Ca antagonists in animal experiments, v. Witzleben, Frey, Keidel, and Fleckenstein (1980) treated spontaneously hypertensive rats with daily oral doses of verapamil and nifedipine for 4 months. The therapy was started at the age of 1 month. As can be seen from the upper curve of Figure 182, rats that were not given nifedipine showed an increase in blood pressure of nearly 100% within 4 months, that is up to almost 200 mm Hg. In contrast, rats treated with nifedipine behaved like normotensive control rats of the same age, that is, the blood pressure of the nifedipine-treated rats remained at the low level of 110 mm Hg. Moreover, vascular damage, consisting of progressive calcinosis of the arterial media, was prevented. When, however, the therapy was discontinued, arterial blood pressure rapidly rose, and subsequently the Ca uptake into the arterial smooth musculature was also intensified. In another series of experiments on spontaneously hypertensive rats, verapamil was used for the control of blood pressure. The efficiacy of verapamil was practically identical to that of nifedipine (see Fleckenstein-Grün and Fleckenstein, 1981). The growth rate of the rats treated with nifedipine was not retarded in comparison with that of untreated hypertensive rats. Normalization of high blood pressure by chronic treatment with nifedipine was also observed in Na-loaded salt-sensitive Dahl rats (Garthoff and Kazda, 1981). Similarly, conscious renal-hypertensive dogs are rather responsive to Ca antagonists. As shown by Hiwatari and Taira (1979), an acute fall of blood pressure could be obtained in these animals with a single oral dose of 1 to 3 mg niludipine/kg. Diltiazem too proved to be effective in the treatment of spontaneously hypertensive, renal-hypertensive and desoxycorticosterone/saline-loaded hypertensive rats (Kiyomoto, 1978/1979). Thus it is not surprising that the Ca antagonists are useful drugs also for practical antihypertensive therapy (see Section 7.4).

In conclusion, the powerful vasodilator action of Ca antagonists is not restricted to the coronary bed, since other types of vascular smooth muscle originating from aorta and the pulmonal, cerebral, renal, mesenteric, femoral, or ear arteries are responsive as well. As schematically illustrated in Figure 183, contraction of all types of vascular smooth muscle basically depends on the availability of free Ca ions for the activation of myofibrillar ATPase. The Ca ions are either supplied from extracellular sources through potential-dependent or receptor-operated Ca channels that are opened by electric, mechanical, or pharmacological stimuli, or alternatively, released from cellular storage sites by nonelectric mechanisms. Regardless of certain peculiarities of the coronary vasculature, the scheme of Figure 183 summarizes the principles of vascular smooth muscle activation as well as the modes of inhibition in a general way. The Ca antagonists block directly, and most effectively, potential- or receptor-dependent transmembrane Ca supply, but also impair transmembrane replenishment of the cellular stores, an effect that appears often with some delay. But lastly, under the influence of Ca antagonists, every kind of contractile smooth muscle activity can be damped in a dose-related manner.

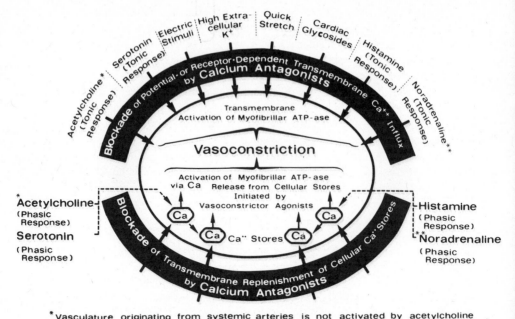

*Vasculature originating from systemic arteries is not activated by acetylcholine

**Noradrenaline produces contraction of extramural coronary vasculature only after previous β-receptor blockade

FIGURE 183. Scheme of the dual source of activator Ca for the tonic and phasic vascular smooth muscle contractions, i.e., (1) potential- or receptor-dependent transmembrane Ca supply for tonic responses, and (2) release of Ca from cellular stores for phasic responses to vasoconstrictor agonists. The Ca antagonists inhibit directly and most effectively transmembrane Ca influx, i.e., pathway 1. However, to a lesser extent, Ca antagonists also interfere with pathway 2, probably indirectly by impairing transmembrane replenishment of cellular Ca stores. The exact anatomical location of these cellular Ca stores is a pending problem (plasma membrane, inner surface of plasma membrane, SR structures?).

6.3.   PROPHYLACTIC ACTIONS OF CALCIUM ANTAGONISTS AGAINST EXPERIMENTAL CALCINOSIS

6.3.1.   Protection by Calcium Antagonists against Arterial Media Calcification (Mönckeberg's Type of Arteriosclerosis Produced by Dihydrotachysterol or Vitamin D)

It is well known from observations on rats and rabbits that a combined treatment with large doses of dihydrotachysterol plus monosodium phosphate as well as intoxication with vitamin D not only produces calcified myocardial necroses, but also causes extensive calcinosis of the arterial media. These experimental vascular alterations are quite similar to Mönckeberg's type of calcifying arteriosclerosis in humans (Herzenberg, 1929; Selye, 1958; Hass, Trucheart, Taylor, and Stumpe,

1958; Eisenstein and Zeruolis, 1964). As already pointed out by Herzenberg (1929), the process of media calcification affects particularly the smooth muscle cells and the elastic fibers. In Herzenberg's experiments on vitamin D–intoxicated rats, calcification of cardiac cells and arterial smooth muscle was always so intimately associated with degenerative processes that it appeared impossible to find out whether calcification or, alternatively, necrotization had to be considered the primary event. However, in the light of our present knowledge of Ca overload as a causative factor in the production of myocardial lesions (see Chapter 3), it was reasonable to assume that in experimental Mönckeberg sclerosis, histological damage also ensues from abundant cellular Ca engulfment.

It was, in fact, not difficult to show that the background of experimental Mönckeberg sclerosis is an enormous intensification of Ca uptake into the arterial walls. For instance, Figure 184A represents experiments in which the net uptake rates of ^{45}Ca into aorta and mesenteric artery were measured during an observation period of 6 hours, both in normal control rats and in rats pretreated for 10 consecutive days with daily oral doses of dihydrotachysterol (0.5 mg DHT/kg) plus monosodium phosphate (20 mmol/kg) (Janke, Hein, Pachinger, Leder, and Fleckenstein, 1971/1972. In the latter animals the speed of vascular ^{45}Ca incorporation was found to be 50 to 70 times greater than normal. In another series of experiments on rats (Figure 184B), vitamin D_3 was administered intramuscularly in the form of a water-soluble cholecalciferol preparation (Vi-De$_3$-Hydrosol®, Wander AG, Bern, Switzerland), in order to avoid the risk of inconstant intestinal D_3 absorption. Here, following one single injection of a high dose of vitamin D_3 (500,000 IU/kg body weight) the rate of net radiocalcium uptake into the wall of the mesenteric artery grew by 35 to 40 times within 3 days. The increase was still 13- to 14-fold when a lower dose of 300,000 IU/kg had been given. The sensitivity of the aortic wall and the ventricular myocardium to vitamin D_3 was somewhat smaller. Nevertheless, even in these tissues, net ^{45}Ca incorporation rose by a factor of 5 to 6 in response to 300,000 IU/kg.

As discussed in Section 3.4, myocardial Ca overload caused by such single vitamin D_3 injections always induces multifocal necrotization in the ventricular wall. Similarly, in the Ca-overloaded vasculature, a rapid disintegration also takes place. Then the electron microscopic appearance of the calcified arterial media is characterized by two morphological alterations (Eisenstein and Zeruolis, 1964):

1. The presence of needlelike crystals, presumably apatite, and fine electron-dense granules in the interior of the smooth muscle cells. In addition, there are vacuoles in the cytoplasm and structural changes in the mitochondria representing further criteria of cellular decay.

2. The occurrence in the extracellular stroma of densely calcified elements such as mineralized elastic fibers and calcific plaques of crystalline structure, mostly in close contact with the plasma membrane of heavily damaged smooth muscle cells.

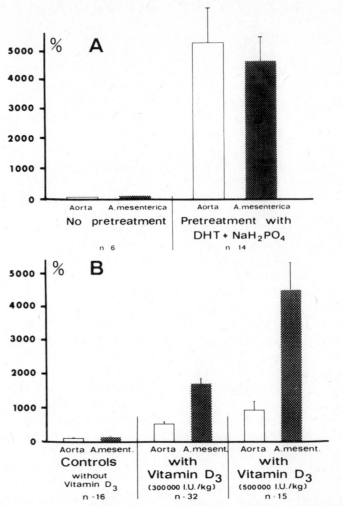

FIGURE 184. Massive increase in net ^{45}Ca uptake into the arterial walls (aorta and mesenteric artery) of rats (A) following pretreatment during 10 consecutive days with daily oral doses of dihydrotachysterol (0.5 mg DHT/kg) plus monosodium phosphate (20 mmol/kg), or (B) produced within 80 hours by a single intramuscular injection of 300,000 or 500,000 IU vitamin D_3 hydrosol/kg. All animals were finally given intraperitoneally 10 μCi ^{45}Ca/kg body weight, and killed 6 hours later for measurements of radioactivity in blood plasma and arterial walls. Then the net radiocalcium uptake into 1 g of fresh arterial tissue was calculated as the percentage of radioactivity simultaneously determined in 1 ml plasma (= 100%). Reproduced from Frey, Keidel, and Fleckenstein (1978/1980).

FIGURE 185. (A) Inhibition of the vitamin-D_3-stimulated net radiocalcium uptake into the right and left ventricular myocardium of rats by subcutaneous or oral administration of verapamil. Following injection of a single intramuscular dose of 300,000 IU vitamin D_3 hydrosol/kg body weight, the ^{45}Ca uptake rate rose within 80 hours by approximately 6 to 7 times. With a daily dose of 2 × 30 mg verapamil/kg body weight subcutaneously or a daily dose of 2 × 100 mg verapamil/kg orally administered for 4 days, the effects of vitamin D_3 were almost completely neutralized. Measurements of the radiocalcium uptake into the myocardium according to the procedure applied in Figure 184 for the arterial walls. From Frey, Keidel, and Fleckenstein (1978/1980). (B) Analogous to (A), however, with the use of an oral dose of 500 mg diltiazem/kg (twice daily) for cardioprotection.

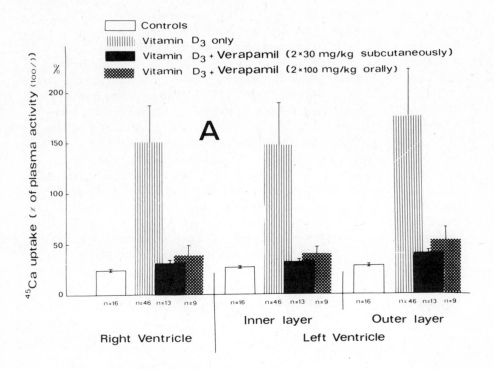

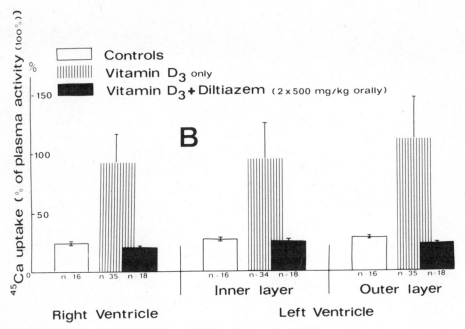

Also in our own experiments with injected vitamin D_3 hydrosol (300,000 IU/kg), all these electron microscopic signs of massive vascular Ca overload regularly appeared (Staubesand, personal communication). Conversely, Ca uptake into bone tissue (ribs) of the same animals was inhibited by roughly 60%.

The efficacy of certain Ca antagonists such as prenylamine and verapamil in preventing experimental vascular Ca overload, was first shown by Janke, Hein, Pachinger, Leder, and Fleckenstein (1971/1972) on rats pretreated with dihydrotachysterol and monosodium phosphate. However, the most impressive results were obtained with the help of verapamil and diltiazem in vitamin-D_3-injected rats. In fact, verapamil and diltiazem can protect the ventricular myocardium and the arterial walls against deleterious Ca overload with virtually equal strength. Figure 185 shows that suitable doses of both substances, applied orally or subcutaneously, reduce the vitamin-D_3-stimulated net radiocalcium uptake of the ventricular myocardium almost to the control level. Simultaneously, in the same vitamin-D_3-treated animals, verapamil and diltiazem suppressed the rate of Ca incorporation into the aortic and the mesenteric walls. Consequently, prophylactic doses of verapamil also prevented the absolute Ca contents of the vitamin-D_3-treated myocardium and arterial walls from a dangerous rise (see Figure 186). The percentages by which the vitamin D_3 effects on both [45]Ca incorporation and absolute Ca content were inhibited by verapamil can be seen from Tables 16 and 17. The data show that, indeed, the

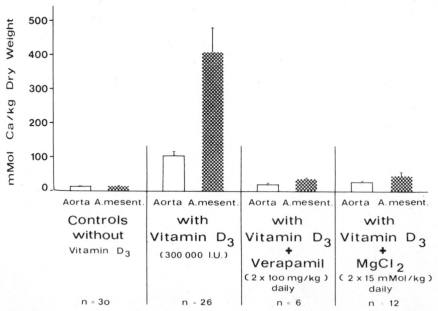

FIGURE 186. Inhibition of vitamin-D_3-induced Ca-overload of the walls of aorta and mesenteric artery of rats by oral administration of verapamil or $MgCl_2$ during 4 days. Determination of tissue Ca contents on the forth day after intramuscular injection of one single dose of 300,000 IU vitamin D_3 hydrosol/kg body weight. From Frey, Keidel, and Fleckenstein (1978/1980).

TABLE 16. Anticalcinotic Efficacy of Verapamil;
Inhibition of Net Vitamin-D_3-Stimulated Myocardial and
Arterial ^{45}Ca Incorporation by Subcutaneous or Oral
Administration of Verapamil[a,b]

	Inhibition by Subcutaneous Verapamil (%)	Inhibition by Oral Verapamil (%)
Right ventricle	94.0 (±2.2)	87.0 (±8.4)
Left ventricle (inner layer)	94.1 (±2.4)	86.5 (±7.7)
Left ventricle (outer layer)	90.5 (±2.5)	80.1 (±9.9)
Aorta	79.4 (±5.9)	71.7 (±11.7)
A. mesenterica sup.	77.9 (±8.7) $N = 13$	87.6 (±5.2) $N = 9$

[a]Experiments on rats. Part of the population received one single intramuscular injection of vitamin D_3 (300,000 IU/kg body weight) on the first day. The other animals were injected with the same dose of vitamin D_3, but received in addition on the first and on 3 subsequent days, a daily dose of 2 × 30 mg verapamil/kg subcutaneously or a daily dose of 2 × 100 mg verapamil/kg orally. On the 4th day, the net radiocalcium uptake rates into heart muscle and arterial walls were measured in all animals during an observation time of 6 hours following intraperitoneal administration of 10 μCi ^{45}Ca/kg. Then the vitamin-D_3-induced rise in Ca-uptake rate (in comparison with normal control animals) and the inhibition of this rise by verapamil (expressed as a percentage; complete inhibition = 100%) were calculated.
[b]From Frey, Keidel, and Fleckenstein (1978/1980).

protection by subcutaneous or oral verapamil against vitamin-D_3-stimulated Ca overload figures in the same range of 80 to 95% for both myocardium and arteries. Diltiazem not only interferes with vitamin-D_3-induced aortic and mesenteric calcinosis, but also with that of the colon (flexura dextra) and renal cortex (see Figure 187).

Similarly, arterial radiocalcium uptake and rise in Ca content was diminished in vitamin-D_3-poisoned rats by oral administration of $MgCl_2$ (see Figure 186 and Table 18). The latter results correspond with observations of Selye (1958), who described a prophylactic effect of $MgCl_2$ against the histological alterations of the arteries of rats treated with dihydrotachysterol plus monosodium phosphate. However, the influence of this prophylaxis on the arterial Ca incorporation was not analyzed by this author. Conversely, alimentary Mg deficiency seems to favor the development

TABLE 17. Anticalcinotic Efficacy of Verapamil; Inhibition of Vitamin-D$_3$-Stimulated Ca Overload of Myocardium and Arterial Walls of Rats by Subcutaneous or Oral Administration of Verapamil[a,b]

	Inhibition by *Subcutaneous* Verapamil (%)	Inhibition by *Oral* Verapamil (%)
Right ventricle	88.5 (±3.8)	81.9 (±6.8)
Left ventricle (inner layer)	86.2 (±4.0)	72.7 (±11.2)
Left ventricle (outer layer)	84.6 (±4.4)	78.3 (±8.5)
Aorta	81.4 (±9.0)	91.7 (±3.3)
A. mesenterica sup.	81.5 (±9.5)	93.8 (±1.2)
	$N = 14$	$N = 6$

[a]Determination of tissue Ca contents by atom absorption spectrometry on the 4th day after intramuscular injection of a single dose of 300,000 IU vitamin D$_3$ hydrosol/kg body weight. Dosage scheme and calculation of the inhibitory effects of verapamil as in Table 16.
[b]From Frey, Keidel, and Fleckenstein (1978/1980).

TABLE 18. Anticalcinotic Efficacy of Magnesium Salts; Inhibition of Vitamin-D$_3$-Induced Rise in ^{45}Ca-Incorporation Rate and in Absolute Ca Content of Myocardium and Arterial Walls of Rats by Oral Treatment with MgCl$_2$[a,b]

	Inhibition of rise ^{45}Ca Incorporation (%)	Inhibition of rise Ca Content (%)
Right ventricle	91.9 (±8.2)	85.6 (±7.2)
Left ventricle (apical region)	83.2 (±15.0)	81.7 (±9.3)
Aorta	92.4 (±4.9)	85.9 (±4.4)
A. mesenterica sup.	95.0 (±3.0)	92.5 (±3.5)
	$N = 13$	$N = 12$

[a]Determination of ^{45}Ca uptake and absolute Ca contents on the 4th day after intramuscular injection of a single dose of 300,000 IU vitamin D$_3$ hydrosol/kg body weight with or without additional MgCl$_2$ (oral administration of a daily dose of 2 × 15 mmol/kg on the first and on three subsequent days). Calculation of the inhibitory effects of MgCl$_2$ as in Tables 16 and 17.
[b]From Frey, Janke, and Fleckenstein, unpublished.

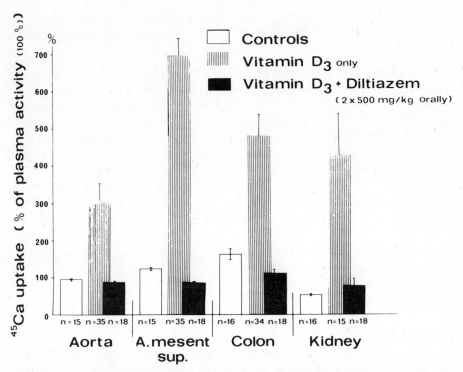

FIGURE 187. Inhibition of vitamin-D$_3$-stimulated net radiocalcium uptake into the walls of rat aorta and mesenteric artery by treatment with oral diltiazem. Simultaneously with inhibition of arterial ^{45}Ca incorporation, the vitamin-D$_3$-induced calcinosis of renal cortex and colon (flexura dextra) is totally prevented. The specimens of myocardium, aorta, mesenteric artery, kidney, and colon analyzed for ^{45}Ca uptake in Figures 185*B* and 187 originated from the same animals.

of arterial media calcinosis. This appears from observations on the occurrence of Mönckeberg's arteriosclerosis in herbivore domestic animals such as horse, cattle, sheep, and goat (Moore, Hallman, and Sholl, 1938; Pueschner and Gussman, 1970). Severe arterial calcinosis produced by a diet low in Mg was also found in experimental studies on rats (Merker and Guenther, 1970) and on dogs (Syllm-Rapoport and Strassburger, 1956; Vitale, Hellerstein, Nakamura, and Lown, 1961). In both vitamin-D$_3$-poisoned and Mg-deficient animals, calcification affected primarily vascular smooth muscle, elastic fibers in the arterial media, and the myocardium. Fragmentation and degeneration of mineralized elastic fibers was frequently seen. As clearly shown by our measurements, all these earlier morphological observations can now be backed by precise quantitative data. Obviously, Ca overload, induced by vitamin-D$_3$-poisoning or by a Mg-deficient regimen, starts a common pathogenic mechanism that leads to both myocardial necrotization and calcinotic arterial media destruction. On the other hand, treatment with Ca antagonists such as verapamil or diltiazem supported by an adequate alimentary Mg supply represents new means for preservation of myocardial and vascular integrity.

6.3.2. Prevention by Verapamil of Arterial Calcium Overload and Concomitant Lenticular Calcification Causing Cataracts in Alloxan-Diabetic Rats

In human pathology, Mönckeberg's type of arterial media calcinosis is a rather frequent complication of diabetes mellitus. Therefore, we have also examined in alloxan-diabetic rats whether such animals might possibly provide another suitable model for experimental investigations on vascular calcinosis and its prevention (Fleckenstein, v. Witzleben, Frey, and Milner, 1981). In these studies, alloxan (80 mg/kg) was intravenously administered to 2-month-old rats so that the blood sugar level rose to a steady value of around 420 mg% for an observation period of $6^1/_2$ months. During this time, the Ca content of the aortic and mesenteric artery walls did not rise dramatically, since there was only an increase in Ca of about 25% above normal. However a much more exciting observation was the following:

1. The majority of the alloxan-diabetic rats developed eye cataracts after a time lapse of about 3 months (Figure 188).

2. In alloxan-diabetic rats treated with verapamil, the occurrence of cataracts was minimal.

Thus without verapamil, 70 lenses out of 113 (= 62%) had become totally opaque after $6^1/_2$ months (see Figure 189). On the other hand, with a daily dose of 25 mg verapamil/kg body weight, given by means of a stomach tube, a loss of lense transparency was only discernible in 1 out of 26 eyes (= 3.9%). As shown in Figure 190, the Ca content of the diabetic lenses without verapamil treatment rose enormously, since in this series there was a 10-fold increase from 1.08 (± 0.02) to 10.89 (± 0.85) mmol Ca/kg dry weight on average. However, with verapamil, the lenticular mean Ca content of the diabetic animals remained in a low range of 3.46 (± 0.61) mmol/kg dry weight. Moreover, the rise in arterial Ca was completely prevented by this treatment. There was a highly significant correlation between Ca overload of the lenses and opacification, in that cataracts developed if the Ca content of the lenses exceeded a threshold value of 7 to 8 mmol/kg dry weight (see Figure 191). Verapamil, by keeping the Ca content of the diabetic lenses below this critical level, preserved transparency.

Untreated diabetic rats also exhibited a marked decrease in lenticular K concentration (from 18 to 2 to 3 mmol/kg dry weight) and a rise in Na content (from 110 to 155 mmol/kg dry weight), whereas the Mg level (7.5 mmol/kg dry weight) did not change within the observation period of $6^1/_2$ months. In addition, there was a progressive hydration of the untreated diabetic lenses when they became opaque. This tumescence was again clearly correlated with excessive lenticular Ca uptake (Figure 192). Verapamil, apart from protecting the diabetic lenses against Ca overload, also prevented, in proportion, these additional alterations in lenticular ion composition and water content.

The possible role of excessive lenticular Ca incorporation as an etiological factor in the development of cataracts is by no means a new problem. Thus the lenticular

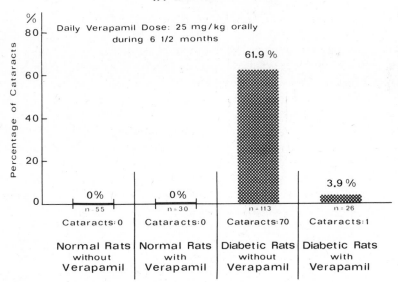

Occurrence (%) of Cataracts in Diabetic Rats

Without Verapamil

70 %

60 %

50 %

Daily Verapamil Dose: 25 mg/kg orally during 6 1/2 months

40 %

30 %

20 %

Alloxan

With Verapamil

0 %

| 0 | 1 | 2 | 3 | 4 | 5 | 6 |

Duration of alloxan diabetes (months)

Occurrence (%) of Cataracts in Diabetic Rats

Percentage of Cataracts

%
80

Daily Verapamil Dose: 25 mg/kg orally during 6 1/2 months

61.9 %

60

40

20

0

0%
n = 55
Cataracts: 0

0%
n = 30
Cataracts: 0

n = 113
Cataracts: 70

3.9 %
n = 26
Cataracts: 1

Normal Rats without Verapamil

Normal Rats with Verapamil

Diabetic Rats without Verapamil

Diabetic Rats with Verapamil

FIGURE 188. The first cataracts developed in alloxan-diabetic rats after a latency period of 3 months. Thereafter, more and more lenses became opaque. After 6½ months, 62% of the lenses of diabetic animals exhibited cataracts. However, chronic oral administration of verapamil fully protected transparency with the exception of only 1 lens. No cataracts were seen in nondiabetic rats, whether they were chronically treated with verapamil or not.

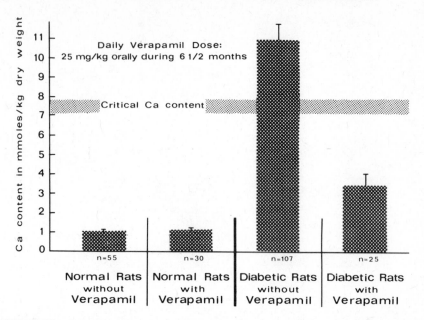

FIGURE 190. Prevention of lenticular Ca overload in alloxan-diabetic rats by long-term administration of verapamil. The columns represent means ± SE of the mean.

Ca content in senile human cataracts has often been shown to be markedly elevated (Burge, 1909; Adams, 1929; Salit, 1933; Duncan and Bushell, 1975). Salit, for instance, reported that the Ca-content of cataractous lenses does indeed show a 10-fold increase on the average. Similarly, in an extensive study of Jedziniak, Nicoli, Yates, and Benedek (1976), the mean Ca content of a total of 60 cataract lenses was, with 90% confidence, 2 to 13 times higher than the mean Ca concentration of normal lenses. As pointed out by Duncan and Bushell (1975), the Ca levels are usually very high in mature cataracts with cortical involvement, whereas conversely, the K content is far below normal in these cases. Obviously, diabetic cataracts correspond with this cortical type (Brooks, 1975). Pure nuclear cataracts, on the other hand, did not show such pronounced shifts in ion composition (Duncan and Bushell, 1975). However, in bovine lenses, the Ca content rises with increasing age in both the cortical region and the lens nucleus (Rink, Münnighoff, and Hockwin, 1977). There is also no doubt that any uptake of Ca, even in modest amounts, leads to a loss of lenticular transparency (Adams, 1929; Jedziniak, Kinoshita, Yates, Hocker, and Benedek, 1972; Spector and Rothschild, 1973; Spector, Adams, and Krul 1974). The Ca binding by the lenticular proteins, especially α-crystallin, results in the formation of high-molecular-weight aggregates that act as scattering centers for light and so produce clouding of the lens. In addition, it has been shown that accumulation of Ca by the lens creates concentrations that are much higher than those in the surrounding media, suggesting specific binding sites for Ca. Accordingly, in normal human lenses only 20% of the Ca was irremovable by long-term

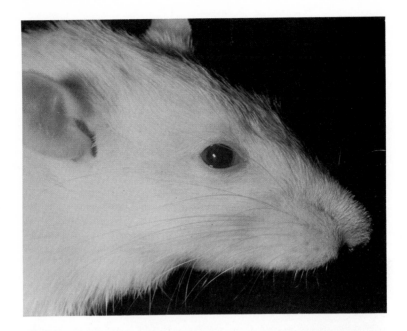

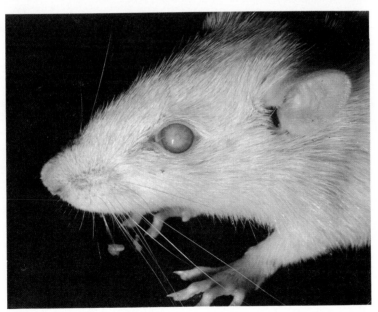

FIGURE 189. Once the critical Ca concentration is reached, the transition from normal transparency to the cataractous state of the diabetic lenses takes merely a few days. Only fully developed cataracts, as shown in this figure, were counted for statistical evaluation. The non-cataractous lenses were completely transparent.

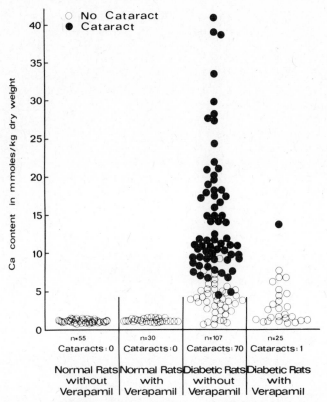

FIGURE 191. Quantitative correlation between lenticular Ca overload and development of cataracts in alloxan-diabetic rats with and without chronic oral administration of verapamil (25 mg/kg daily for 6½ months). Verapamil, by preventing excessive increases in lenticular Ca content, inhibited cataract formation.

dialysis, whereas in completely opaque lenses almost 70% of the Ca remained fixed within them (Racz and Kellermayer, 1978).

Thus the regulation of Ca concentration in the lens is an important factor in maintaining its high degree of transparency. Observations on freeze-fractured bovine lenses clearly indicate that the lenticular epithelium is a most effective barrier to abundant Ca entry (Duncan and Bushell, 1976) and possibly also eliminates Ca from the lens by active extrusion (Iwata, 1974). Hence when the epithelium is damaged, Ca accumulates and causes lenticular opacity. As shown by Fagerholm (1979), isolated subepithelial lens fiber bundles obtained from decapsulated rat and rabbit lenses rapidly swell and break down in the presence of Ca concentrations equivalent to those present in aqueous humor. Only a Ca content of the incubation media that did not exceed 0.05 mM proved to be innocuous under the phase contrast microscope. At a Ca content of 1 mM, swelling and an almost total disruption of the lens fibers took place within 6 hours, whereas lens fiber disintegration was

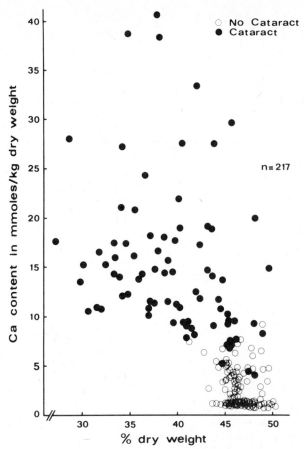

FIGURE 192. Correlation between lenticular Ca overload, cataract occurrence, and hydration in both alloxan-diabetic and normal rats with or without chronic verapamil treatment. Due to swelling, the relative dry weights of cataractous lenses declined considerably compared with the fresh weights, (the maximum decrease being a fall from 50 to 25%). The tumescence of cataractous lenses is obviously another consequence of excessive Ca uptake, since verapamil also prevented this hydration. Thus verapamil stabilized the lenticular dry weights always above 40%.

completed within 2 hours only if the Ca content of the surrounding medium had been elevated to 2 mM. A low Ca content of aqueous humor, as in cases of latent hypoparathyroidism or manifest tetany, seems to impair the barrier function of the lens epithelium or the lens cell membranes (Clark, Mengel, Bagg, and Benedek, 1980). But even in this case, enough Ca is still present to allow excessive lenticular Ca uptake and opacification. Accordingly, there is no significant difference in the Ca content of hypocalcemic cataracts and senile cataracts (see Brooks, 1975).

Although the formation of cataracts in alloxan-diabetic rats has been described (Charalampous and Hegsted, 1950; Patterson, 1953), no data concerning a possible involvement of Ca were hitherto available. Thus the observations of Fleckenstein,

v. Witzleben, Frey, and Milner (1981) were the first to demonstrate (1) the key role of lenticular Ca overload also in the pathogenesis of experimental diabetic cataracts and (2) the possibility of inhibiting the development of such Ca-induced cataracts by preventing lenticular Ca overload with the help of suitable Ca antagonists such as verapamil. Verapamil enters the aqueous humor but does not influence, according to our analyses on diabetic rats, the Ca content or the elevated glucose concentration in the anterior eye chamber. Whether verapamil acts by tightening the lens epithelium against a pathologic permeability increase to Ca or more directly by inhibiting the Ca deposition on the lenticular fibers is still an open question. However, the protective action on the lens is not a common property of all Ca antagonists since in contrast with verapamil, the 1,4-dihydropyridine compounds such as nifedipine as well as diltiazem were nearly ineffective in this respect. This is possibly due to insufficient penetration of these drugs into the aqueous humor.

CHAPTER SEVEN

The Practical Significance
of Calcium Antagonists in
Cardiovascular Therapy

7.1. GENERAL CONSIDERATIONS

Calcium antagonism is a unifying concept that offers a common denominator for a multitude of pharmacological effects on myocardium, cardiac pacemakers, and smooth muscle cells. Also the term *calcium antagonist,* proposed by us in 1969 as a novel drug designation, represents more than a sophisticated scientific name, since it yields an explanation of the multifaceted practical consequences arising from the nowadays worldwide application of these agents. In fact, as can be concluded from the extensive research work depicted in the preceding chapters, the administration of Ca antagonists as antianginal, antiarrhythmic, antihypertensive, or cardioprotective drugs makes use of different manifestations of one and the same elementary membrane action. Thus the elucidation of the involvement of Ca in various physiological and pathophysiological processes has made the pharmacology of Ca antagonists and the wide scope of their therapeutic actions easily understandable.

In principle, all Ca antagonists when systemically administered in a sufficiently high dosage range, will exert the following basic effects:

On the myocardium, the Ca antagonists restrict Ca-dependent contractile tension and oxygen requirement. Moreover, they are capable of protecting the heart against the deleterious consequences of intracellular Ca overload that otherwise would lead to myocardial necrosis. *On the cardiac pacemakers,* the fundamental action of Ca antagonists consists of damping Ca-dependent nomotopic and particularly ectopic automaticity. Moreover, reentry pathways may be blocked. *On vascular smooth muscle,* Ca-dependent tone is reduced and spastic contractions abolished. Accordingly, all Ca antagonists are able to relax the smooth musculature from coronary and other arteries. They also dilate the resistance vessels in systemic circulation, thereby acting as antihypertensive drugs.

However, these particular effects on myocardium, cardiac pacemakers, and vascular smooth muscle are differently accentuated depending on the individual Ca antagonist used (see the scheme of Figure 193). For instance, *verapamil* exerts its influence on myocardium, pacemakers, and vasculature with comparable intensity. On the other hand, *nifedipine* and its derivatives *niludipine* and *nimodipine* preferentially suppress vascular contractility, whereas, at least in humans, their influence on the cardiac pacemaker functions is modest. As for *diltiazem,* the vasodilator actions of this drug are also more pronounced than its inhibitory influence on cardiac tension development and pacemaker activity. Due to these peculiarities, *nifedipine* and its derivatives have to be considered the Ca antagonists with the most powerful vasodilator efficacy. Conversely, *verapamil* is particularly useful for direct cardioprotection, as in the case of cardiomyopathies and for antidysrhythmic purposes. *Diltiazem,* however, although more related to verapamil than to nifedipine, has a position somewhere in between.

There is no doubt that verapamil, nifedipine, and diltiazem represent the Ca-antagonistic principle of action in its purest form. For this reason, the following discussion about the therapeutic use of Ca antagonists focuses on these three top drugs. Table 19, reproduced from a review article of Henry (1980), contains a compilation of pertinent data concerning dosage, absorption, bioavailability, therapeutic plasma concentrations, metabolism, excretion, and so forth, in a condensed form. In the proposed oral dosage range for humans, all three Ca antagonists exert

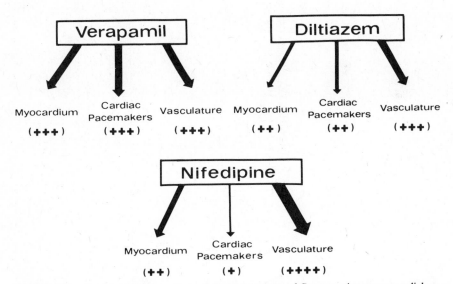

FIGURE 193. Potential inhibitory effects of therapeutic doses of Ca antagonists on myocardial contractility, SA-node automaticity, and AV conduction as well as on vascular smooth muscle tone and spasms, particularly in coronary stem arteries. However, these potential negative inotropic, chronotropic, and dromotropic actions of systemically administered Ca antagonists are usually subject to considerable attenuation by sympathetic cardiovascular reflexes. Conversely, baroreceptor-mediated increases in sympathetic drive contribute additionally to extramural coronary vasodilation.

TABLE 19. Pharmacokinetics of Ca Antagonists[a,b]

	Nifedipine	($\pm$) Verapamil	Diltiazem
Dosage			
Oral (mg/8 h)	10–20	80–160	60–90
Intravenous (μg/kg)	5–15	150	75–150
Absorption			
Oral (%)	>90	>90	>90
Bioavailability (%)	65–70	10–22	20–40
Onset of action			
Sublingual (min)	3		
Oral (min)	<20	<30	<30
Therapeutic plasma concentration (ng/ml)	25–100 (7×10^{-8}–2×10^{-7} M)	15–100 (3.2×10^{-8}–2×10^{-7} M)	30–130 (7×10^{-8}–3×10^{-7} M)
Protein binding (%)	90	90	80

Plasma half-time			
Initial fast (α) (min)	150–180	15–30	20
Slow (β) (h)	5	3–7	4
Metabolism	Extensively metabolized to an inert free acid and lactone	Extensive 1st pass hepatic extraction (70% of oral dose)	Extensively deacetylated
Excretion			
Renal (%)	70 1st day (80 total)	50 1st day (70 total)	35 (total)
Fecal (%)	<15	15	65

[a]Reproduced from Henry (1980) with slight modifications.
[b]Detailed data concerning the pharmacokinetics of the three main Ca antagonists were published by the following researchers.
Verapamil: Schomerus, Spiegelhalder, Stieren, and Eichelbaum, 1976; Eichelbaum, Ende, Remberg, Schomerus, and Dengler, 1978; Remberg, Ende, Eichelbaum, and Schomerus, 1980; Eichelbaum, Birkel, Grube, Gütgemann, and Somogyi, 1980; Eichelbaum, Somogyi, v.Unruh, and Dengler, 1981; Eichelbaum, Dengler, Somogyi, and v.Unruh, 1981.
Nifedipine: Horster, 1975 a,b; Patzschke, Duhm, Maul, Medenwald, and Wegner, 1975; Schlossmann, Medenwald, and Rosenkranz, 1975; Raemsch, 1981.
Diltiazem: Rovei, Gomeni, Mitchard, Larribaud, Blatrix, Thebault, and Morselli, 1980; Kinney, Moskowitz, and Zelis, 1981; Piepho, Bloedow, Lacz, Runser, Dimmit, and Browne, 1982; Zelis and Kinney, 1982; Kölle, Ochs, Thomann, and Neurath, 1982.

distinct vasodilator effects in coronary and systemic circulation, whereas their inhibitory influences on myocardial contractility, SA-node automaticity, and AV conduction are usually smaller or even indiscernible. This obvious lack of strong cardiodepression by the proposed therapeutic oral doses is explained by the fact that a reflex augmentation of endogenous sympathetic drive (in response to the drug-induced fall in blood pressure) may neutralize the direct Ca-antagonistic effects on myocardium and nodal cells more or less completely. Thus nifedipine, the strongest vasodilator but weakest inhibitor of the nodal functions, may even give rise to an overshooting reflex increase in heart rate and AV conduction velocity. On the other hand, the direct inhibitory pacemaker effects of verapamil are so pronounced that they are less easily masked by endogenous sympathetic reflex activity. Nevertheless, even here, the full impact of the verapamil-induced depression of the SA- and AV-nodal functions becomes apparent only after β-receptor blockade. Hence β-blockers and verapamil may potentiate each other with respect to their nodal actions to a sometimes dangerous extent, particularly if verapamil is injected intravenously after previous β-receptor blockade. Simultaneously, in man, an exaggerated negative-inotropic effect may also be provoked by this inappropriate drug combination (Seabra-Gomes, Rickards, and Sutton, 1976). More details concerning the interactions of Ca antagonists and β-adrenergic neurotransmitters have been compiled in Section 4.2.3.

7.2. EFFICACY OF CALCIUM ANTAGONISTS IN THE TREATMENT OF EXERTIONAL ANGINA

7.2.1. Verapamil

Several Ca antagonists have been introduced primarily for the treatment of coronary disease without a distinct scientific label, or even under a false designation. For instance, verapamil (Iproveratril, Isoptin®) was launched in 1963 by the Knoll Pharmaceutical company, Ludwigshafen, Germany, as an antianginal drug with coronary vasodilator actions and a putative β-receptor-blocking activity on the myocardium. Therefore, the researchers who studied verapamil first in clinical trials attributed its therapeutic effects partially to nitroglycerin-like influences and partially to propranolol-like influences. Nevertheless, it became quite clear as early as around the mid-1960s that verapamil opened a hopeful new way in the management of angina (Tschirdewahn and Klepzig, 1963; Fischer, 1965; Strässle and Burckhardt, 1965; Neumann and Luisada, 1966; Wette, Heimsoth, and Jansen, 1966; Benda, Doneff, Lujf, and Moser, 1967; Kaltenbach and Zimmermann, 1968; Hofmann, 1968; Sandler, Clayton, and Thornicroft, 1968). Although the doses applied by the first clinical investigators were relatively small, 60 to 80% of the patients with severe exertional or postinfarct angina responded with subjective relief of pain and objective signs of improvement in the ECG under a standardized work load. When compared with β-blockers (propranolol, pindolol) or nitrites (nitroglycerin, isosorbide dinitrate), the antianginal efficacy of verapamil appeared to be virtually equal

(Kaltenbach, 1970; de Ponti, Mauri, Ciliberto, and Caru, 1979). Confirmatory results were obtained in double-blind crossover therapeutic trials against a placebo. Thus verapamil (120 mg thrice daily) and propranolol (100 mg thrice daily) proved to be of equal potency in exercise-tolerance tests as assessed by the alleviation of the ischemic ST-segment depression (Livesley, Catley, Campbell, and Oram, 1973). The two drugs were more effective than a placebo both in reduction of daily attacks ($P < 0.01$) and the prolongation of exercise tests ($P < 0.05$). When compared with a placebo in a Danish multicenter study, even a lower dose of verapamil (80 mg three times daily) significantly decreased the incidence of attacks and the nitroglycerin consumption by approximately 25% (Andreasen, Boye, Christoffersen, Dalsgaard, et al., 1975). In another comparative double-blind crossover study with verapamil (80 mg three times daily) or practolol (100 mg three times daily) against a placebo over 4 weeks, Fagher, Persson, and Svensson, 1977 observed the best results in the verapamil-treated group of patients. Verapamil appeared to be the most efficient drug in reducing attack frequency and nitroglycerin consumption as well as in augmenting physical working capacity. Nevertheless, oral medication with the higher dose of 120 mg verapamil three times daily seems to be more appropriate for an antianginal standard therapy. Clinical reports have emphasized that this dose regularly diminished ST-segment depression, invariably increased anginal threshold, and eliminated pain completely in less severe cases without any significant side effects (Bala Subramanian, Khanna, Narayanan, and Hoon, 1976; Bala Subramanian, Lahiri, Paramasivan, and Raftery, 1980). As shown directly in resting patients (Rudolph, Kriener, and Meister, 1971), as well as in patients undergoing standardized ergometer tests (Roskamm, Fröhlich, and Reindell, 1966), verapamil is able to diminish cardiac oxygen requirement as concluded from a reduced coronary oxygen extraction.

However, the beneficial influence of verapamil in coronary patients is probably complex, because several therapeutically important factors, analyzed in the preceding chapters, seem to work together:

1. Direct reduction of myocardial energy expenditure during exercise, thus lowering oxygen demand.

2. Indirect decrease in cardiac oxygen requirement by facilitation of heart work at a reduced level of arterial blood pressure (diminution of afterload).

3. Improvement of oxygen supply to the myocardium due to vasodilator or spasmolytic effects, particularly on extramural coronary vessels (stem arteries, collaterals, anastomoses).

4. Cellular cardioprotection, that is, increase in ischemic tolerance by prevention of precipitous Ca engulfment into the hypoxic or anoxic myocardium.

In addition, verapamil can inhibit exercise-induced ectopic ventricular beats. All clinical effects of verapamil described above were obtained with racemic ($\pm$)-verapamil. The strong ($-$)-enantiomer of verapamil is nearly exclusively responsible for this drug activity, whereas the contribution of the much weeker ($+$)-enantiomer is practically negligible.

7.2.2. Nifedipine

The introduction into coronary therapy of nifedipine (Bay a 1040; trade name: Adalat®), developed in the Bayer Laboratories, Elberfeld, Germany, largely profited from the previous research work with the Ca antagonists verapamil and D 600. Thus early in 1970 we could inform the clinical investigators during a business meeting of this company that nifedipine represented another highly potent member of the Ca antagonist family (see Fleckenstein, 1970/1971a, b). This preliminary communication was conducive to a better orientation of the clinical research projects on nifedipine, which were at that time already under way. Then in 1972 a first series of coordinated publications on nifedipine appeared. The papers dealt with pharmacology (Vater, Kroneberg, Hoffmeister, et al., 1972; Hashimoto, Taira, Chiba, Hashimoto, Jr., et al., 1972; Raff, Kosche, and Lochner, 1972), with the fundamental Ca-antagonistic actions on heart muscle (Fleckenstein, Tritthart, Döring, and Byon, 1972) and vasculature (Grün and Fleckenstein, 1972), and with the therapeutic aspects (Loos and Kaltenbach, 1972; Kaltenbach, Becker, Kober, and Loos, 1972; Hayase, Hirakawa, Hosokawa, Mori, Kanyama, and Iwasa, 1972; Kochsiek and Neubaur, 1972; Kobayashi, Ito, and Tawara, 1972). Since many of the pharmacological and clinical investigations had been carried out in Japan, the first international symposium on nifedipine was held in Tokyo in autumn 1973. The proceedings, edited by Hashimoto, Kimura, and Kobayashi and printed by University of Tokyo Press, appeared in 1975. This volume presented, apart from a multitude of additional pharmacological data (Kroneberg, 1975; Hashimoto, Taira, Ono, Chiba, et al., 1975; Imai, 1975; Kanazawa, 1975; Nakamura, Etoh, Hamanaka, Kuroiwa, et al., 1975), a comprehensive report on the hemodynamic effects of nifedipine in humans and on its antianginal properties. Thereby, further research work about the practical use of Ca antagonists was enormously stimulated.

7.2.2.1. Hemodynamic Findings with Nifedipine.

Single acute doses of nifedipine injected intravenously (0.015 to 0.03 mg/kg within 90 to 180 sec) or given sublingually (10 to 20 mg) were shown to reduce systolic and diastolic blood pressure, left ventricular systolic pressure (LVSP) and enddiastolic pressure (LVEDP) as well as systemic peripheral resistance. Simultaneously, there was an increase in coronary flow and coronary venous oxygen saturation. On the other hand, because of sympathetic reflex stimulation in response to the fall in blood pressure, stroke volume, cardiac output, and particularly heart rate at rest exhibited a slight or even marked tendency to rise (Cherchi, Fonzo, and Bina, 1975; Lydtin, Lohmöller, Lohmöller, and Walter, 1975; Lichtlen, 1975; Ekelund, Atterhög, and Melin, 1975; van den Brand, Remme, Meester, Tiggelaar-de Widt, de Ruiter, and Hugenholtz, 1975). Likewise, Just, v. Mengden, Kersting, and Krebs (1979) observed a baroreceptor-dependent 24% increase in left ventricular contractility, as assessed with ultrasound cardiography 30 min after ingestion of 20 mg of nifedipine. An analogous reflex enhancement of cardiac performance occurred following ingestion of 10 mg of isosorbide dinitrate (13%) or 2.5 mg of nitroglycerin (18%). If, however, nifedipine is applied directly to the heart via intrabypass injections, the basic negative-inotropic action, necessarily connected with Ca antagonism, is also unmasked on human myocardium *in situ* (Serruys, Brower, Ten Katen, Bom, and Hugenholtz, 1981). Under these conditions, a small amount of nifedipine (0.1 mg = 1.4 to 2 μg/kg) intracoronarily infused during 10 sec at a pacing rate of 90 beats/min profoundly altered regional myocardial wall motion. Thus in the musculature directly supplied by the selectively injected bypasses, the onset of shortening was delayed, the shortening rate diminished, and the extent of shortening decreased to 67% of the control values within a few seconds. There was a gradual return to normal after 2 min. In summary, nifedipine exerts a direct negative-inotropic effect when regionally administered, but after intravenous or oral administration, this effect is overridden by reflex increases in contractility and in heart rate as a result of lowered systemic arterial pressure.

7.2.2.2. Acute Antianginal Efficacy. The above doses of nifedipine systemically administered to coronary patients in exercise tests increased the working capacity and the threshold for pain consistently as found by all investigators. To exclude the inaccuracy of subjective statements, the remarkable antianginal potency of nifedipine was further assessed by extensive ECG studies under standardized work loads (see Loos and Kaltenbach, 1972; Kobayashi, Ito, and Tawara, 1972; Kaltenbach, 1975; Stein, 1975; Cherchi, Fonzo, and Bina, 1975). Thus a highly significant reduction by nifedipine of the ST-segment depression could be demonstrated. The hemodynamic correlate consisted of an inhibitory effect of nifedipine on exercise-induced elevation of LVEDP and V_{max} similar to that of nitroglycerin (Kurita, 1975; Kaltenbach, 1975; Kaltenbach, Schulz, and Kober, 1979). Moreover, nifedipine (20 mg sublingually) improved the tolerance of coronary patients to cardiac pacing at higher rates (120 to 140/min). Accordingly, under the influence of nifedipine, the threshold frequencies for pain, ST-segment depression, and, most interestingly, for cardiac lactate production rose (Schaefer, Schwarzkopf, Schoettler, and Wilms, 1975a, b).

7.2.2.3. Antianginal Long-Term Therapy. Long-term observations with nifedipine on patients suffering from stable exertional angina were even more impressive than the results of short trials, since the antianginal efficacy increased with continuation of the nifedipine therapy. Thus it was found in an open multicenter study on 147 thoroughly supervised outpatients from 15 hospitals that the number of anginal attacks, as well as the daily nitroglycerin consumption, progressively declined during a 6-month treatment with nifedipine (minimal oral dose: thrice 10 mg daily). At the end of this study, attack frequency and nitroglycerin intake had been diminished in comparison with the prenifedipine period by 75 and 80% respectively (Braasch and Ebner, 1975). There was obviously no sign of tachyphylaxis. Ebner (1975a), in summarizing observations on 418 nifedipine-treated coronary patients from 16 research groups in Japan and Germany, calculated a mean success rate of 70.6%. This average is based on the decrease in (1) frequency and severity of attacks and (2) nitroglycerin consumption. The high success rate is also backed by a host of ECG examinations. Later evaluations of the long-term treatment with nifedipine on 714 patients (Ebner, 1975b) and finally on 3668 patients (Ebner and Dünschede, 1976) showed even a slight increase in success rate up to 72.0 and 76.95% respectively. These positive figures can possibly be further improved by the use of a standard dose of three times 20 mg nifedipine daily, which, according to more recent experiences, seems to guarantee a therapeutic optimum.

7.2.2.4. Comparison of Nifedipine with Other Coronary Drugs. Nifedipine was found in exercise-tolerance tests to be of similar acute potency as nitroglycerin, intravenous doses of nitroglycerin (0.35 mg) and nifedipine (1.0 mg) being roughly equivalent (Cherchi, Fonzo, and Bina, 1975). However, the antianginal action of one single intravenous dose of 1 mg nifedipine was more protracted since it lasted for at least 90 min, the maximum duration being 150 min. Accordingly, Kaltenbach, Schulz, and Kober (1979), by simultaneous assessment of the nifedipine effects (1.0 mg intravenously) on coronary flow and ST-segment depression, revealed a large discrepancy in patients with stable exertional angina between the surprisingly long duration of the antianginal activity in the ECG and the only short-lived augmentation of coronary flow that rapidly expired within 6 min. Thus the antianginal potency of nifedipine seemed to be more attributable in stable angina to "an alteration of the Ca-mediated myocardial contraction process leading to reduced oxygen requirements or to increased tolerance of ischemia of the heart," rather than to coronary vasodilation (Kaltenbach, Schulz, and Kober, 1979). There is no doubt that a simple dilation of the cardiac resistance vessels by dipyridamol is lacking any therapeutic value in exercise tests (Kaltenbach, 1975). Also pentaerythritol tetranitrate proved to be much less efficient than nifedipine (Maggi, 1975; Maggi and Piscitello, 1975).

7.2.2.5. Combination of Nifedipine with β-Blockers. Chronic oral administration of nifedipine lowers cardiac afterload and in coronary patients with hyperdynamic circulatory state may lead to a similar improvement as treatment with β-blockers does. However, the reflex increase in sympathetic tone brought about by the nifedipine-induced reduction in blood pressure is often a limiting factor if nifedipine is given alone. Thus the appropriate therapy for angina complicated with hyperkinetic cardiovascular disorders may preferably consist of a combined administration of nifedipine and a β-blocker. Whereas in the case of verapamil the superposition of Ca-antagonistic effects upon β-receptor blockade has to be considered dangerous, the combined application of nifedipine with reasonable doses of β-blockers such as propranolol or metoprolol seems to be rather advantagous (Lydtin, Lohmöller, Lohmöller, and Walter, 1975; Itoh, Tawara, and Itoh, 1975; Ekelund, Atterhög, and Melin, 1975; Ekelund and Atterhög, 1975; Grandjean and Valenti, 1979; Lynch, Dargie, Krikler, and Krikler, 1980).

7.2.3. Diltiazem

Diltiazem is the last highly specific Ca antagonist introduced into coronary therapy. Hence the number of reports concerning its effects on exercise-inducible chronic stable angina is still relatively small. However, there is no doubt that diltiazem

shares a distinct beneficial influence on exertional angina with the other Ca antagonists of group A (Pool, Seagren, Bonanno, Salel, and Dennish, 1980; Kober,
Berlad, Hopf, and Kaltenbach, 1981; Hossack and Bruce, 1981). The antianginal
potency of diltiazem is as dose-dependent as that of verapamil and nifedipine. For
instance, placebo-controlled double-blind randomized crossover studies at three dose
levels (120, 180, and 240 mg diltiazem/day) have shown that the greatest dose
produces the statistically best results with respect to exercise tolerance and ischemic
ECG improvement (Pool et al.). Adverse side effects were lacking.

   As to the hemodynamic changes associated with the systemic administration of
diltiazem in humans, there is also a principal correspondence with those of verapamil
and nifedipine. Thus a significant rise in coronary venous oxygen saturation and a
fall in left ventricular oxygen extraction has been observed during intravenous
infusion of 30 μg diltiazem/kg/min for 10 minutes. Simultaneously, a slight decrease
in systolic, diastolic, and mean aortic pressures, as well as in systemic vascular
resistance occurred (Bourassa, Cote, Theroux, Tubau, Genain, and Waters, 1980).
Heart rate tended to decline when systemic vascular resistence changed little. But
if systemic blood pressure dropped, the direct negative chronotropic effect of diltiazem was again neutralized by endogenous sympathetic reflex activity. However,
these hemodynamic repercussions following administration of diltiazem, seem to
be somewhat less pronounced than those produced by nifedipine.

   A first comprehensive survey of the pharmacological and clinical features of
diltiazem was presented in 1978 on the occasion of a symposium in Hakone, Japan.
The proceedings edited by R.J. Bing, appeared in 1979. The qualitative and quantitative data on the diltiazem actions thoroughly evaluated in comparison with
verapamil and nifedipine, clearly indicated that diltiazem shares, indeed, the cardinal
properties of the major Ca antagonists (see Bing, Weishaar, Rackl, and Pawlik,
1978/1979; Schwartz, Nagao, and Matlib, 1978/1979; Taira, 1978/1979). This is
now generally accepted.

7.2.4.   Calcium Antagonists of Group B (Prenylamine, Fendiline, Perhexiline Maleate)

Prenylamine, classified by us as a Ca antagonist of group B, exerts similar hemodynamic effects as the compounds of group A do, however, with a lesser intensity.
Thus after systemic administration of prenylamine, blood pressure may also decline
and coronary vasodilation develop. This is again correlated with a reciprocal reflex
stimulation of heart rate and an increase in cardiac contractile performance. For
instance, Arntz, Kreuzer, Bostroem, and Gleichmann (1968) were able to show in
healthy humans that an intravenous dose of 0.43 mg prenylamine/kg acutely lowered
systolic and diastolic blood pressure by 10 and 12% because of a reduction of
peripheral resistance by 40%, whereas heart rate, stroke volume, cardiac output,
and dp/dt_{max} rose by 9, 14, 20, and 34% respectively. Also most other cardiovascular
effects of prenylamine fit equally well into the usual pattern of Ca-antagonist actions
(Lindner, 1971). As to the antianginal potency of daily oral doses of 180 to 300
mg prenylamine, numerous studies testify to the therapeutic usefulness of this

treatment from the early 1960s onward (Overkamp, 1960; Kerridge, Mazurkie, and Verel, 1961; Baumgarten, 1962; Anderson, 1963). Subsequent double-blind cross-over studies against a placebo confirmed these positive results (Luisada and Neumann, 1963; Donat and Schlosser, 1966; Cardoe, 1970, 1971; Winsor, Bleifer, Cole, Goldman, Karpman, Kaye, Oblath, and Stone, 1971; Sepaha, Jain, and Jain, 1971; Tucker, Carson, Bass, and Massey, 1974). Likewise, *fendiline,* a chemical analogue of prenylamine, has also been reported to be of benefit in angina pectoris. This conclusion was based on exercise tests (Spiel and Enenkel, 1976) and on open trials (Lüthy, 1978). However, detailed observations on the hemodynamic actions of fendiline in healthy humans or coronary patients are practically lacking.

Perhexiline maleate, on the other hand, has been scrutinized much more intensely. This drug too, in accordance with its fundamental Ca-antagonistic properties (Fleckenstein-Grün, Fleckenstein, Byon, and Kim, 1976/1978), exerts the typical triad of damping effects on myocardium, cardiac pacemakers, and vasculature. Corresponding to its negative inotropic influence on isolated myocardium (see Figure 27), perhexiline also reduces left ventricular work and myocardial oxygen consumption in intact dogs and humans when systemically administered (Hudak, Lewis, and Kuhn, 1970; Hudak, Lewis, Lucas, and Kuhn, 1973; Cho, Belej, and Aviado, 1970). Moreover, perhexiline diminishes the rate of impulse discharge from the SA-nodal cells by decreasing both the slope of spontaneous diastolic depolarization and the upstroke velocity of the pacemaker action potentials (Matsuo, Cho, and Aviado, 1970). This negative chronotropic effect also manifests itself in a reduction of exercise-induced tachycardia (Grupp, Bunde, and Grupp, 1970; Pepine, Schang, and Bemiller, 1973, 1974). Furthermore, perhexiline prolongs AV-conduction time and exhibits certain antiarrhythmic properties in animals and in coronary patients (Sukerman, 1973; Drake, Singer, Haring, and Dirnberger, 1973). The negative chronotropic effects of perhexiline were shown to be exerted directly, that is to say, without stimulation of parasympathetic reflex mechanisms or blockade of nodal β-receptors.

As to the influence of the drug on coronary flow, most data were obtained from dogs. The observations indicate that perhexiline produces vasodilation not only of the coronary bed, but also in pulmonary and systemic circulation (Cho, Belej, and Aviado, 1970). Numerous studies have shown symptomatic improvement by perhexiline in patients with angina pectoris (Hirshleifer, 1969; Winsor, 1970; Burns-Cox, Chandrasekhar, Ikram, Peirce, Pilcher, Quinlan, and Russell Rees, 1971). Daily oral doses of 300 to 400 mg perhexiline maleate also proved to be effective in carefully controlled exercise tests (Gitlin and Nellen, 1973; Morledge, 1973; Cherchi, Bina, Fonzo, and Raffo, 1973; Cawein, Lewis, Hudak, and Hoekenga, 1973; Morledge, Adams, Hudak, Powell, and Kuzma, 1976/1978; Ferlemann, Krehan, and Kaltenbach, 1979). Hence perhexiline is undoubtedly a rather potent antianginal agent. However, the above authors, except Ferlemann et al., were not aware of the Ca-antagonistic mechanism of action.

Unfortunately, perhexiline maleate, at least in the high dosage range of 400 mg daily, is not free from unpleasant side effects such as dizziness, weight loss, headache (Datey, Bagri, Kelkar, Varma, Bhootra, and Amin, 1973; de Oliveira,

Loyola, and Da Cunha Chaves, 1973; Hoekenga, Bunde, Cawein, Kuzma, and Griffin, 1973; Gitlin, 1973), and even peripheral neuropathies (Laplane, Bousser, Bouche, and Touboul 1976/1978). A perhexiline-induced rise in serum transaminase levels (SGOT, SGPT) has also frequently been observed (Garson, Gülin, and Phear, 1973; Armstrong, 1973; Pilcher, Chandrasekhar, Russell Rees, Boyce, Peirce, and Ikram, 1973). Hence periodic liver-function tests are advisable in all patients under long-term perhexiline treatment.

7.3. OUTSTANDING ANTIANGINAL POTENCY OF CALCIUM ANTAGONISTS IN VASOSPASTIC CORONARY DISEASE

7.3.1. Prinzmetal's Variant Angina

The scientific basis of the nowadays worldwide use of Ca antagonists for the treatment of spastic forms of angina was provided in the early 1970s by a coincidence of three achievements, namely:

1. The demonstration, in our laboratory, of the extreme power and almost universal scope of Ca antagonists such as nifedipine, D 600, and verapamil in suppressing all types of spasms of extramural coronary vasculature directly, that is, beyond the receptor level (Fleckenstein 1970/1971b; Grün, Fleckenstein, and Byon, 1971b; Grün and Fleckenstein, 1971, 1972; see Sections 6.2.2 and 6.2.4).

2. The discovery by Japanese clinicians, also engaged in the examination of nifedipine, of the dramatic responsiveness of Prinzmetal's "variant" angina to the Ca-antagonist treatment.

3. The definite verification of a spastic origin of variant angina and of a major spastic component in unstable angina and in angina at rest.

The typical variant angina, characterized by ST-segment elevation according to Prinzmetal's first description (Prinzmetal, Kennamer, Merliss, Wada, and Bor, 1959), is a relatively seldom phenomenon, at least in Europe and in the United States. In Japan, however, the occurrence of variant angina is by no means rare. Consequently, the collective of Japanese patients first treated with nifedipine in the years 1970 to 1973 also included a considerable number of cases with Prinzmetal's disease. Due to this fortunate constellation, several Japanese cardiologists became rapidly aware of the particularly high efficacy of nifedipine in such Prinzmetal patients and in patients with angina at rest (see Mabuchi, Kishida, and Suzuki, 1975; Hosoda, Kasanuki, Miyata, Endoh, and Hirosawa, 1975; Fukuzaki, Okamoto, Yokoyama, and Tomomatsu, 1975; Itoh, Tawara, and Itoh, 1975; Niitani and Fujimaki, 1975). These papers were part of the first international symposium on nifedipine in Tokyo in 1973 and nourished the hypothesis of Ca-antagonist-sensitive spasms as the decisive factor in the etiology of variant angina.

Indeed, just in the same years, multiple reports on the occurrence of coronary arterial spasms during attacks of Prinzmetal's angina appeared, primarily based on angiographic evidence (Dhurandar, Watt, Silver, Trimble, and Adelman, 1972; King, Zir, Kaltman, and Fox, 1973; Froment, Normand, and Amiel, 1973; Oliva, Potts, and Pluss, 1973; Applefield and Roman, 1974; Kerin and MacLeod, 1974; Schroeder, Silverman, and Harrison, 1974; Hart, Silverman, and King, 1974). Hence in summarizing these results, Meller, Pichard, and Dack stated in 1976 that the causative role of coronary arterial spasm in Prinzmetal's variant angina should be accepted as *"a proved hypothesis."* In all probability, the typical ST-segment elevation signifies transmural ischemia of spastic origin. This could be further substantiated by myocardial thallium scintigraphy since simultaneously with ST-segment elevation massive transmural deficits in myocardial perfusion appeared (Maseri, Parodi, Severi, and Pesola, 1976). The ischemic episodes in cases of variant angina were unrelated to preceding hemodynamic changes that are known to raise cardiac oxygen demand such as sympathetic stimulation of heart rate and myocardial contractile performance or increases in blood pressure (Parodi, Severi, Maseri, and Biagini, 1978). Thus in contrast with exertional angina, which is "secondary" to an augmentation of cardiac oxygen requirement, Prinzmetal's variant angina represents a "primary" type of inadequate coronary perfusion that occurs preferentially at rest.

In the absence of any discernible narrowing of the coronary stem arteries during the attack-free intervals, Prinzmetal's spastic angina may result from purely functional disorders of the coronary vasculature. However, more frequently the ischemic episodes seem to be due to spasms superimposed on atherosclerotic stenoses. As shown in Figure 194, in a considerable percentage of cases, the atherosclerotic processes develop eccentrically. This means that the smooth muscle motility of the media can fully persist in the nonaffected parts of the coronary arterial wall. Moreover, the eccentrically located atheromatous lesions seem to sensitize the intact parts of the media to sudden spastic reactions, which then dramatically impair coronary flow. There is reason to believe that many patients with variant angina suffer from such eccentric stenoses of major branches of the coronary arterial tree. On the other hand, stable exertional angina seems to be a consequence of rigid concentric stenoses with no residual responsiveness to any vasoconstrictor or vasodilator influence.

Furthermore, the characteristic interventions that were found in our experiments to produce spasms of the extramural porcine coronary vasculature, also proved to be capable of causing attacks of variant angina in humans. This is particularly true of the following provocative tests, used for unveiling latent forms of Prinzmetal's disease:

1. *Administration of cholinergic agents.* As previously demonstrated on isolated pig coronary strips (see Section 6.2.6 Figures 167 and 168), acetylcholine is a very potent coronary vasoconstrictor. Accordingly, Yasue, Touyama, Shimamoto, Kato, Tanaka, and Akiyama (1974) and Endo, Hirosawa, Kaneko, Hase, Inoue, and Konno (1976) induced coronary spasm and ischemic attacks in patients with

Eccentric Stenoses

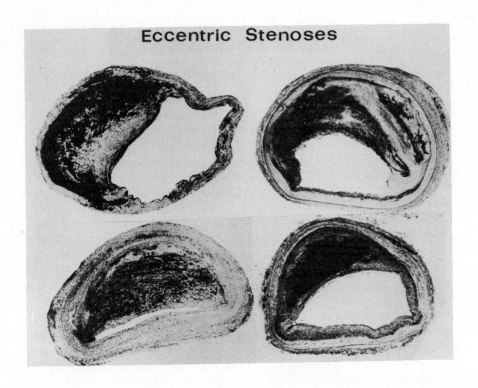

Concentric Stenoses

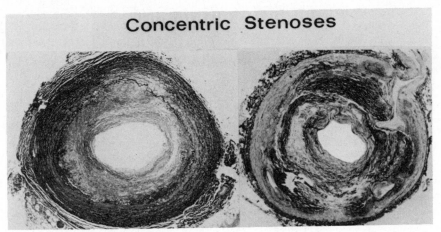

FIGURE 194. Collection of eccentric and concentric stenoses of human coronary stem arteries. Reproduced from Bäurle (1951), Pathological Institute, Freiburg, with permission of F. Büchner, and from Stolte (1981).

variant angina by injection of *methacholine*. Interestingly enough, the spontaneous ischemic episodes in typical Prinzmetal's disease also usually occur at night, during sleep, or after opulent meals, that is, under parasympathetic domination. *Atropine* stopped spontaneous attacks in approximately 80% of the patients (Yasue, 1980).

2. *Selective adrenergic α-receptor stimulation.* According to our results, reported in Section 6.2.6 (see Figure 169), adrenergic β-receptor blockade with pindolol will unmask hidden α-receptors, which then mediate massive coronary vasoconstrictor responses when stimulated with adrenaline or noradrenaline. These observations too are consistent with those of Yasue, Touyama, Kato, Tanaka, and Akiyama (1976), who provoked attacks of variant angina by injecting adrenaline after β-blockade with propanolol. In these clinical experiments on patients with variant angina, propranolol was not only ineffective, but rather aggravated the attacks, in contrast with its beneficial influence in cases of exertional angina (Yasue, 1980). Indeed, after β-receptor blockade, both sympathetic and parasympathetic neurotransmitters produce extramural coronary vasoconstriction unidirectionally. Therefore, β-blockers should not be used in the treatment of variant angina. Propranolol in large doses may sometimes alleviate the ischemic episodes in certain patients with Prinzmetal's disease (Guazzi, Magrini, Fiorentini, and Polese, 1971). But this modest efficacy is probably due to the pronounced Ca-antagonistic side effects of propranolol, which have, however, often been ignored by clinical investigators (see Section 2.1.1). Ergonovine represents another coronary vasoconstrictor drug (Stein, 1949) with selective α-receptor stimulating properties that is frequently used for provocation of attacks of variant angina (Heupler, Proudfit, Siegel, Shirey, Razavi, and Sones, 1975; Schroeder, Bolen, Quint, Clark, Hayden, Higgins, and Wexler, 1977; Curry, Pepine, Sabom, Feldman, Christie, and Conti, 1977; Curry, Pepine, Sabom, and Conti, 1979; Gerry, Achuff, Becker, Pond, and Greene, 1979). Again, isolated pig coronary vasculature reacts identically.

3. *Alkalotic shift of blood pH by hyperventilation and Tris-buffer infusion.* Ca-dependent tone and contractility of isolated porcine coronary vasculature were greatly potentiated in our studies by lowering the intracellular concentration of the naturally Ca-antagonistic H ions by means of an alkaline Tris-buffer solution (see Section 6.2.3, Figures 145, 146, 149). Thus it was not surprising that Tris-buffer infusions combined with hyperventilation were also later shown to provoke coronary spasm in patients with variant angina (Yasue, Nagao, Omote, Takizawa, Miwa, and Tanaka, 1978).

Moreover, sudden vasoconstriction of the altered coronary arteries may also be due to mechanical irritation resulting from friction or stretch by the introduced catheter tip or from extension of the arterial wall by rapidly injected contrast material (Chahine, Raizner, Ishimori, Luchi, and MacIntosh, 1975). Thus a variety of stimuli are able to elicit coronary spasm of Prinzmetal's type. But the final common reaction, regardless of the special stimulatory or conditioning factors, seems to consist of an *exaggerated transmembrane Ca influx* into hyperexcitable coronary smooth muscle cells. This type of transmembrane Ca supply to the contractile system is most effectively inhibited by Ca antagonists (see the scheme of Figure 183).

In fact, the Ca antagonists have completely fulfilled in clinical practice the great therapeutic expectations that arose from their efficacy against coronary *in vitro* spasms (see Section 6.2.4). *Nifedipine* was the first Ca antagonist successfully used by Japanese cardiologists in patients with variant angina during the period between 1970 and 1973. Further evidence of an outstanding therapeutic efficacy of nifedipine rapidly accumulated in the following years. Thus Hosoda and Kimura (1976) presented a report on the nifedipine treatment of 47 patients with variant angina at a dose level of 40 mg daily. Thirty cases (64%) responded excellently in that there was a complete cessation of the anginal attacks, whereas in a further 10 cases (21%), frequency and severity of the episodes were significantly reduced, a success rate of 85%.

A similarly high efficacy of nifedipine in the treatment of variant angina was also found by other clinical research groups (Endo, Kanda, Hosoda, Hayashi, Hirosawa, and Konno, 1975; Muller and Gunther, 1978; Heupler and Proudfit, 1979; Goldberg, Reichek, Wilson, Hirshfeld, Muller, and Kastor, 1979). In 1980, a most convincing report on the nifedipine therapy for coronary artery spasm appeared from the Cardiovascular Division, Peter Bent Brigham Hospital, Harvard Medical School, and eight cooperating hospitals. Also in this multicenter study, which summarized the results obtained in 127 patients with coronary spasm, a *"prompt, dramatic, and sustained decrease in attack frequency was observed during nifedipine treatment"* (Antman, Muller, Goldberg, MacAlpin, Rubenfire, Tabatznik, Liang, Heupler, Achuff, Reichek, Geltman, Kerin, Neff, and Braunwald, 1980). In the majority of patients, conventional antianginal therapy including nitrates and β-adrenergic blockers had failed. Daily oral doses of 40 to 160 mg nifedipine significantly reduced the mean weekly rate of anginal attacks from 16 to 2 ($P <$ 0.001). In 63% of the patients, complete control of anginal attacks was achieved, and in 87% the frequency of angina was reduced by at least 50%.

Verapamil given in sufficient doses (320 to 480 mg/day) to patients with variant angina seems to act as beneficially as nifedipine does (Solberg, Nissen, Vlietstra, and Callahan, 1978; Fischer Hansen and Sandøe, 1978; Parodi, Maseri, and Simonetti, 1979; Freedman, Dunn, Richmond, and Kelly, 1979; Johnson, Mauritson, Willerson, Cary, and Hillis, 1981). The same is true of *diltiazem* (Yasue, Omote, Takizawa, Nagao, Miwa, and Tanaka, 1979; Schroeder, Rosenthal, Ginsburg, and Lamb, 1980). According to the report of Schroeder and his associates, diltiazem caused a 90% reduction in pain episodes, with many patients becoming pain-free on a 240-mg daily dose. Regarding these data and the lack of adverse side effects, the prophylactic treatment with *diltiazem* was also judged to be *"dramatically effective"* (Schroeder et al.).

Quite recently, in a review of Kimura and Kishida (1981), data from 11 cardiology institutes in Japan were evaluated to determine the effectiveness of drug therapy, particularly with Ca antagonists, in a total of 286 patients with frequent attacks of variant angina (11.7 ± 1.0 per week before drug application). In fact, anginal attacks disappeared completely in 115 (77.2%) out of 149 patients treated with *nifedipine* (30 to 60 mg daily). In 25 patients (16.8%), attack frequency decreased to less than half. Similar results were obtained in 87 patients treated with daily doses of 90 to 240 mg *diltiazem*. Thus the efficacy rates of *nifedipine, diltiazem,* and *verapamil* were 94, 90.8, and 85.7%, respectively. With a combination of *nifedipine plus diltiazem,* administered to 15 patients, a 100% efficacy rate could be reached. The figure of 85.7% effectiveness of the treatment with *verapamil* has been calculated from a relatively small group of 28 patients, who were given an average dose of 228 mg of the drug per diem. Usually a higher daily oral dose of 320 to 480 mg of verapamil is recommended to obtain an *optimal* therapeutic response. In a follow-up study of Waters, Szlachcic, and Theroux (1981) on 100 patients with variant angina over an average time of 17.6 months, nifedipine, diltiazem, and verapamil appeared to be equally effective. Of 24 patients treated with nifedipine, 21 were asymptomatic. Of 12 patients, treated with diltiazem, 11 were attack-free. Of 14 patients taking verapamil, 13 had no further episodes. Myocardial infarction or cardiac death did not occur in any patient while taking nifedipine, diltiazem, or verapamil. Chronic administration of perhexiline maleate was effective in only 64% of the patients.

Kimura and Kishida (1981) indicated that coronary lesions were discernible in 92 of 162 patients (56.7%) who underwent coronary angiography. However, regardless of the presence or absence of such organic coronary processes, the three Ca antagonists nifedipine, diltiazem, and verapamil were effective in 92.3% of the patients with normal or nearly normal coronary arteries, and in 82.6% of those with stenosis of more than 50% of the luminal diameter. In sharp contrast with this high therapeutic success rate of Ca antagonists, the effectiveness of β-blockers was rather poor, since in only 11.1% of the patients with Prinzmetal's spastic angina did the latter drugs exert a positive effect. Although long-acting nitrates, such as isosorbide dinitrate, given orally were often used for the prevention of attacks of variant angina, these drugs too are far less effective than Ca antagonists (Yasue, 1980). This is in full agreement with our observations on isolated coronary vasculature, where the spasmolytic action of nitrates was always incomplete and transient (see Section 6.2.4; Figures 153, 154, 162, 163).

Interestingly enough, Ca antagonists are not only able to prevent spontaneous attacks of variant angina, but also suppress the vasoconstrictor responses to provocative tests. For instance, *diltiazem* has been shown to neutralize the effects of Tris-buffer infusion and hyperventilation (Yasue, Nagao, Omote, Takizawa, Miwa, and Tanaka, 1978). *Verapamil,* injected intravenously in a dose of 10 mg, neutralized ergonovine-induced ischemic episodes with 100% efficacy as realized with [201]thallium scintigraphy (Mathey, Montz, Hanrath, Kuck, and Bleifeld, 1980). Intravenous injection of 0.8 mg nitroglycerin, on the other hand, acted only weakly. In another study on 23 patients with typical variant angina, the inhibitory effects of *nifedipine* (80 mg/day), *diltiazem* (360 mg/day), *verapamil* (480 mg/day), and *perhexiline* (400 to 1000 mg/day) upon ergonovine-induced pain and ST-segment elevation were compared (Waters, Theroux, Dauwe, Crittin, Affaki, and Mizgala, 1979). Nifedipine, diltiazem, and verapamil consistently increased the threshold doses of ergonovine at which symptoms of myocardial ischemia occurred. During long-term treatment with nifedipine, 18 patients out of the total of 23 became completely protected against coronary spasm induced by 0.4 mg ergonovine. One single dose of 20 mg nifedipine (buccal absorption) can even acutely neutralize the coronary vasoconstrictor effect of 0.2 mg of ergonovine (Goldberg, Reichek, Wilson, Hirshfeld, Muller, and Kastor, 1979). In this study, coronary spasm due to α-adrenergic stimulation by means of the "cold-pressor test," could also be prevented with nifedipine. Gunther, Green, Muller, Mudge, and Grossman (1981) reported corresponding results obtained with 10 mg nifedipine (buccal absorption) in 10 patients. Here too, the pathological coronary vasoconstrictor reactions to cold were completely normalized. It has to be further clarified whether this nifedipine effect is due to an influence more on the cardiac resistance vessels than on the great subepicardial trunk arteries.

In summarizing this host of clinical observations, the most specific Ca antagonists nifedipine, verapamil, and diltiazem, classified by us as Ca antagonists of category A, also proved to be of outstanding coronary spasmolytic potency in patients with Prinzmetal's variant angina. Nifedipine, verapamil, and diltiazem, the strongest inhibitors of Ca-dependent contractile activation of extramural coronary vasculature in pigs and rabbits (Figure 150 and 151), obviously keep this top position in humans also.

7.3.2. Angina at Rest, Unstable Angina, Coronary Infarction

It has been convincingly demonstrated by Maseri and his colleagues that the "variant" form of angina with typical ST-segment elevation represents only one extreme of a continuous spectrum of acute transient ischemia caused by vasospasm (see the review of Maseri, Severi, De Nes, L'Abbate, Chierchia, Marzilli, Ballestra, Parodi, Biagini, and Distante, 1978). These researchers showed in their scintigraphic studies with thallium-201 on patients with angina at rest that regional reduction of coronary blood supply by vasospasm is not necessarily associated with ST-segment elevation, but may also manifest itself by ST-segment *depression*. In fact, spontaneous ischemic episodes characterized by ST-segment elevation or depression may alternate even in the same patient within a few minutes (Jouve, Guiran, Viallet, Gras, Blanc, Arnoux, Rouvier, and Brunel, 1969; van Ekelen and Robles de Medina (1978). As generally accepted, ST-segment elevation signifies *transmural* myocardial ischemia, whereas ST-segment depression occurs when ischemia affects primarily the subendocardial parts of the left ventricular wall. Thus the direction of the ST-segment deviation is certainly no mark of distinction between different pathogenic mechanisms. It rather indicates differences in the extent and location of the ischemic regions.

Vasospastic myocardial ischemia can occur in the absence of discernible arterial lesions or in the presence of an extremely variable degree of coronary atherosclerosis. Hence in coronary patients, spastic angina at rest may even develop in addition to typical exertional angina so that in severe cases, both classic exercise-induced and spastic angina at rest may coexist. Moreover, coronary vasospasm of increasing intensity probably plays a major etiological role in the pathogenesis of unstable "crescendo" angina. This spasm may evolve into acute myocardial infarction and even sudden death. In 37 of Maseri's patients who manifested acute myocardial infarction, the location corresponded to the areas of electrocardiographic changes during previous anginal attacks at rest. In a number of cases, direct evidence of severe vasospasm had previously been obtained also by thallium-201 scintigraphy or coronary angiography of the corresponding arterial branches that supplied the infarcted zone (Maseri, L'Abbate, Baroldi, Chierchia, Marzilli, Ballestra, Severi, Parodi, Biagini, Distante, and Pesola, 1978). Similar observations were reported by Johnson and Detwiler (1977). However, apart from cases with evident angina at rest or instable angina, spasm may cause infarction or contribute to infarction in other patients as well. For instance, Oliva and Breckinridge (1977) demonstrated the occurrence of coronary spasm in 6 of 15 patients (40%) studied within 12 hours following the onset of infarction. But the total incidence of spasm was possibly higher because there is no guarantee that initial spasm was still present in all cases at the time of angiography many hours later. Thus Maseri and his colleagues as well as Hillis and Braunwald (1978), Braunwald (1978, 1980, 1981), and Bleifeld (1980) emphazised in recent years the need to reconsider the traditional concept of angina that had concentrated nearly exclusively on the causative role of an increase in myocardial oxygen demand in the presence of rigid permanent coronary obstruction. Now all these authors agree that blood supply can also be critically restricted by transient coronary vasospasm without any previous augmentation of cardiac energy expenditure. Indeed, there is a broad spectrum of clinical manifestations of coronary artery spasm, including *"not only Prinzmetal's variant angina, the prototypical syndrome, but also some forms of exercise-induced angina, unstable angina, acute myocardial infarction, typical angina pectoris, and sudden death"* (Braunwald, 1981). And this author continues, *"Thus coronary artery spasm may have a far more important role in the pathogenesis of the clinical manifestations of ischemic heart disease than had been thought previously."*

Needless to say, if the occurrence of coronary vasospasm is not restricted to Prinzmetal's variant angina, the Ca antagonists may represent the drugs of choice also for other manifestations of functional coronary insufficiency. This applies particularly to the administration of Ca antagonists in cases of instable "crescendo" angina to prevent imminent infarction. There are several vascular and nonvascular effects of Ca antagonists that can, in such instances, beneficially cooperate, namely:

1. Suppression of superimposed arterial spasm in atherosclerotic coronary stem arteries.
2. Increase in collateral flow to the ischemic region.
3. Antihypertensive action in systemic circulation, thus relieving the heart indirectly.
4. Cellular cardioprotection by reducing cardiac oxygen requirement and shielding hypoxic myocardium from detrimental Ca overload (see Section 2.10 and Chapter 3).
5. Elimination of ventricular arrhythmias and conduction disturbances arising from "slow-channel activity" of the partially depolarized ischemic region (see Chapter 5 and Section 7.5.1).

The ability of Ca antagonists to protect ischemic myocardium is well known from animal experiments. Many observations have been carried out in anesthetized open-chest dogs with the left descending coronary artery or its main branches acutely ligatured. In all these cases, infarct size, structural or ECG changes, and enzyme (CK) losses were shown to be significantly decreased by appropriate treatment with Ca antagonists. Simultaneously, collateral flow to the ischemic area and to the surrounding regions as well as local contractile performance improved. The rate of postoperative survival also rose. This happened irrespective of whether *verapamil* (Wende, Bleifeld, Meyer, and Stühlen, 1975; Smith, Singh, Nisbet, and Norris, 1975; Reimer, Lowe, and Jennings, 1977), *diltiazem* (Nakamura, Kikuchi, Senda, Yamada, and Koiwaya, 1980), or *nifedipine* (Welman, Carroll, Scott Lawson, Selwyn, and Fox, 1978; Henry, Shuchleib, Clark, and Perez, 1979) were administered to the dogs for cardioprotection. A considerable increase in collateral flow by *diltiazem* has also been established with the microsphere technique in anesthetized pigs after ligature of three or four terminal branches of the left anterior descending coronary artery (Millard, 1980). Similarly, *nifedipine* administered at the onset of coronary infarction to chronically instrumented conscious dogs augmented collateral blood flow to the ischemic zone and reduced enzyme loss from this region (Clark, Christlieb, Henry, Fischer, Nora, Williamson, and Sobel, 1979). In other studies on awake dogs, collaterals were allowed to develop during progressive occlusion of the left circumflex coronary artery, produced by an implanted ameroid constrictor. Under these conditions, underperfusion and functional impairment of the collateral-dependent myocardial area could be seen only during treadmill exercise or rapid pacing. Again, acute improvement of regional contractile function by *verapamil* (Osakada, Kumada, Gallagher, Kemper, and Ross, 1981) and an increase in collateral blood flow by *diltiazem* (Franklin, Millard, and Nagao, 1980) could be demonstrated.

Animal experiments of the foregoing type represent a model of human exercise-induced angina. They resemble studies of Lichtlen, Engel, Wolf, and Pretschner (1979) and of Lichtlen, Engel, Wolf, and Hundeshagen (1979) with *nifedipine* in patients showing fixed $\geq 75\%$ stenosis of one or two of the three main coronary trunk arteries. When nifedipine was given sublingually in a 20-mg dose at rest, the average increase in regional myocardial blood flow (measured with the precordial Xenon-clearance technique) amounted to 18.4% in the poststenotic area ($p < 0.05$), and to 11% in the normally supplied myocardium ($p < 0.05$). Atrial pacing without nifedipine led to a greater rise in regional perfusion of the normal than in that of the poststenotic area. However, with nifedipine, poststenotic perfusion during pacing was further enhanced ($p < 0.01$) so that here too the higher flow intensities of the normally supplied myocardium could be finally attained. This happened in spite of a significant fall in mean aortic pressure ($p < 0.0025$).

All results indicate that the Ca antagonists verapamil, diltiazem, and nifedipine are capable of improving collateral blood supply to poststenotic regions in canine, porcine, and human hearts in a similar manner. Accordingly, Ca antagonists may preserve jeopardized myocardium in the border zone of infarction, thereby reducing the definite size of the necrotizing area, or even totally prevent infarction if coronary vasospasm is the major determinant of critical ischemia. First encouraging observations on reduction of infarct size in humans with the help of verapamil infusions have been reported by Wolf, Habel, Witt, Nötges, Everling, and Hochrein (1977).

7.4. USE OF CALCIUM ANTAGONISTS IN THE TREATMENT OF HYPERTENSION

In normotensive individuals, blood pressure always tends to decrease if high doses of verapamil, nifedipine, or diltiazem are administered. This effect is partially due to a negative inotropic action, but results primarily from a decrease in systemic vascular resistance (Section 6.2.9). The Ca antagonists reduce Ca-dependent vascular smooth muscle tone by direct interference with transmembrane Ca supply and thereby counteract every kind of contractile tension development of the vascular wall. However, the higher the wall tension is elevated above normal, the easier relaxation is induced by a given Ca-antagonist concentration. This means that the Ca antagonists are powerful antihypertensive drugs at high blood pressure levels, but act much weaker in the normotensive range.

7.4.1. Verapamil

The first detailed reports calling attention to the beneficial influence of verapamil in hypertensive emergencies (systolic blood pressure 230 to 300 mm Hg) showed that one single intravenous injection of 5 mg verapamil consistently decreases systolic and diastolic blood pressure by 20 to 25% within 1 to 2 min (Brittinger, Schwarzbeck, Wittenmeier, Twittenhoff, Stegaru, Huber, Ewald, v. Henning, Fabricius, and Strauch, 1970; Bender, 1970). According to observations on roughly 100 patients with massive renal or essential hypertension, the effect of a single intravenous dose of verapamil slowly subsides with a half-time of about 30 min. But the reduction in blood pressure could be fully maintained over several hours with continuous verapamil infusions (0.07 to 1.5 mg verapamil/min intravenously). Critical hypertension in children with advanced renal failure also responded satisfactorily to single intravenous doses of verapamil (0.1 mg/kg) or to intravenous infusions (Diekmann and Hösemann, 1974; Schärer, Alatas, and Bein, 1977). Furthermore, dramatic normalization of blood pressure with verapamil has been achieved in preeclampsia (Brittinger et al.).

Recently, clinical interest has more concentrated on the control of hypertension by *chronic oral administration* of verapamil. Also with this mode of medication, a significant antihypertensive efficacy of verapamil could be established (Lewis, Morley, Lewis, and Bones, 1978; Lederballe Pedersen, 1978; Spies, Koch, Appel, Palm, and Kaltenbach, 1978). Further confirmation came from two randomized, double-blind, crossover trials (Midtbø and Hals, 1980; Anavekar, Christophidis, Louis, and Doyle, 1981). Continuous monitoring of intraarterial blood pressure showed that verapamil (dose range 120 to 160 mg TDS) given over 6 weeks produced a consistent antihypertensive effect throughout the 24-hour cycle (Gould, Stewart Mann, Kieso, Bala Subramanian, and Raftery, 1981).

Hemodynamic investigations revealed that verapamil lowered blood pressure of hypertensive patients by producing a fall in total peripheral vascular resistance, whereas in doses up to 160 mg thrice daily, stroke volume and renal blood flow were not influenced. Blood pressure control by verapamil could be achieved without reflex tachycardia and without clinically significant fluid retention. No changes in plasma renin activity, aldosterone content, and total amount of catecholamines occurred (de Leeuw, Smout, Willemse, and Birkenhäger, 1981). The absence of undesired side effects in verapamil-treated hypertensive patients has also been stressed by other clinical investigators (Muiesan, Agabiti-Rosei, Alicandri, Beschi, Castellano, Corea, Fariello, Romanelli, Pasini, and Platto, 1981). Verapamil also exerted no influence upon plasma Na, K, bicarbonate, creatinine, uric acid, blood glucose, serum lipids, and high-density lipoprotein. In 75 hypertensive patients, given verapamil (80 or 160 mg TDS) for 1 year, tolerance did not develop (Lewis, Stewart, Lewis, Bones, Morley, and Janus, 1981).

The efficacy of verapamil in the long-term treatment of hypertension is similar to that of β-blockers. This conclusion has also recently been substantiated by two randomized double-blind crossover studies against a placebo. In these trials, *verapamil* (120 to 160 mg thrice daily) was compared (1) with *propranolol* (60 to 80 mg thrice daily) (Leonetti, Pasotti, Ferrari, and Zanchetti, 1981) and (2) with *pindolol* (7.5 mg twice daily) (Doyle, Anavekar, and Oliver, 1981). At these dose levels, the antihypertensive effectiveness of the three drugs was roughly equal. However, there is a distinct advantage of verapamil over the β-blockers at an advanced age, in that hypertension of old patients is much more responsive to verapamil than to β-blockade (Bühler, Hulthen, Kiowski, and Bolli, 1982; see Figure 195). Furthermore, β-blockers should be avoided in patients with acute or chronic asthma or impairment of peripheral blood circulation. However, verapamil is not only innocuous in obstructive airways disease (Ringqvist, 1974), but may even be therapeutically useful in these cases, since it can prevent, in contrast with β-blockers, exercise-induced asthma (Patel, 1981). Moreover, verapamil is able to improve arterial blood flow to the extremities. Other Ca antagonists, for instance nifedipine (Cerrina, Denjean, Alexandre, Lockhart, and Duroux, 1981) or perhexiline (Feinsilver, Cho, and Aviado, 1970), also exhibit both vasodilator and bronchodilator activities.

7.4.2. Nifedipine

It is well known that nifedipine injected intravenously also induces a rapid fall of systolic and diastolic blood pressure both in animals and in normotensive or hypertensive humans. However, observations on the practical use of nifedipine as an antihypertensive drug are hitherto scarce. Nevertheless, it has become quite clear from a few recent studies that nifedipine, even after oral administration, is at least as potent as verapamil in hypertensive emergencies (Olivari, Bartorelli, Polese,

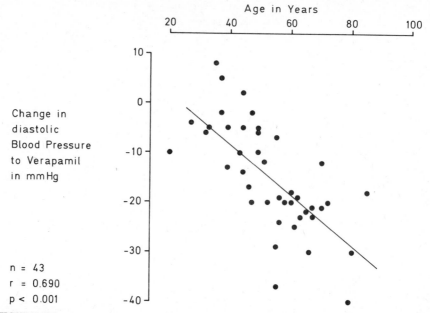

FIGURE 195. Age and diastolic blood pressure in response to verapamil. Daily oral doses of 240 to 720 mg verapamil (427 ± 158 mg/day) were given as monotherapy for an average of 93 days to 43 patients with essential hypertension. From Bühler, Hulthen, Kiowski, and Bolli (1982).

Fiorentini, Moruzzi, and Guazzi, 1979; Ueda, Kuwajima, Ito, Kuramoto, and Murakami, 1979; Magometschnigg and Pichler, 1981; MacGregor, Markandu, Bayliss, Brown, and Roulston, 1981). The onset of action following sublingual application of 10 to 20 mg nifedipine is rapid since a significant decrease in blood pressure of hypertensive patients could regularly be seen after 10 min, with a maximum at 30 to 60 min. Most patients receiving 20 mg nifedipine still showed a discernible therapeutic response after 6 to 8 hours (Lederballe Pedersen and Mikkelsen, 1978). Nifedipine proved to be dramatically effective even in cases of severe intractable hypertension that could not be managed by monotherapy or combined therapy with thiazide, α-methyldopa, β-blockers, or hydralazine. Patients in acute hypertensive crisis with disturbed consciousness (mean blood pressure 237/110 mm Hg) could also be successfully treated with one single oral dose of 10 mg nifedipine (see Figure 196). There was in these patients a deep acute fall of blood pressure and an improvement of clinical symptoms for at least 3 hours (Ueda et al.). The responsiveness of hypertensive subjects to nifedipine is unphysiologically high, since blood pressure of normotensive individuals was almost refractory to 10 to 20 mg nifedipine (Lederballe Pedersen, Christensen, and Rämsch, 1980; MacGregor, Markandu, Bayliss, Brown, and Roulston, 1981). If compared with oral administration of verapamil (160 mg), blood pressure reduction by nifedipine (10 to 20 mg) in hypertensive patients occurs faster and therefore stimulates sympathetic reflex

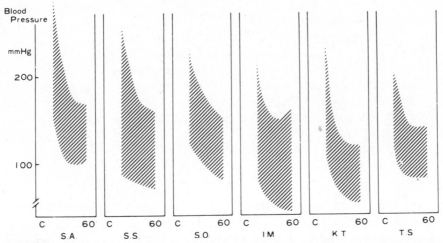

FIGURE 196. Effects of nifedipine on systolic and diastolic blood pressure of 6 patients, 3 males and 3 females aged from 64 to 77 years, in acute hypertensive crisis. Three patients took 10 mg nifedipine orally. Three patients with disturbances of consciousness and convulsions received 10 mg of the drug dissolved in 10 ml water via a gastric tube. With the fall of blood pressure, all patients showed improvement of their clinical symptoms without adverse reactions attributable to nifedipine. From Ueda, Kuwajima, Ito, Kuramoto, and Murakami (1979).

activity to a greater extent. Thus with patients in the standing position, nifedipine produced a moderate increase in heart rate and a rise in plasma catecholamines by more than 100% (Muiesan et al.). However, the researchers did not find a change in plasma renin activity, in plasma and urinary aldosterone, and in plasma volume following the nifedipine application. These results differ slightly from observations of Japanese clinicians who found increases in plasma renin activity of normotensive and hypertensive subjects, at least after sublingual administration of the relatively high dose of 30 mg nifedipine (Aoki, Kondo, Mochizuki, Yoshida, Kato, Kato, and Takikawa, 1978). However, if nifedipine (30 mg) was administered simultaneously with propranolol (0.2 mg/kg body weight intravenously), not only the nifedipine-induced reflex increase in heart rate but also the rise in plasma renin activity could be completely neutralized. On the other hand, the antihypertensive effect of nifedipine was enhanced and prolonged by propranolol. Thus the administration of nifedipine combined with β-receptor blockade appeared to be particularly satisfactory in the management of hypertension, because of increased efficacy and minimized adverse drug effects.

7.4.3. Diltiazem

Since 1975 an abundant number of publications in Japanese have delt with the therapeutic use of diltiazem in patients with essential hypertension. Regarding the antihypertensive efficacy of verapamil and nifedipine, it was in fact not surprising that diltiazem too exhibited this property, although in a mitigated form. A survey in English, containing the results collected from 15 Japanese cardiology institutes, was published by Ikeda (1979). These studies had been carried out over 6 weeks on 97 hypertensive patients according to a double-blind crossover protocol against a placebo. Diltiazem proved to be useful for the control of mild and moderate forms of hypertension at a daily oral dose of 180 mg, particularly in combination with thiazide. The effect of a single oral dose of 60 mg diltiazem on blood pressure of hypertensive subjects was still discernible after 6 hours (Maeda, Takasugi, Tsukano, Tanaka, and Shiota, 1981). Recent observations from European cardiologists are consistent with those of the Japanese investigators (Klein, 1982; Brandt and Klein, 1982). In the study of Klein, the antihypertensive potency of a daily oral dose of 180 to 270 mg diltiazem was equivalent to 30 to 60 mg of nifedipine.

In summarizing the essence of these studies, verapamil, nifedipine, and diltiazem act as useful antihypertensive drugs, via a decrease in peripheral vascular resistance. Sympathetic reflex activity is rather pronounced after administration of nifedipine, but weak or indiscernible when the patients receive diltiazem or verapamil. However, the most striking phenomenon that deserves a special comment is the extraordinary power of verapamil and nifedipine in relieving critical hypertension. Indeed, acute hypertensive episodes can be interrupted so dramatically with Ca antagonists that this effect points to a particular action of Ca antagonists on a special Ca-dependent vasopressor mechanism responsible for overshooting tension development. *This mechanism is possibly identical with vasoconstrictive autoregulation.* As discussed in Section 6.2.8, and Section 6.2.9, autoregulatory vasoconstriction represents a positive feedback mechanism that in hypertensive crisis may escape control (see Figure 197). In this case, an initial stimulus evokes contraction of the vascular wall and a blood pressure rise. Thereby, further autoregulatory vasoconstriction is elicited that in turn increases intravascular pressure additionally, leading to the development of even more active tension in the vascular wall, and so on. Whatever the primary stimulus may be, the most efficient way to interrupt this vicious circle is a blockade of Ca-dependent autoregulatory vasoconstriction with the help of Ca antagonists (see Figures 176 to 181). According to our experimental studies, autoregulatory vasoconstriction is in fact one of the easiest suppressible vascular reactions, even at low Ca-antagonist concentrations.

The acute reduction by Ca antagonists of left ventricular afterload may cause dramatic improvement in cases of critical hypertension complicated by congestive heart failure. However, there is also a considerable decrease by Ca antagonists of pulmonary hypertension, particularly in patients with alveolar hypoxia. A dose of 10 mg intravenous verapamil (Reuben and Kuan, 1980), 20 mg sublingual nifedipine (Simonneau, Escourrou, Duroux, and Lockhart, 1981), or 10 mg of intravenous diltiazem (Kambara, Fujimoto, Wakabayashi, and Kawai, 1981) were again very effective when pulmonary hypertension was pronounced, but they acted weakly in the normal pulmonary pressure range. Thus Ca antagonists meet the therapeutic requirements also with respect to pulmonary circulation.

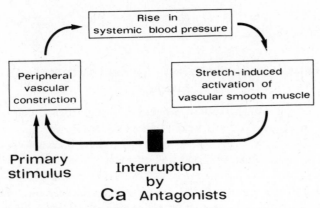

FIGURE 197. Scheme of the positive-feedback mechanism arising from autoregulatory pressure-induced vasoconstriction. Interruption of the vicious circle, possibly underlying hypertensive crises, can probably be effectuated with the help of Ca antagonists. The Ca-dependent autoregulatory vasoconstriction is much more sensitive to the action of Ca antagonists than is vasoconstriction directly produced by vasoconstrictive agonists such as noradrenaline (Grün and Fleckenstein, 1972). For physiological details see Sections 6.2.8 and 6.2.9.

7.5. THERAPEUTIC SIGNIFICANCE OF CALCIUM ANTAGONISTS IN CARDIAC ARRHYTHMIAS

The Ca antagonists as research tools have enormously contributed during the last decade to the elucidation of the crucial role of Ca ions in nomotopic and ectopic pacemaker activity. As depicted in Chapter 5, ectopic ventricular automaticity can depend completely on a slow-channel-mediated transmembrane Ca–K exchange, which is, of course, most susceptible to the inhibitory influence of Ca antagonists. But, conversely, other forms of spontaneous ectopic impulse discharge, particularly from Purkinje fibers, depend more on an electrogenic inward current of Na ions. In this case, Na-antagonistic agents, such as quinidine, procaine, lidocaine, and so forth, are consequently the more promising antiarrhythmic agents. The decisive determinant of whether ectopic automaticity depends more on the transmembrane influx of Na or Ca ions consists of the absolute height of the diastolic membrane potential at which the pacemaker cells operate. But unfortunately, the heart of a patient is still inaccessible to the necessary measurements. Thus despite of all recent advances in basic knowledge, the medical management of ectopic atrial and ventricular automaticity with Na antagonists or Ca antagonists remains a matter of clinical empiricism. According to some medical reviewers, verapamil, the prototypical Ca antagonist with antiarrhythmic potency, appears to be more useful for the treatment of atrial than ventricular ectopic automaticity. But this generalization is probably premature (Coumel, Attuel, and Leclercq, 1981). However, there are two clearly defined situations in which Ca antagonists are by far superior to other antiarrhythmic drugs, namely (1) ischemia-induced ventricular automaticity of vasospastic origin, and (2) supraventricular reentry tachycardia.

7.5.1. Ectopic Ventricular Tachycardia and Fibrillation in Vasospastic Angina

Ischemia-induced ventricular autorhythmicity is a phenomenon that occurs in its purest form in patients with Prinzmetal's variant angina. However, it is particularly remarkable that ectopic ventricular automaticity usually does not develop during the ischemic episodes, characterized by ST-segment elevation, but afterward, upon resolution of the attacks, when the patients exhibit deep negative T waves (Maseri, L'Abbate, Chierchia, Parodi, Severi, Biagini, Distante, Marzilli, and Ballestra, 1979). Thus in these cases ventricular tachycardia and even fibrillation are not directly connected with complete spastic vascular occlusion, but rather coincide with reperfusion of previously blocked coronary arterial branches. Similar observations were reported by Braunwald (1981). He also stated that the ventricular arrhythmias in patients with Prinzmetal's variant angina develop or are most intense after the ST-segment elevation has returned to baseline, *"suggesting that they are precipitated by reperfusion of the myocardium after relief of spasm."* As depicted in Section 3.5.4, the onset of reperfusion after temporal standstill of coronary circulation is the very moment at which an "avalanche" of Ca ions invades the myocardial fibers at a still reduced membrane potential. Obviously, tachyarrhythmia and ventricular fibrillation are the electrophysiological manifestations of this transmembrane intrusion of Ca, in exchange for K (see Sections 5.3.3 and 5.3.4). In accordance with observations on ischemic animal hearts, Ca antagonists are also able to block such dysrhythmias in humans. Two particularly dramatic cases of variant angina, complicated by recurrent ventricular fibrillation, have been reported by Mizuno, Tanaka, Honda, and Kimura (1979). One patient developed 21 episodes of transient ST-elevation and 12 attacks of ventricular fibrillation within 10 hours in spite of continuous intravenous infusion of lidocaine (2 to 4 mg/min). And DC defibrillation was required three times. Finally, the fibrillation could be completely suppressed with one single intravenous dose of 0.2 mg of nifedipine. In the second case of similar severity, lidocaine was again ineffective. But intravenous injection of 0.4 mg of nifedipine stopped the series of attacks of ventricular fibrillation also in this patient. Therapy was continued successfully with a daily oral dose of 30 mg nifedipine.

Clearly, the Ca antagonists not only suppress symptomatic attacks of ventricular fibrillation arising from coronary vasospasm, but also abolish or prevent coronary spasm itself, thus eliminating the primary reason for dangerous ventricular automaticity. The observations suggest a more intense use of Ca antagonists as antiarrhythmic agents also in cases of unstable angina and acute myocardial infarction with respect to possible involvement of a vasospastic component. In a recent study of Fazzini, Marchi, Pucci, Ledda, and Mugelli (1981), 50 patients with acute myocardial infarction, 3 of them presenting ventricular tachycardia and 47 showing ventricular premature beats, were injected a single intravenous dose of 0.1 mg verapamil/kg in 2 min under continuous ECG and blood pressure monitoring. The treatment was effective in 42 patients (= 84%) who showed complete cessation of arrhythmia within 90 to 180 seconds. The group of responders comprised the 3 patients with ventricular tachycardia and 39 with ventricular premature beats. Thus the beneficial effects of verapamil in human infarction were analogous to those reported in dogs after coronary artery ligation (Kaumann and Aramendia, 1968) or temporary coronary occlusion (Fondacaro, Han, and Yoon, 1978). Here too, verapamil prevented ventricular tachycardia and fibrillation with particularly high efficacy.

7.5.2. Paroxysmal Supraventricular Tachycardia

Bender, Kojima, Reploh, and Oelmann in 1966 introduced verapamil into human therapy for antiarrhythmic purposes. Inspired by successful animal experiments (see Section 5.2.2), Bender and his colleagues injected a standard dose of 5 mg verapamil intravenously. Thereby, in 21 patients with atrial fibrillation and in 4 patients with atrial flutter, the ventricular rate was significantly slowed. Subsequent clinical investigations of Bender (1967, 1970), Brichard and Zimmermann (1970), Schamroth (1971) and Schamroth, Krikler, and Garrett (1972) definitely established this new therapy. In the latter study, verapamil was administered intravenously in a dose of 10 mg over 15 to 30 sec to 181 patients. Of 115 patients suffering from atrial fibrillation, 111 responded with ventricular slowing and 71 with regularization. Eighteen patients had atrial flutter, conversion to sinus rhythm being obtained in 4, and a decrease in the ventricular response in 11. However, the highest efficacy rate of intravenous verapamil was observed in 20 patients with paroxysmal supraventricular tachycardia, since they all were promptly converted to sinus rhythm.

There are in principle two basic effects of verapamil that could possibly explain this striking result, namely:

1. Slowing or suppression by verapamil of supraventricular ectopic foci.
2. Retardation by verapamil of AV impulse conduction and prolongation of the AV-node recovery time. Thereby the maximum frequency of atrial impulses that effectively reach the His-Purkinje system is lowered.

The final answer came from further extensive studies, particularly of Krikler and his associates, using intracardiac recordings of electric activity and programmed electric stimulation of the heart (Krikler, 1974a, b; Spurrell, Krikler, and Sowton, 1974a, b). According to their observations, it is primarily the mechanism (2), that is, the inhibitory influence of verapamil on AV-node conduction that matters (see Section 4.2.1).

Paroxysmal supraventricular tachycardia is either due to a reciprocating mechanism within the AV node or related to an intranodal reentry pathway or to an AV circus movement associated with an anomalous bypass tract as in patients with the Wolff-Parkinson-White (WPW) syndrome. In the latter case, the anterograde pathway of the reentry loop mostly consists of the normal conduction system (AV node,

His-Purkinje fibers), whereas the retrograde impulses use the anomalous AV bypass tract for return. Verapamil, by counteracting impulse conduction through the AV node, can dramatically interrupt such circus movements. The drug depresses Ca-dependent excitation of the central region (N zone) of the AV node and thereby damps a decisive section of the reentry pathway, regardless of whether reciprocation depends on an intranodal circuit or an accessory AV connection.

Krikler and Spurrell (1974), in continuation of their studies, were able to restore sinus rhythm with 100% efficiency in 32 patients suffering from paroxysmal supraventricular tachycardia by a single rapid intravenous injection of 10 mg verapamil. Identical results were obtained in a further 10 patients with AV tachycardias associated with the WPW syndrome. In a separate group of 18 patients in whom AV junctional tachycardias were induced during intracardiac electrography, conversion to sinus rhythm was achieved in 15 patients, with prolongation of the cycle length in the others. Circus-movement tachycardias were induced in 8 patients with the WPW syndrome, and conversion to sinus rhythm occurred in 7. Interestingly enough, the results were less consistent in patients with ectopic atrial tachycardia and flutter, although even in these cases the elevated atrial or ventricular rates usually tended to decline under the verapamil treatment. Intravenous *nifedipine* (7.5 μg/kg), on the other hand, does not significantly impair AV conduction and consequently never terminated paroxysmal supraventricular tachycardia (Rowland, Evans, and Krikler, 1979; Dargie, Rowland, and Krikler, 1981). *Diltiazem* too reduces AV-node conduction rather mildly. Thus verapamil has hitherto kept its primacy in the armamentarium of antiarrhythmic drugs used for the treatment of supraventricular reentry tachycardias. Indeed for this indication, verapamil has found worldwide acceptance. The intravenous administration of 5 to 10 mg verapamil in adults is safe provided the patient is not under the influence of reserpine or a β-blocker. Verapamil is absolutely contraindicated in the presence of a "sick sinus syndrome." After successful conversion to sinus rhythm, recurrence of supraventricular tachyarrhythmias could be prevented in 75% of the patients with oral doses of verapamil alone (240 to 480 mg daily) or in combination with quinidine [Karnell and Köhler (see Krikler 1974b)].

7.6. CARDIOPROTECTION BY CALCIUM ANTAGONISTS AGAINST HYPERCONTRACTILE DISORDERS

7.6.1. Cardiac Hypertrophy and Structural Damage as Consequences of Catecholamine-Induced Myocardial Calcium Overload; Prophylaxis with Calcium Antagonists

As depicted in Chapter 3, excessive β-adrenergic stimulation of heart muscle induces a transient hypercontractile state, followed by high-energy-phosphate exhaustion and irreversible mitochondrial damage, finally leading to disseminated or confluent myocardial necrotization. This happens in rats if a single high dose of a β-adrenergic agent, for instance 30 mg isoproterenol/kg body weight injected subcutaneously, multiplies the normal cytoplasmic Ca concentration in the ventricular tissue. If, however, in our experiments small doses of isoproterenol (1 mg/kg daily) were administered over a week, the myocardial Ca content grew only moderately, and the predominant morphological phenomenon consisted of *ventricular hypertrophy* (Fleckenstein, Fréy, and Keidel, 1980/1982). In 157 experiments of the latter type, we found a rise of the ratio of ventricular weight (expressed in milligrams) over body weight (expressed in grams) from 0.56 to 0.8 (right ventricle) and from 2.02 to 2.65 (left ventricle). Moreover, after 7 days, scarce disseminated necroses in the state of healing were discernible in the apical region of the left ventricle. This was accompanied by an increase in the apical hydroxyproline titer, an observation that is indicative of a proliferation of connective tissue that replaces necrotic cardiac fibers, hydroxyproline representing 13% of the collagen mass.

Cardiomegaly as a consequence of chronic administration of low doses of isoproterenol has repeatedly been described (Rakusan, Tietzova, Turek, and Poupa, 1965; Stanton, Brenner, and Mayfield, 1969; Alderman and Harrison, 1971; Pfitzer, Knieriem, Dietrich, and Herbertz, 1972). But this myocardial fiber hypertrophy can obviously be accompanied by degenerative processes in the subendocardial and apical areas and by formation of fibrous scars. Thus the histological appearance of the chronically isoproterenol-treated rat hearts resembled, in some extent, that of *"hypertrophic cardiomyopathy"* of other origin, that is, hereditary cardiomyopathy of Syrian hamsters, or even hypertrophic obstructive cardiomyopathy in man.

However, the most important finding was that the same Ca-antagonist treatment that prevented acute isoproterenol-induced myocardial necrotization, that is, administration of verapamil, KCl, or $MgCl_2$, also inhibited isoproterenol-induced cardiac hypertrophy. Table 20 represents a quantitative evaluation of our results. The figures represent the degree of inhibition (expressed in percent) of the isoproterenol effects on ventricular weight (in relation to body weight) and on the apical hydroxyproline content. As can easily be seen from these data, verapamil alone (daily doses of 15 mg/kg subcutaneously administered for 7 days) inhibited the isoproterenol-induced growth of the relative ventricular mass by 65.7% ($\pm$ 3.2%), and the concomitant increase in the hydroxyproline content by 79.8% ($\pm$ 12.1%). However, the most efficient treatment consisted of combining the subcutaneous administration of verapamil with oral doses of KCl or $MgCl_2$ twice daily for 7 days. With this regimen, the isoproterenol-induced left ventricular hypertrophy and the rise in hydroxyproline could be completely prevented in most cases. The inhibition of left ventricular hypertrophy by 118.6% ($\pm$ 9.9%) (!) that was observed in the isoproterenol-treated rats under the therapy with verapamil plus $MgCl_2$ means that in this series the relative ventricular weights were found to be even smaller than those of the control animals without any drug application. The right ventricles too responded favorably to the Ca-antagonistic therapy, although the efficacy did not reach the 100% mark.

The experiments indicate that both ventricular necroses and hypertrophy produced by an exaggerated sympathetic drive are different consequences of the same myocardial alteration, that is, intracellular Ca overload. Moderate chronic increases in myocardial Ca content following application of relatively small doses of isoproterenol lead to potentiation of contractile force and ventricular hypertrophy, whereas

TABLE 20. Inhibition of Both Isoproterenol-Induced Cardiac Hypertrophy and Isoproterenol-Induced Increase in Apical Hydroxyproline Content of Rats by Simultaneous Prophylactic Administration of Verapamil in Combination with KCl or MgCl$_2$[a,b]

Cardioprotective Treatment	Inhibition of Isoproterenol-Induced Ventricular Hypertrophy		Inhibition of Isoproterenol-Induced Increase in Hydroxyproline Content (apex) (%)
	Right (%)	Left (%)	
With verapamil	34.5 (± 4.3)	65.7 (± 3.2)	79.8 (± 12.1)
With verapamil + KCl	58.5 (± 14.2)	106.5 (± 9.0)	110 (± 23.5)
With verapamil + MgCl$_2$	88.6 (± 8.6)	118.6 (± 9.9)	82.6 (± 8.6)

[a]All rats received a daily subcutaneous dose of 1 mg isoproterenol/kg body weight for 7 consecutive days.
[b]The figures indicate the percentage inhibition by which the isoproterenol effects could be reduced with the help of verapamil and the Ca-antagonistic salts. Verapamil was administered in the form of daily subcutaneous doses of 15 mg/kg body weight for a period of 7 days simultaneously with isoproterenol, at different injection sites. However, KCl (twice daily 5 mmol/kg) and MgCl$_2$ (twice daily 12.5 mmol/kg) were administered during the 7-day period with a stomach tube. (Janke, Fleckenstein, and Frey, 1978.)

higher degrees of acute Ca overload produce necrotization. In keeping with this, isoproterenol-induced hypertrophy and myocardial lesions can be prevented, at least in part, by verapamil, KCl, or MgCl$_2$, because these agents counteract excessive myocardial Ca uptake. However, most effective is a combined application of verapamil together with these salts. These observations gave an important hint for practical therapy also.

There is no doubt that the widespread medical use of β-adrenergic catecholamines for tocolytic purposes (inhibition of premature labor) in gynecology and as broncholytic drugs in the therapy of asthma increasingly implicates the risk of cardiotoxic side effects. Apart from a multitude of subjective complaints such as anger, palpitation, retrosternal discomfort, dizziness, heat sensation, and so forth, objective signs of myocardial damage also evidence the need for sufficient cardioprotection. Thus casuistic reports have clearly shown that during tocolytic therapy with β-mimetic agents (mostly fenoterol or ritodrine), the mothers may react under unfavorable circumstances with ST-segment depression, myocardial enzyme (CK) loss, left ventricular contractile failure, pulmonal edema, and occasionally with sudden death (Bender, Goeckenjan, Meger, and Müntefering, 1977; Ries, 1979; Bass, Friedemann, and Künzli, 1979). A detailed description of 12 cases with pulmonal edema was presented by Curtius, Goeckenjan, Steyer, and Hust (1980). All these 12 patients had, however, additionally received corticosteroids, which possibly aggravated the cardiotoxicity of β-adrenergic catecholamines (see Section 3.3). Perhaps intense tocolytic therapy may also affect the fetus, since Hillemanns and Trolp (1977) observed cardiomegaly, endocardial fibrosis, or fresh myocardial necroses in three newborns whose mothers had previously undergone this treatment. Similarly, Kurland, Williams, and Lewiston (1979) called attention to the eventuality of severe myocardial damage and untoward death of isoproterenol-treated asthmatics. The unfortunate patient of their case report, an 18-year-old girl, received a continuous infusion of 0.16 μg/kg/min of isoproterenol, again with supplementary intravenous *hydrocortisone* (200 mg every 6 hours). Following further treatment with *calcium* gluconate, *epinephrine,* and *sodium bicarbonate,* idioventricular rhythm, tachycardia, and finally cardiac standstill developed. This occurred 38 hours after admission to the hospital. Histological examination revealed multiple small areas of necrosis throughout the ventricular myocardium. Needless to say, hydrocortisone, calcium gluconate, epinephrine, and alkalization were liable to *enhance* this lethal isoproterenol intoxication.

There is, in fact, clear evidence (see Sections 3.3 and 3.5) that dramatic manifestations of the latent cardiotoxicity of β-adrenergic agents can be evoked by the following:

1. Direct increase in plasma Ca concentration produced by administration of Ca salts.
2. Relative preponderance of Ca over the H, K, and Mg ions that normally have to act as an equilibrating counterpoise; hence, K or Mg deficiency as well as alkalization can enormously potentiate catecholamine-induced myocardial damage.
3. Agents that facilitate Ca supply to the heart (dihydrotachysterol) or produce a negative K balance (corticosteroids, certain diuretics).

In order to minimize the hazards arising from the tocolytic or broncholytic therapy with β-adrenergic compounds, we not only recommended paying attention to the incompatibilities 1 to 3, but also suggested a prophylactic Ca-antagonist treatment with verapamil plus K and Mg salts, simultaneously administered with the β-adrenergic stimulants (Fleckenstein, Grün, Tritthart, and Byon, 1971; Fleckenstein, Janke, Fleckenstein-Grün, 1978; Janke and Fleckenstein 1978). Our proposals have willingly been accepted by most German gynecologists in that they have preferably been using for almost 10 years a combination of β-adrenergic agents plus verapamil as standard tocolytic therapy (Weidinger and Wiest, 1971, 1973a, b; Mosler, 1972; Weidinger, Wiest, Dietze, and Witzel, 1973; Hüter and Lammers, 1973; Koepcke and Seidenschnur, 1973; Neubüser, 1974; Weidinger, 1976). In contrast with the vivid sensations of discomfort arising from the monotherapy with fenoterol, simultaneous intravenous infusions of fenoterol (1 to 4 μg/min) plus verapamil hydrochloride in a dose ratio of 1 part fenoterol to 40 parts verapamil are usually well tolerated without subjective complaints and without objective signs of cardiac impairment. It is a pending problem whether verapamil at this dose level is also able to contribute to the suppression of premature labor in analogy with its tocolytic efficacy on uterine muscle *in vitro* (see Section 6.1).

7.6.2. Calcium-Antagonist Treatment of Human Hypertrophic Cardiomyopathy

Human hypertrophic obstructive cardiomyopathy seems to consist, in essence, of a primary hypercontractile dysfunction of the heart with secondary ventricular hypertrophy and eventual obstruction of the left (and sometimes also the right) ventricular outflow tract. The syndrome has been thoroughly described by several authors as *"asymmetrical hypertrophy"* (Teare, 1958), *"muscular subvalvular aortic stenosis"* (Menges, Brandenburg, and Brown, 1961, *"idiopathic hypertrophic subaortic stenosis"* (Braunwald, Lambrew, Rockoff, Ross, and Morrow, 1964), *"hypertrophic hyperkinetic cardiomyopathy"* (Criley, Lewis, White, and Ross, 1965), or *"hypertrophic obstructive cardiomyopathy"* (van Noorden, Olsen, and Pearse, 1971). All authors agreed upon the particular importance of asymmetric hypertrophy of the interventricular septum and of the free left ventricular wall. In such hearts the total muscular mass may occasionally grow to fourfold above normal. Hence even during diastole, the width of the left ventricular cavity is rather narrow, while its axis is elongated. However, upon onset of systole, the greatly hypertrophied septum bulges into the left ventricular outflow tract so that the small residual passage between the enlarged septum and the thick ventricular wall is further compressed. In addition to obstruction of ventricular outflow, hypertrophic cardiomyopathy is complicated by an abnormally low ventricular compliance, an important consequence of which is impedance of ventricular filling (Braunwald, Lambrew, Rockoff, Ross, and Morrow, 1964).

Furthermore, there are some functional characteristics, indicative of the hypercontractile state that probably underlies hypertrophy, such as the following:

1. A high rate of left ventricular systolic pressure rise (dp/dt_{max}).
2. An elevated left ventricular peak systolic pressure.
3. An augmentation of the left ventricular ejection fraction.
4. An overcontraction of the sarcomeres as directly evidenced by electron-microscopic examinations (Harmjanz and Reale, 1981).
5. A delayed decay of contractile tension during diastole, thus causing the above-mentioned stiffness of the ventricle that compromises refilling (Harmjanz, Böttcher, and Schertlein, 1971).

These functional peculiarities are attributable, in the light of current knowledge, to an increased availability of Ca to the contractile system. Thus it is not surprising that rapidly acting cardiac glycosides and other drugs that potentiate Ca-dependent contractile tension usually intensify the outflow obstruction. This is particularly true of isoproterenol, which consistently diminishes the size of the stenotic orifice if acutely administered (Braunwald, Lambrew, Rockoff, Ross, and Morrow, 1964;

Criley, Lewis, White, and Ross, 1965). Moreover, our observations on the development of cardiomegaly in chronically isoproterenol treated rats (see the preceding section) also suggest the possibility that the development of stenosing hypertrophy is related to an exaggerated transmembrane Ca supply, however of longer duration.

Whatever the ultimate etiological roots may be, the assessment of hypercontractility in human hypertrophic cardiomyopathy delivered the key to an appropriate management. There were, in fact, two rational therapeutic alternatives to be studied, namely treatment with β-blockers or with Ca antagonists. As to the therapy with β-blockers, most clinical research groups used nethalide or propranolol (Harrison, Braunwald, Glick, Mason, Chidsey, and Ross, 1964; Cohen and Braunwald, 1967; Swan, Bell, Oakley, and Goodwin, 1971; Adelman, Wigle, Ranganathan, Webb, Kidd, Bigelow, and Silver, 1972). However, the results were not satisfactory because more than transient symptomatic improvement was seldom obtainable. Thus in 1975, Kaltenbach, Hopf, and Keller tried the second possibility, that is, the use of Ca antagonists. The researchers, inspired by the outstanding cardioprotective efficacy of verapamil in catecholamine-poisoned rats and cardiomyopathic hamsters (see Chapter 3), administered this drug in a high daily oral dose of 480 mg to 20 patients with hypertrophic obstructive cardiomyopathy for an average of 12 months. Beforehand, the medication with propranolol or pindolol (mean duration 20 months) had been discontinued.

The results of the verapamil treatment were impressive. Apart from subjective improvement in 15 patients, there was a statistically significant regression of the cardiac volume and the electrocardiographic signs of left ventricular hypertrophy (Kaltenbach, Hopf, and Keller, 1976). According to a subsequent report based on a total of 22 (and finally 39) patients, subjective discomfort disappeared or lessened considerably in two thirds of the patients who had been symptomatic on β-blocker treatment (Kaltenbach, Hopf, Kober, Bussmann, Keller, and Petersen, 1979). Usually it took several weeks of treatment with verapamil before this improvement could be noticed. After an average of 15 months, the objective criteria of left ventricular hypertrophy, such as increases in heart volume, left ventricular muscle mass, Sokolow index (sum of maximal S and R deflections in leads V_1 to V_5), and coronary artery dimension also exhibited a clear trend toward normalization. Confirmatory reports came from different cardiology centers. For instance, in a study of Troesch, Hirzel, Jenni, and Krayenbühl (1979), a daily oral dose of 240 mg verapamil was administered over a test period of 4 to 9 months to 28 patients with asymmetric septal hypertrophy (22 of them exhibiting outflow obstruction). This treatment led to subjective relief, and significantly diminished the abnormal thickness of the interventricular septum as evidenced with m-mode echocardiography. Patients receiving daily oral doses of 480 mg verapamil for 3.5 to 6 months, also exhibited considerable improvement of their exercise capacity (Rosing, Kent, Maron, and Epstein, 1979). The beneficial influence of verapamil even manifested in acute hemodynamic studies, where the drug, after intravenous infusion, caused an immediate increase in the effective orifice size of the left ventricular outflow tract, reflected in a diminution of the basal left ventricular outflow tract gradient (Schmid, Pavek, and Klein, 1979; Rosing, Kent, Borer, Seides, Maron, and Epstein, 1979).

This widening of the orifice is primarily due to a verapamil-induced reduction of systolic peak tension. However it turned out that such acute hemodynamic tests with intravenous verapamil do not allow any prognostication about the therapeutic long-term effects of oral verapamil in individual patients.

Probably the long-term benefit of oral verapamil is more related to chronic improvement of ventricular compliance and diastolic filling than to a spectacular acute decrease in the systolic contractility parameters. In fact, recent observations of several clinical research groups have consistently shown that the main effect of oral verapamil is an improvement of the diastolic function, rather than an attenuation of contractile force. Accordingly, Bonow and Epstein (1981) as well as Bonow, Rosing, Bacharach, Green, Lipson, Condit, Kent, and Epstein (1981) found an accelerated onset of diastolic relaxation and an increased left ventricular peak filling rate (both $P < 0.001$) after oral verapamil (320 to 640 mg/day), whereas the left ventricular ejection fraction, peak ejection rate, or ejection time did not change. Similarly, Raff, Brundage, Ports, and Chatterjee (1981) noticed an increase in end-diastolic volume as the clearest effect of orally administered verapamil during a mean follow-up period of 9.8 months. Thus the regression of hypertrophy, the reduction of septal and parietal ventricular stiffness, as well as the trend to normalization of diastolic filling seem to be the most important therapeutic factors during long-term administration of verapamil. In this respect, verapamil differs from propranolol, which leaves hypertrophy and the diastolic filling parameters unaffected (Bonow and Epstein, 1981).

In summary, verapamil provides a new approach for the medical treatment of patients with hypertrophic cardiomyopathy. The overall success rate recently calculated by Hopf, Kaltenbach, and Kober (1981) from a total of 50 patients amounts to 82%. There was improvement in 57% and complete cessation of symptoms in 25% of the cases. Apart from hemodynamic benefit, verapamil may also afford protection against complicating ventricular arrhythmias (Goodwin and Krikler, 1976). In consequence, a cogent indication for surgical treatment of hypertrophic cardiomyopathy (ventricular septal myotomy-myectomy) in cases of refractoriness to β-blockers no longer exists.

CHAPTER EIGHT

Prospective Topics in Calcium-Antagonist Research

The Ca antagonists are exemplary of a rapid and successful exploitation of basic physiological, pathophysiological, and pharmacological research work for multiple therapeutic purposes. In fact, most of the beneficial cardiovascular effects of Ca antagonists in humans were predictable or at least easily explainable on the basis of previous experimental studies. However, regarding the nearly universal involvement of Ca in cellular life, it is natural that a number of Ca-dependent functions were hitherto not sufficiently examined with respect to their susceptibilities to Ca-antagonistic agents. However, apart from a number of open questions of basic nature, some promising new developments in the clinical field also deserve particular attention.

8.1. SOME UNSOLVED FUNDAMENTAL PROBLEMS

As to basic research, more detailed information is, for instance, needed about the possible inhibitory influence of Ca antagonists on Ca-dependent platelet aggregation as the initial step in coronary thrombosis. Thus epinephrine (10^{-6} M) can induce aggregation by massive α-receptor-mediated stimulation of transmembrane Ca uptake into human platelets, whereas verapamil (5×10^{-5} M) blocks both Ca influx and the formation of platelet clusters (Owen, Feinberg, and Le Breton, 1980). It is not known whether this experimental observation also matters in practice, or whether verapamil shares this property with other, possibly more effective, Ca antagonists.

Furthermore, the eventual interference of Ca antagonists with Ca-dependent release of coronary vasoconstrictor agonists such as serotonin and thromboxane A_2 from platelets or release of histamine from mast cells has not yet been studied in sufficient detail. Obviously, the concentrations of Ca antagonists that suppress coronary smooth muscle contractility in a direct way are low, whereas those that block liberation of endogenous vasoconstrictor agonists are considerably stronger. Nevertheless, present knowledge does not yet allow us to decide whether blockade of endogenous vasoconstrictor release by Ca antagonists is totally irrelevant with respect to suppression of coronary spasm, or alternatively may represent an auxiliary mechanism. Since the release of thromboxane A_2 from platelets seems to be capable of inducing coronary arterial smooth muscle contractions, this substance certainly deserves particular interest (Ellis, Oelz, Roberts, Payne, Sweetman, Nies, and Oates, 1976).

Lastly, the proper biochemical or biophysical identification of the presumptive Ca receptors, representing the targets of the Ca-antagonist actions, should be one of the major aims of future research. In fact, it is still unknown whether these Ca-binding sites in the excitable membranes of myocardial fibers, SA- or AV-nodal cells, vascular smooth muscle, and even in platelets are uniform with respect to their molecular configuration, or whether they rather represent a population of related receptor groups for superficial Ca accumulation and transmembrane inward Ca transport. Unexplained species differences as well as certain peculiarities in the action of different Ca antagonists may cast some doubt on a strict "Ca receptor" homogeneity. Possible differences in chemical structure of "Ca receptors" or discrimination between individual Ca antagonists with respect to binding on distinct types of "Ca receptors" have to be taken into consideration. In any case, the somewhat modified aspects of specific Ca antagonism, represented by verapamil, diltiazem, or nifedipine (see Fig. 193), exclude an absolute conformity in the pattern of "Ca receptor" blockade. There is here a wide field of speculation, which now needs experimental examination and concretization.

8.2.   FUTURE USE OF CALCIUM ANTAGONISTS FOR INFARCT PROPHYLAXIS AND IN CARDIAC SURGERY

As to the clinical use of Ca antagonists, one can predict on the basis of present knowledge that these drugs will further enrich the therapeutic armamentarium in various respects. One important new indication, particularly for nifedipine (or other 1,4-dihydropyridines), will probably arise from their convincing effectiveness in preventing imminent infarction in cases of "crescendo angina." An exemplary report on 52 patients admitted to the coronary care unit because of impending infarction, has recently been published by Serruys, Steward, Booman, Michels, Reiber, and Hugenholtz (1980). All these 52 patients, in spite of receiving maximal doses of β-blockers and nitrates at bedrest, had remained symptomatic, so that, nifedipine was administered in addition. The effect was dramatic, since complete cessation of the ischemic episodes took place within 2 hours in 42 patients, and there was no relapse under a daily oral dose of 60 mg nifedipine. Of the 10 nonresponders, all with extensive multivessel disease, 2 died within 24 hours from acute infarction, and 8 received urgent coronary bypass grafting in an effort to alleviate their symptoms. All had severe three-vessel disease in contrast with the responders, in whom one- or two-vessel disease was predominant. Angiographic measurements of the diameters of stenotic, poststenotic, and normal left extramural coronary artery segments revealed that intracoronary administration of nifedipine (0.15 mg) to these patients produced statistically significant vasodilation. For instance, the increase in diameter of stenosed coronary artery sections was between 4 and 30%. The results showed that nifedipine will produce decisive circulatory improvement in many cases of life-threatening coronary ischemia, thus preventing infarction or possibly contributing to reduction of infarct size, as in animal experiments, when the ischemic tissue breakdown is already in progress. The results are undoubtedly conducive to intensified studies on the usefulness of Ca antagonists in such cardiac emergencies.

Another fact, clearly established by experimental work, is acute cellular cardioprotection by Ca antagonists based on prevention of Ca overload (see Chapter 3). Following more than one decade of laboratory investigations with different Ca antagonists, clinical interest now concentrates on nifedipine, which provides excellent preservation of ischemic myocardium in dogs and, as recently demonstrated, also in man. As could be expected from previous animal experiments (Henry, Schuchleib, Borda, Roberts, Williamson, and Sobel, 1978; Henry, Clark, and Williamson, 1978/1980; Henry, Shuchleib, Clark, and Perez, 1979; Clark, Christlieb, Henry, Fischer, Nora, Williamson, and Sobel, 1979), addition of nifedipine to cardioplegic solutions considerably improves postoperative recovery of myocardial contractile function (Clark, Christlieb, Ferguson, Weldon, Marbarger, Sobel, Roberts, Henry, Ludbrook, Biello, and Clark, 1981). Thus of 38 cardiac high-risk patients treated with nifedipine dissolved in cold cardioplegic solution, 35 survived severe surgical interventions, the average cardiac ischemic time being 80 min at a myocardial temperature of 14°C. In contrast with 40 control patients undergoing heart surgery of similar severity but without addition of nifedipine, the use of the Ca antagonist in the 35 test patients totally prevented the dangerous *"low cardiac output syndrome,"* which otherwise often develops at the cessation of cardiopulmonary bypass. Accordingly, under the beneficial influence of nifedipine, the cardiac and stroke work indexes returned to normal within 36 hours. Moreover, when cardioplegia had been performed in the presence of nifedipine, the need for mechanical (i.e., intra-aortic balloon pumping) and pharmacologic circulatory support was minimized and the postischemic death poll reduced to practically zero. The introduction of nifedipine as a potent adjunct for myocardial preservation in cardioplegic solutions certainly represents an important approach to more safety in future cardiac surgery.

It should also be kept in mind that in analogy to the "calcium paradox" model, the moment of resuming normal coronary blood circulation has to be considered a most critical stage, particularly if a cardioplegic solution with a reduced Ca content had previously been administered. Even with respect to this possible complication, cardioprotection with a Ca antagonist is advisable as shown by Ruigrok, Boink, Zimmerman, and Meijler (1978/1980) using verapamil.

8.3. PROGRESSIVE CALCIUM OVERLOAD OF AGING HUMAN ARTERIES; CAN CALCIUM ANTAGONISTS RETARD VASCULAR SENESCENCE?

For more than 50 years human pathology has emphasized the decisive role of arterial lipid accumulation, particularly cholesterol, in the pathogenesis of arteriosclerosis, whereas the concomitant calcinosis is mostly considered a phenomenon of secondary importance. However, our studies with dihydrotachysterol and vitamin D_3 on ventricular myocardium (see Chapter 3) and arterial smooth muscle (see Sections 6.3.1 and 6.3.2) have established that excessive incorporation of Ca can represent the primary cause of cardiac necrotization and severe arteriosclerotic lesions. Thus overdoses of dihydrotachysterol and vitamin D_3 regularly produce calcinosis of the arterial media resembling Mönckeberg's type of human arteriosclerosis, characterized by ultrastructural arterial smooth muscle damage, elastic-fiber breakdown, and formation of calcific plaques in the extracellular stroma. Conversely, verapamil and diltiazem by preventing exaggerated Ca uptake in the arterial walls are able to preserve functional and structural integrity. The observations indicated that at least in certain types of arteriosclerosis, the etiological significance of Ca overload of the arterial media is not inferior to that of cholesterol accumulation.

Arteriosclerosis, whether symptomatic or not, is an inevitable consequence of advanced age. For instance, in a recent study of Nauth, Hort, and Hubinger (1979), the incidence of sclerotic lesions of the coronary stem arteries amounted to 92% at an average age of 65 years in 100 unselected autopsies. Both arterial Ca overload and augmentation of wall cholesterol seem to be the latent precursors of overt arteriosclerosis. Figure 198 represents exemplary observations of Bürger (1939) showing consistent increases in the Ca and cholesterol contents of senescent human aortas, over an age span from 10 to 70 years. The rise in Ca content seems to be even steeper than that in cholesterol. Interestingly enough, the aortic walls of 1- to 36-year-old horses also exhibited the same typical correlation between the rises in Ca and cholesterol contents, although there is no appreciable alimentary cholesterol intake in such herbivores (Bürger, 1957).

To obtain more-detailed data about the age-dependent changes in Ca (and Mg)

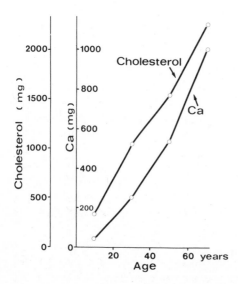

FIGURE 198. Human aortic wall; age-dependent increases in Ca and cholesterol contents, expressed in mg/100 g dry tissue. From Bürger (1939).

content of *normal human arteries,* we have examined arterial wall tissue that mostly originated from forensic autopsies, covering the whole lifespan from 1 to 90 years. The analyses were carried out on the descending branch of the left coronary artery ($N = 86$), the superior mesenteric artery ($N = 134$), and aortic tissue ($N = 141$). *All artery segments with visible plaques were discarded.* In fact, as illustrated in Figures 199 to 201, the senescence of human arteries is reflected in a dramatic augmentation of their Ca content. Thus in 81- to 90-year-old humans, the absolute amounts of arterial Ca (mmol Ca/kg dry tissue) were by 7 times (coronary artery), 20 times (mesenteric artery), and nearly 100 times (aorta) higher than those in the respective infantile arteries, age 0 to 10 years. In surprising contrast with the arterial wall, the myocardial fibers are exempt from any age-induced change in absolute Ca content or Ca:Mg ratio. Thus 122 papillary muscles (see Figure 202) excised together with the arterial specimens from the same autopsies had a Mg content that was always twice to fourfold that of Ca, regardless of whether at 10 or 90 years.

Our results demonstrate that the steady rise in arterial Ca content during lifetime is a most characteristic criterion of age. *In all probability, progressive age-induced vascular Ca overload represents the decisive inherent risk factor that predisposes senescent arteries to arteriosclerotic degeneration.* Only during the first decade of human life is the Ca content of the arterial walls smaller than the Mg content. However, from this time onward, arterial Ca disproportionally rises. For instance in the aorta, the amounts of Ca already surpass those of Mg at an age of 10 to 20 years. Above 30 years, Ca predominates in all arterial walls. Beyond the age of 60, Ca overload is speeded up dramatically in the mesenteric and aortic walls, and above 80 years it reaches in these arteries the deleterious range that is well known from our animal experiments with dihydrotachysterol or vitamin D_3. Only in the coronary arteries (see Figure 199) does progressive Ca uptake seem to be slowed down beyond the age of 60. But this mysterious phenomenon is probably due to a statistical selection effect of coronary calcinosis in the population beyond 60 years, skimming away the coronary "high-calcium carriers" by precipitous coronary death. A number of sporadic observations of our laboratory indicate that the natural process of age-dependent arterial calcinosis proceeds faster than normal in heavy cigarette smokers and diabetics. We think that this is the cause rather than the consequence of premature arteriosclerotic vascular damage.

Apart from calcinosis there are a number of other typical signs of vascular senescence that are possibly attributable to the influence of progressive arterial Ca accumulation, namely:

1. Rarefaction of intact smooth muscle cells in the media, probably resulting from Ca-induced mitochondrial destruction.

2. Loss of vascular elasticity due to Ca-induced mineralization and degeneration of elastic fibers.

3. Inclination to increases in systolic and diastolic blood pressure as a consequence of elevated Ca-dependent peripheral vascular tone.

Human Coronary Artery

FIGURE 199

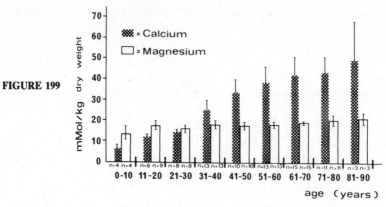

Human Mesenteric Artery

FIGURE 200

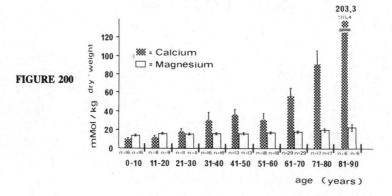

Human Aorta

FIGURE 201

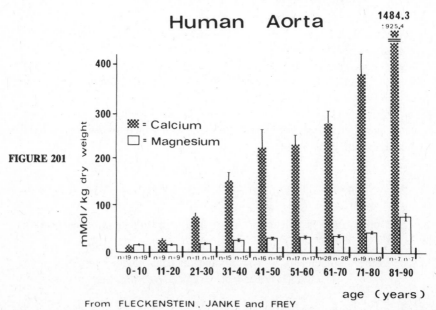

From FLECKENSTEIN, JANKE and FREY

Human Papillary Muscle

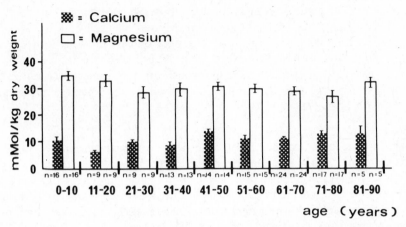

FIGURE 202. Absence of age-dependent changes in Ca and Mg content of 122 papillary muscles from the same autopsies as in Figures 199 to 201.

The Ca antagonists were hitherto used for functional vasodilation and spasmolytic purposes. Apart from the coronary system, this indication can probably be extended to vasospasms in pulmonary and systemic circulation (glycoside-induced mesenteric artery spasm, cerebral artery spasm, Raynaud's syndrome, etc.). *However, in the present context, it is a question of much greater medical significance whether these drugs are also capable of providing long-term protection of the arterial wall against age-dependent Ca overload or premature calcinosis in smokers and diabetics.* This would mean that the Ca antagonists not only afford symptomatic improvement, but also interfere with the fundamental pathogenetic process of arterial calcinosis. Although direct clinical evidence is still lacking, there are several observations in favor of this assumption:

1. According to clinical experience on coronary patients, the therapeutic peak effect of Ca antagonists is attainable in many cases only by *chronic* treatment over several weeks or even months.

FIGURE 199–201. Progressive arterial Ca overload and increase in the ratio Ca:Mg with advanced age. Tissue samples were taken from the descending branch of the left coronary artery ($N = 86$), the superior mesenteric artery ($N = 134$), and the aorta ($N = 141$). The arteries mostly originated from autopsies of traffic victims. Only artery segments without visible plaques were analyzed using atom absorption spectrometry. Data from Fleckenstein, Fleckenstein-Grün, Janke and Frey (1977); See Fleckenstein-Grün and Fleckenstein (1978/1980).

2. If this long-term therapy with Ca antagonists is discontinued, there is in many cases no relapse to the antetreatment stage, a finding that indicates a distinct improvement of the basic arterial disease.

3. There is a particularly high susceptibility of old hypertensive patients to Ca antagonists, the maximum antihypertensive efficacy being reached at an age of around 80 years (see Figure 195 from Bühler, Hulthen, Kiowski, and Bolli, 1982). These results, as well as distinct beneficial effects of Ca antagonists in cases of intermittent claudication, prove that even in the most advanced age groups, vascular Ca overload is still responsive to Ca-antagonist treatment.

Thus Ca-antagonists continue to be a challenge to clinical medicine. Table 21 summarizes our results regarding the anticalcinotic potency of different Ca antagonists. Obviously, the strength of anticalcinotic vascular long-term protection is not predictable from acute Ca-antagonistic vasodilator potency. For instance in rats, the somewhat weaker Ca-antagonistic vasodilators verapamil and diltiazem exert more pronounced anticalcinotic long-term effects than nifedipine does. An additional administration of Mg salts proved to be able to further promote the verapamil or diltiazem action. All these observations point to the possibility of an eventual

TABLE 21. Anticalcinotic Potency of Different Ca Antagonists in Various Rat Tissues[a]

Type of Calcinosis	Verapamil	Diltiazem	Nifedipine
Dihydrotachysterol (arteries)	+	+	−
Vitamin D_3 (arteries)	+	+	−
Vitamin D_3 (kidney and colon)	+	+	−
Spontaneous hypertension (arteries)	+	+	+
Alloxan-diabetes (arteries)	+	+	−
Alloxan-diabetes (lens cataracts)	+	−	−

[a]Definitions: (+) = anticalcinotic efficacy. (−) = no discernible or slight anticalcinotic influence.

retardation of the Ca-dependent arterial aging process (and of secondary circulatory complications) by a suitable Ca antagonist therapy. Regarding the fact that human life-span is decisively determined by arterial senscence, any further progress in this field would be of utmost scientific and practical importance. Hence, a definite clarification of the *possible significance of Ca antagonists in geriatrics* is certainly one of the most fascinating topics of future research.

References

Abderhalden, E., and Gellhorn, E. 1920. Das Verhalten des Herzstreifenpräparates (nach Loewe) unter verschiedenen Bedingungen. *Pflügers Arch. ges. Physiol.* **183,** 303–332.

Adams, D. R. 1929. The role of calcium in senile cataracts. *Biochem. J.* **23,** 902–912.

Adelman, A. G., Wigle, E. D., Ranganathan, N., Webb, G. D., Kidd, B. S. L., Bigelow, W. G., and Silver, M. D. 1972. The clinical course in muscular subaortic stenosis: a retrospective and prospective study of 60 hemodynamically proved cases. *Ann. Intern. Med.* **77,** 515–525.

Affolter, H., Chiesi, M., Dabrowska, R., and Carafoli, E. 1976. Calcium regulation in heart cells. The interaction of mitochondrial and sarcoplasmic reticulum with troponin-bound calcium. *Eur. J. Biochem.* **67,** 389–396.

Akiyama, T., and Fozzard, H. A. 1979. Ca and Na selectivity of the active membrane of rabbit A. V. nodal cells. *Am. J. Physiol.* **236,** C1–C8.

Alanis, J., Lopez, E., Mandoki, J. J., and Pilar, G. 1959. Propagation of impulses through the atrio-ventricular node. *Am. J. Physiol.* **197,** 1171–1174.

Alderman, E. L., Harrison, D. C. 1971. Myocardial hypertrophy resulting from low dosage isoproterenol administration in rats. *Proc. Soc. Exp. Biol. Med.* **136,** 268–270.

Allela, A. 1958. Steuerung der Coronardurchblutung, in *Probleme der Coronardurchblutung,* Bad Oeynhausener Gespräche, Springer, Berlin-Göttingen-Heidelberg, Vol. 2.

Allen, G. S., and Banghart, S. B. 1979. Cerebral arterial spasm: In vitro effects of nifedipine on serotonin-, phenylephrine- and potassium-induced contractions of canine basilar and femoral arteries. *Neurosurgery* **4,** 37–42.

Anavekar, S. N., Christophidis, N., Louis, W. J., and Doyle, A. E. 1981. Verapamil in the treatment of hypertension. *J. Cardiovasc. Pharmacol.* **3,** 287–292.

Anderson, D. E. 1963. Prenylamine "Segontin" in angina of effort. *Med. J. Aust.* **50,** 149–150.

Anderson, N. C., Ramon, F., and Snyder, A. 1971. Studies on calcium and sodium in uterine smooth muscle excitation under current-clamp and voltage-clamp conditions. *J. Gen. Physiol.* **58,** 322–339.

Andersson, K. E., and Ulmsten, U. 1978. Effects of nifedipine on myometrial activity and lower abdominal pain in women with primary dysmenorrhoea. *Brit. J. Obstet. Gynaecol.* **85,** 142–148.

Andreasen, F., Boye, E., Christoffersen, E., Dalsgaard, P., Henneberg, E., Kallenbach, A., Ladefoged, S., Lillquist, K., Mikkelsen, E., Norderø, E., Olsen, J., Pedersen, J. K., Bruun Petersen, G., Schroll, J., Schultz, H., and Seidelin, J. 1975. Assessment of verapamil in the treatment of angina pectoris. *Eur. J. Cardiol.* **2,** 443–452.

Anrep, G. V. 1926. The regulation of the coronary circulation. *Physiol. Rev.* **6,** 596–629.

Antman, E., Muller, J., Goldberg, S., MacAlpin, R., Rubenfire, M., Tabatznik, B., Liang, C., Heupler, F., Achuff, S., Reichek, N., Geltman, E., Kerin, N. Z., Neff, R. K., and Braunwald, E. 1980. Nifedipine therapy for coronary-artery spasm. Experience in 127 patients. *N. Engl. J. Med.* **302**, 1269–1273.

Antoni, H. 1961. Elektrophysiologische Studien zum Problem der Flimmer-Entstehung und Flimmer-Beseitigung, in *Beiträge zur Ersten Hilfe und Behandlung von Unfällen durch elektrischen Strom.* Edited by R. Hauf, pp. 38–53. Verlags- und Wirtschaftsgesellschaft der Elektrizitätswerke, Frankfurt.

Antoni, H. 1972. Some theoretical notes about induction and interruption of atrial or ventricular fibrillation by electrical current. *Herz/Kreislauf* **4**, 324–331.

Antoni, H., and Engstfeld, G. 1961. Restitutive Wirkungen der sympathischen Übertragerstoffe auf die elektrische und mechanische Aktivität des Kalium-gelähmten Myokards. *Verh. Deutsch. Ges. Kreisl.-Forsch.* **27**, 232–237.

Antoni, H., Engstfeld, G., and Fleckenstein, A. 1960. Inotrope Effekte von ATP und Adrenalin am hypodynamen Froschmyokard nach elektromechanischer Entkoppelung durch Ca^{++}-Entzug. *Pflügers Arch. ges. Physiol.* **272**, 91–106.

Antoni, H., Herkel, K., and Fleckenstein, A. 1963. Die Restitution der automatischen Erregungsbildung in Kalium-gelähmten Schrittmacher-Geweben durch Adrenalin. Elektrophysiologische Studien am isolierten Sinusknoten (Meerschweinchen, Rhesusaffe) sowie am Purkinje-Faden (Rhesusaffe). *Pflügers Arch. ges. Physiol.* **277**, 633–649.

Antoni, H., and Oberdisse, E. 1965. Elektrophysiologische Untersuchungen über die Barium-induzierte Schrittmacher-Aktivität im isolierten Säugetiermyokard. *Pflügers Arch. ges. Physiol.* **284**, 259–272.

Antoni, H., and Rotmann, M. 1968. The negative inotropic mechanism of acetylcholine in the isolated frog's myocardium. *Pflügers Arch. ges. Physiol.* **300**, 67–86.

Antoni, H., and Zerweck, T. 1967. Besitzen die sympathischen Übertragerstoffe einen direkten Einfluss auf die Leitungsgeschwindigkeit des Säugetiermyokards? Elektrophysiologische Untersuchungen an isolierten Papillarmuskeln und Purkinjefäden des Rhesusaffen. *Pflügers Arch. ges. Physiol.* **293**, 310–330.

Aoki, K., Kondo, S., Mochizuki, A., Yoshida, T., Kato, S., Kato, K., and Takikawa, K. 1978. Antihypertensive effect of cardiovascular Ca^{2+}-antagonist in hypertensive patients in the absence and presence of beta-adrenergic blockade. *Am. Heart J.* **96**, 218–226.

Applefield, M. M., and Roman, J. A. 1974. Prinzmetal's angina with extensive spasm of the right coronary artery. *Chest* **66**, 721–722.

Armstrong, M. L. 1973. A comparative study of perhexiline, beta-adrenergic blocking agents and placebos in the management of angina pectoris. *Postgrad. Med. J.* **49** (April suppl.), 108–111.

Arntz, B., Kreuzer, H., Bostroem, B., and Gleichmann, U. 1968. Die Wirkung von Prenylamin auf Herzminutenvolumen, Herzfrequenz, Blutdruck und dp/dt bei Herzgesunden. *Pharmacol. Clin.* **1**, 67–71.

Aronson, R. S., and Cranefield, P. F. 1974. The effect of resting potential on the electrical activity of canine cardiac Purkinje fibres exposed to Na-free solution or to ouabain. *Pflügers Arch. ges. Physiol.* **347**, 101–116.

Bäurle, W. 1951. Die Coronarsklerose bei Hypertonie. *Beitr. path. Anat.* **111**, 108–124.

Bailey, K. 1948. Tropomyosin: a new asymmetric protein component of the muscle fibril. *Biochem. J.* **43**, 271–278.

Bajusz, E. 1963. *Conditioning Factors for Cardiac Necroses*, Karger-Verlag, Basel-New York.

Bajusz, E., Baker, J. R., and Nixon, C. W. 1966. Effects of catecholamines upon cardiac and skeletal muscles of dystrophic hamsters. *Fed. Proc.* **25**, 475.

Baker, P. F. 1972. Transport and metabolism of Calcium ions in nerve, in *Progress in Biophysics and Molecular Biology*, Edited by J. A. V. Butler and D. Noble, **24**, 177–223. Pergamon, Oxford-New York.

Bala Subramanian, V., Khanna, P. K., Narayanan, G. R., and Hoon, R. S. 1976. Verapamil in ischaemic heart disease—quantitative assessment by serial multistage treadmill exercise. *Postgrad. Med. J.* **52**, 143–147.

Bala Subramanian, V., Lahiri, A., Paramasivan, R., and Raftery, E. B. 1980. Verapamil in chronic stable angina—A controlled study with computerised multistage treadmill exercise. *Lancet* **1980/ I**, 841–844.

Barcroft, J. 1927. *Die Atmungsfunktion des Blutes*. Springer, Berlin, Vol. 1.

Barzu, T., Dam, D. T., Cuparencu, B., Dancea, S., and Böhm, B. 1979. Ultrastructural and biochemical investigations on the effect of calcium overload in the rat heart. *Aggressologie* **20**, 149–154.

Bass, O., Friedemann, M., and Künzli, H. 1979. Ein Fall von akuter Linksherzinsuffizienz unter Tokolyse mit β-Stimulation. *Schweiz. Med. Wschr.* **109**, 1427–1430.

Bassett, A. L., and Gelband, H. 1974. Nicotine and the action potential of cat ventricle. *J. Pharmacol. Exp. Ther.* **188**, 157–165.

Baumgarten, A. 1962. The clinical effects of a new anti-anginal agent, prenylamine ("Segontin"). *Med. J. Aust.* **49**, 429–431.

Bayliss, W. M. 1902. On the local reactions of the arterial wall to changes of internal pressure. *J. Physiol.* (Lond.) **28**, 220–231.

Beck, O. A., Witt, E., Lehmann, H. -U., and Hochrein, H. 1978. Die Wirkung von Gallopamil (D 600) auf die intrakardiale Erregungsleitung und Sinusknotenautomatie beim Menschen. *Z. Kardiol.* **67**, 522–526.

Beeler, G. W., and Reuter, H. 1970a. Membrane calcium current in ventricular myocardial fibres. *J. Physiol.* (Lond.) **207**, 191–209.

Beeler, G. W., and Reuter, H. 1970b. The relation between membrane potential, membrane currents and activation of contraction in ventricular myocardial fibres. *J. Physiol.* (Lond.) **207**, 211–229.

Belardinelli, L., Harder, D., Sperelakis, N., Rubio, R., and Berne, R. M. 1979. Cardiac glycoside stimulation of inward Ca current in vascular smooth muscle of canine coronary artery. *J. Pharmacol. Exp. Ther.* **209**, 62–66.

Benaim, M. E. 1972. Asystole after verapamil. *Brit. Med. J.* **2**, 169–170.

Benda, L., Doneff, D., Lujf, A., and Moser K. 1967. Experimentelle und klinische Untersuchungen mit α-Isopropyl-α-((N-methyl-N-homoveratryl)-γ-aminopropyl)-3,4-dimethoxyphenylacetonitril (Iproveratril). *Wien. Med. Wschr.* **117**, 829–838.

Bender, F. 1967. Isoptin zur Behandlung der tachykarden Form des Vorhofflatterns. *Med. Klin.* **62**, 634–636.

Bender, F. 1970. Die Behandlung der tachykarden Arrhythmien und der arteriellen Hypertonie mit Verapamil. *Arzneimittelforschung (Drug Res.)* **20**, 1310–1316.

Bender, H. G., Goeckenjan, G., Meger, C., and Müntefering, H. 1977. Zum mütterlichen Risiko der medikamentösen Tokolyse mit Fenoterol (Partusisten®). *Geburtsh. Frauenheilk.* **37**, 665–674.

Bender, F., Kojima, N., Reploh, H., and Oelmann, G. 1966. Behandlung tachykarder Rhythmusstörungen des Herzens durch Beta-Rezeptorenblockade des Atrioventrikular-gewebes. *Med. Welt* **17**, 1120–1123.

Bender, F., and Zimmerhof, K. 1967. Wenckebach Periode als Zeichen der Überdosierung eines Mittels mit sympathikolytischer Herzwirkung. *Med. Welt* **18**, 1585.

Bendixen, H. H., Laver, M. B., and Flacke, W. E. 1963. Influence of respiratory acidosis on circulatory effect of epinephrine in dogs. *Circ. Res.* **13**, 64–70.

Bennett, M. R. 1967. The effect of cations on the electrical properties of the smooth muscle cells of the guinea-pig vas deferens. *J. Physiol.* (Lond.) **190**, 465–479.

Bennett, M. R., and Burnstock, G. 1966. Application of the sucrose-gap method to determine the ionic basis of the membrane potential of smooth muscle. *J. Physiol.* (Lond.) **183**, 637–648.

Benson, E. S., Evans, G. T., Hallaway, B. E., Phibbs, C., and Freier, E. P. 1961. Myocardial creatine phosphate and nucleotides in anoxic cardiac arrest and recovery. *Am. J. Physiol.* **201**, 687–693.

Bernard, C. 1975. Establishment of ionic permeabilities of the myocardial membrane during embryonic development of rats, in *Developmental and Physiological Correlates of Cardiac Muscle. Edited by M. Lieberman and T. Sano, pp. 169–184, Raven Press, New York.*

Berne, R. M., Belardinelli, L., Harder, D. R., Sperelakis, N., and Rubio, R. 1978/1980. Response of large and small coronary arteries to adenosine, nitroglycerin, cardiac glycosides, and calcium-antagonists, in *Calcium-Antagonismus,* Edited by A. Fleckenstein and H. Roskamm, Proceedings of an International Symposium 1978 in Frankfurt, pp. 208–220, Springer-Verlag, Berlin-Heidelberg-New York, 1980.

Betz, E. 1975. Experimental production of cerebral vascular disorders, In *Handbook of Experimental Pharmacology,* Edited by G. V. R. Born, O. Eichler, A. Farah, H. Herken, A. D. Welch, and J. Schmier, Vol. 16/3. pp. 183–232, Springer-Verlag, New York-Berlin-Heidelberg.

Bevan, J. A., Garstka, W., Su, C., and Su, M. O. 1973. The bimodal basis of the contractile response of the rabbit ear artery to norepinephrine and other agonists. *Europ. J. Pharmacol.* **22**, 47–53.

Bianchi, C. P., and Shanes, A. M. 1959. Calcium influx in skeletal muscle at rest, during activity, and during potassium contracture. *J. Gen. Physiol.* **42**, 803–815.

Biedert, S., Barry, W. H., and Smith, T. W. 1979. Inotropic effects and changes in sodium and calcium contents associated with inhibition of monovalent cation active transport by ouabain in cultured myocardial cells. *J. Gen. Physiol.* **74**, 479–494.

Biedl, A., and Reiner, M. 1900. Studien über Hirncirculation und Hirnödem, II. Zur Frage der Innervation der Hirngefässe *Pflügers Arch. ges. Physiol.* **79**, 158–194.

Bier, C. B., and Rona, G. 1979. Mineralocorticoid potentiation of isoproterenol-induced myocardial injury: Ultrastructural equivalent. *J. Mol. Cell. Cardiol.* **11**, 961–966.

Bilek, I., Laven, R., Peiper, U., and Regnat, K. 1974. The effect of verapamil on the response to noradrenaline or to potassium-depolarization in isolated vascular strips. *Microvasc. Res.* **7**, 181–189.

Bilek, I., and Peiper, U. 1973. The influence of verapamil on the noradrenaline activation of the isolated aorta and portal vein of the rat. *Pflügers Arch. ges. Physiol.* **343** (Suppl.), R 57.

Bing, O. H. L., Brooks, W. W., and Messer, J. V. 1973. Heart muscle viability following hypoxia: protective effect of acidosis. *Science* **180**, 1296–1297.

Bing, R. J., Weishaar, R., Rackl, A., and Pawlik, G. 1978/1979. Antianginal drugs and cardiac metabolism, in *New Drug Therapy with a Calcium Antagonist, Diltiazem,* Hakone Symposium, 1978, Edited by R. J. Bing, pp. 27–37, Excerpta Medica, Amsterdam–Princeton, 1979.

Bleifeld, W. 1980. Koronararterien-Spasmus. *Dtsch. Med. Wschr.* **105**, 1233–1234.

Böhm, C., Schlepper, M., and Witzleb, E. 1960. Eine neue Koronargefäss-erweiternde Substanz. *Dtsch. Med. Wschr.* **85**, 1405–1408.

Bohr, D. F. 1963. Vascular smooth muscle; Dual effect of calcium. *Science* **139**, 597–599.

Bohr, D. F. 1964. Electrolytes and smooth muscle contraction. *Pharmacol. Rev.* **16**, 85–111.

Bonow, R. O., and Epstein, S. E. 1980/1981. Effects of verapamil on left ventricular filling in patients with hypertrophic cardiomyopathy, in *Calcium Antagonism in Cardiovascular Therapy,* International Symposium, Florence, October, 1980, Edited by A. Zanchetti and D. M. Krikler, pp. 363–364, Excerpta Medica, Amsterdam-Oxford-Princeton, 1981.

Bonow, R. O., Rosing, D. R., Bacharach, S. L., Green, M. V., Lipson, L. C., Condit, J. R., Kent, K. M., and Epstein, S. E. 1981. Long-term effects of verapamil on left ventricular diastolic filling in patients with hypertrophic cardiomyopathy. *Am. J. Cardiol.* **47**, 409.

Boothby, C. B., Garrard, C. S., and Pickering, D. 1972. Verapamil in cardiac arrhythmias. *Brit. Med. J.* **2**, 348–349.

Bossert, F., and Vater, W. 1971. Dihydropyridine, eine neue Gruppe stark wirksamer Coronartherapeutika. *Naturwissenschaften* **58**, 578.

Boulet, L., and Boulet, M. A. 1945. Effets antagonistes du baryum et du potassium sur le coeur. *C.R. Soc. Biol.* (Paris) **139**, 1106–1107.

Bourassa, M. G., Cote, P., Theroux, P., Tubau, J. F., Genain, C., and Waters, D. D. 1980. Hemodynamics and coronary flow following diltiazem administration in anesthetized dogs and in humans. *Chest* **78** (Suppl. 1), 224–230.

Bozler, E. 1941. Influence of estrone on electrical characteristics and motility of uterine muscle. *Endocrinology* **29**, 225–227.

Bozler, E. 1942. The activity of the pacemaker previous to the discharge of a muscular impulse. *Am. J. Physiol.* **136**, 543–552.

Bozler, E. 1943. Tonus changes in cardiac muscle and their significance for the initiation of impulses. *Am. J. Physiol.* **139**, 477–480.

Bozler, E. 1947. The response of smooth muscle to stretch. *Am. J. Physiol.* **149**, 299–301.

Bozler, E. 1962. Initiation of contraction in smooth muscle. *Physiol. Rev.* **42**, 179–186.

Braasch, W., and Ebner, F. 1975. Long-term treatment with nifedipine, in *1st International Nifedipine (Adalat) Symposium,* Tokyo, November, 1973, Edited by K. Hashimoto, E. Kimura, and T. Kobayashi, pp. 200–204, University of Tokyo Press, 1975.

Braasch, W., and Fleck, D. 1961. Die Beeinflussung der Coronardurchblutung und Sauerstoffversorgung des Herzmuskels durch *N*-(3′-Phenyl-propyl-(2′)-1,1-diphenyl-propyl-(3)-amin. *Arzneimittelforschung (Drug Res.)* **11**, 336–339.

Brading, A. F., Bülbring, E., and Tomita, T. 1969. The effect of sodium and calcium on the action potential of the smooth muscle of the guinea pig taenia coli. *J. Physiol.* (Lond.) **200**, 637–654.

van den Brand, M., Remme, W. J., Meester, G. T., Tiggelaar-de Widt, I., de Ruiter, R., and Hugenholtz, P. G. 1975. Hemodynamic effect of nifedipine (Adalat) in patients catheterized for coronary artery disease, in *2nd International Nifedipine (Adalat) Symposium,* Amsterdam, October, 1974, Edited by W. Lochner, W. Braasch, and G. Kroneberg, pp. 145–153, Springer-Verlag, Berlin-Heidelberg-New York, 1975.

Brandt, D., and Klein, W. 1982. Dosiswirkungsbeziehung von Diltiazem bei Patienten mit essentieller Hypertonie, in *Calciumantagonisten zur Behandlung der Angina pectoris, Hypertonie und Arrhythmie,* International Symposium on Diltiazem, Copenhagen, June 25–27, 1981, Edited by F. Bender and K. Greeff, pp. 202–209, Excerpta Medica, Amsterdam-Oxford-Princeton, 1982.

Braunwald, E. 1978. Coronary spasm and acute myocardial infarction—New possibility for treatment and prevention. *N. Engl. J. Med.* **299**, 1301–1303.

Braunwald, E. 1980. Introduction: Calcium channel blockers. *Am. J. Cardiol.* **46**, 1045–1046.

Braunwald, E. 1981. Coronary artery spasm. Mechanisms and clinical relevance. *JAMA* **246**, 1957–1959.

Braunwald, E., Lambrew, C. T., Rockoff, S. D., Ross, J., and Morrow, A. G. 1964. Idiopathic hypertrophic subaortic stenosis. *Circulation* **30** (Suppl. 4), 3–119.

van Breemen, C., Farinas, B. R., Gerba, P., and McNaughton, E. D. 1972. Excitation-contraction coupling in rabbit aorta studied by the lanthanum method for measuring cellular calcium influx. *Circ. Res.* **30**, 44–54.

van Breemen, C., and Lesser, P. 1971. The absence of increased membrane permeability during norepinephrine stimulation of arterial smooth muscle. *Microvasc. Res.* **3**, 113–114.

Breithardt, G., Seipel, L., Wiebringhaus, E., and Loogen, F. 1976. Effect of verapamil on sinus node in patients with normal and abnormal sinus node function. *Circulation* (Suppl 2), 19.

Breithardt, G., Seipel, L., Wiebringhaus, E., and Loogen, F. 1978. Effects of verapamil on sinus node function in man. *Eur. J. Cardiol.* **8**, 379–394.

Bretschneider, H. J. 1958. Über den Mechanismus der hypoxischen Coronarerweiterung, in *Probleme der Coronardurchblutung,* Bad Oeynhausener Gespräche, Springer, Berlin-Göttingen-Heidelberg, 1958, Vol. 2.

Brichard, G., and Zimmermann, P. 1970. Verapamil in cardiac dysrhythmias during anaesthesia. *Brit. J. Anaesth.* **42,** 1005–1011.

Brierley, G. P., Murer, E., and Bachmann, E. 1964. The accumulation of calcium and inorganic phosphate by heart mitochondria. *Arch. Biochem. Biophys.* **105,** 89–102.

Briggs, A. H., and Holland, W. C. 1960. K^{42} and Cl^{36} fluxes during acetylcholine-and Ca^{++}-induced atrial fibrillation. *Am. J. Physiol.* **198,** 838–840.

Briggs, F. N., and Portzehl, H. 1957. The influence of relaxing factor on the pH-dependence of the contraction of muscle models. *Biochim. Biophys. Acta* (Amst.) **24,** 482–488.

Bristow, M. R., and Green, R. D. 1977. Effect of diazoxide, verapamil and compound D 600 on isoproterenol and calcium-mediated dose-response relationships in isolated rabbit atrium. *Eur. J. Pharmacol.* **45,** 267–279.

Brittinger, W. D., Schwarzbeck, A., Wittenmeier, K. W., Twittenhoff, W. D., Stegaru, B., Huber, W., Ewald, R. W., v. Henning, G. E., Fabricius, M., and Strauch, M. 1970. Klinisch-experimentelle Untersuchungen über die blutdrucksenkende Wirkung von Verapamil. *Dtsch. Med. Wschr.* **95,** 1871–1877.

Brobmann, G. F., Barth, K., Strecker, E. P., Schmidt-Hieber, M., and Schmidt, H. A. 1975. Die Wirkung von Strophanthin auf die intestinale Durchblutung: ein Beitrag zur Pathophysiologie der hämorrhagischen Enteropathie. *Langenbecks Arch. Chir.* (Suppl Chir. Forum), 291.

Brobmann, G. F., Mayer, M., Grimm, W., and Safer, A. 1978/1980. Aufhebung Herzglycosid-induzierter Spasmen der Mesenterialgefässe durch Calcium-Antagonisten im Hundexperiment, in *Calcium-Antagonismus,* Proceedings of an International Symposium 1978 in Frankfurt, Edited by A. Fleckenstein and H. Roskamm, pp. 230–242, Springer-Verlag, Berlin-Heidelberg-New York, 1980.

Brooks, M. H. 1975. Lenticular abnormalities in endocrine dysfunction, in *Cataracts and Abnormalities of the Lens,* Edited by J. G. Bellows, pp. 285–301, Grune and Stratton, New York-San Francisco-London.

Brooks, C., and Lu, H.-H. 1972. *The Sinoatrial Pacemaker of the Heart,* Charles C. Thomas, Springfield, Ill.

Brown, E. B., and Miller, F. 1952. Tolerance of the dog heart to carbon dioxyde. *Am. J. Physiol.* **170,** 550–554.

Büchner, F., and Iijima, S. 1961., see Büchner, F., Die allgemeine Pathologie des Blutkreislaufs, in Handbuch Allgemeine Pathologie, Edited by F. Büchner, E. Letterer and F. Roulet, Vol. 5, part I, pp 791–954, Springer-Verlag, Berlin-Göttingen-Heidelberg.

Büchner, F., and Onishi, S. 1968. *Der Herzmuskel bei akuter Koronarinsuffizienz im elektronenmikroskopischen Bild.* Urban and Schwarzenberg, Munich.

Büchner, F., and Onishi, S. 1970. *Herzhypertrophie und Herzinsuffizienz in der Sicht der Elektronenmikroskopie.* Urban and Schwarzenberg, Munich-Basel-Vienna.

Büchner, F., Onishi, S., and Wada, A. 1978. *Cardiomyopathy Associated with Systemic Myopathy.* Urban and Schwarzenberg, Baltimore-Munich.

Bühler, F. R., Hulthen, L., Kiowski, W., and Bolli, P. 1982. Greater antihypertensive efficacy of the calcium channel inhibitor verapamil in older and low renin patients, in *Clinical Science* (Suppl. 1), 9th Scientific Meeting of the ISH, Mexico City, February 21–24, 1982.

Bülbring, E. 1955. Correlation between membrane potential, spike discharge and tension in smooth muscle. *J. Physiol.* (Lond.) **128,** 200–221.

Bülbring, E. 1957. Changes in configuration of spontaneously discharged spike potentials from smooth muscle of the guinea-pig's taenia coli. The effect of electronic currents and of adrenaline, acetylcholine and histamine. *J. Physiol.* (Lond.) **135,** 412–425.

Bülbring, E. 1962. Electrical activity in intestinal smooth muscle. *Physiol. Rev.* **42** (Suppl. 5), 160–174.

Bülbring, E., Burnstock, G., and Holman, M. E. 1958. Excitation and conduction in the smooth muscle of the isolated taenia coli of the guinea-pig. *J. Physiol.* (Lond.) **142**, 420–437.

Bülbring, E., and Kuriyama, H. 1963. Effects of changes in the external sodium and calcium concentrations on spontaneous electrical activity in smooth muscle of guinea-pig taenia coli. *J. Physiol.* (Lond.) **166**, 29–58.

Bülbring, E., and Tomita, T. 1967. Properties of the inhibitory potential of smooth muscle as observed in the response to field stimulation of the guinea-pig taenia coli. *J. Physiol.* (Lond.) **189**, 299–315.

Bülbring, E., and Tomita, T. 1970. Calcium and the action potential in smooth muscle, in *Calcium and Cellular Function*, Edited by A. W. Cuthbert, Macmillan, London, pp. 249–260.

Bürger, M. 1939. Die chemischen Altersveränderungen an Gefässen. *Z. Neurol. Psych.* **167**, 273–280.

Bürger, M. 1957. *Altern und Krankheit*. Georg Thieme, Leipzig.

Burge, W. E. 1909. Analyses of the ash of the normal and the cataractous lens. *Arch. Ophthalmol.* **38**, 435–450.

Burns-Cox, C. J., Chandrasekhar, K. P., Ikram, H., Peirce, T. H., Pilcher, J., Quinlan, C. D. M., and Russell Rees, J. 1971. Clinical evaluation of perhexiline maleate in patients with angina pectoris. *Brit. Med. J.* **4**, 586–588.

Burnstock, G., and Prosser, C. L. 1960. Responses of smooth muscles to quick stretch; relation of stretch to conduction. *Am. J. Physiol.* **198**, 921–925.

Busch, W. A., Stromer, M. H., Goll, D. E., and Suzuki, A. 1972. Ca^{2+}-specific removal of Z lines from rabbit skeletal muscle. *J. Cell Biology,* **53**, 367–381.

Byon, Y. K. 1971. Myocardial oxygen consumption in isometric contractions abbreviated by quick release, Abstr. N° 267, in *Proceedings 25th International Congress Physiol. Sciences,* Munich 1971, Vol. 9. p. 93.

Byon, Y. K., and Fleckenstein, A. 1965. Ca^{++}-Effekte auf O_2-Verbrauch und mechanische Spannungsentwicklung isolierter Papillarmuskeln und Froschherz-Streifen bei Ruhe und elektrischer Reizung. *Pflügers Arch. ges. Physiol.* **283**, R15–R16.

Byon, Y. K., and Fleckenstein, A. 1969. Parallele Beeinflussung von isometrischer Spannungsentwicklung und O_2-Verbrauch isolierter Papillarmuskeln unter dem Einfluβ von Ca^{++}-Ionen, Adrenalin, Isoproterenol und organischen Ca^{++}-Antagonisten (Iproveratril, D 600, Prenylamin). *Pflügers Arch. ges. Physiol.* **312**, R8–R9.

Byon, Y. K., and Fleckenstein, A. 1973. Myocardial oxygen consumption at various rates of tension development, in *Das chronisch kranke Herz,* Proceedings International Symposium, Bad Krozingen (Germany), October 18–20, 1972, Edited by H. Roskamm and H. Reindell, pp. 53–57, F. K. Schattauer Verlag, Stuttgart-New York, 1973.

Caldwell, P. C., and Walster, G. 1963. Studies on the micro-injection of various substances into crab muscle fibres. *J. Physiol.* (Lond.) **169**, 353–372.

Calhoun, J. A., and Harrison, T. R. 1931. The effect of digitalis on the potassium content of the cardiac muscle of dogs. *J. Clin. Invest.* **10**, 139–144.

Carafoli, E. 1974. Mitochondria in the contraction and relaxation of heart, in *Recent Advances in Studies on Cardiac Structure and Metabolism,* **4**, 393–406, Edited by N. S. Dhalla, University Park Press, Baltimore.

Carafoli, E. 1975. Mitochondria, Ca^{2+} transport and the regulation of heart contraction and metabolism. *J. Mol. Cell. Cardiol.* **7**, 83–89.

Carafoli, E., Dabrowska, R., Crovetti, F., Tiozzo, R., and Drabikowski, W. 1975. An in vitro study of the interaction of heart mitochondria with troponin-bound Ca^{2+}. *Biochem. Biophys. Res. Commun.* **62**, 908–912.

Carafoli, E., Tiozzo, R., Lugli, G., Crovelti, R., and Kratzing, C. 1974. The release of calcium from heart mitochondria by sodium. *J. Mol. Cell. Cardiol.* **6**, 361–371.

Cardoe, N. 1970. A 2-year study of the efficacy and tolerability of prenylamine in the treatment of angina pectoris. *Postgrad. Med. J.* **46**, 708–711.

Cardoe, N. 1971. The treatment of angina pectoris over a two-year period. A double-blind study of prenylamine (Synadrin; Segontin) in outpatients. *Clin. Trials J.* **8** (Suppl. 1), 18–23.

Carmeliet, E., and Vereecke, J. 1969. Adrenaline and the plateau phase of the cardiac action potential. Importance of Ca, Na and K conductance. *Pflügers Arch ges. Physiol.* **313**, 300–315.

Carmeliet, E., and Zaman, M.Y. 1979. Comparative effects of lignocaine and lorcainide on conduction in the Langendorff-perfused guinea pig heart. *Cardiovasc. Res.* **13**, 439–449.

Casteels, R., and Droogmans, G. 1976. Membrane potential and excitation-contraction coupling in the smooth muscle cells of the rabbit ear artery. *J. Physiol.* (Lond.) **263**, 163–164 P.

Casteels, R., and Kuriyama, H. 1965. Membrane potential and ionic content in pregnant and non-pregnant rat myometrium. *J. Physiol.* (Lond.) **177**, 263–287.

Cawein, M. J., Lewis, R. E., Hudak, W. J., and Hoekenga, M. T. 1973. Clinical evaluation of perhexiline maleate in patients with angina pectoris associated with a positive coronary artery disease index. *Postgrad. Med. J.* **49** (April Suppl.), 121–124.

Cerrina, J., Denjean, A., Alexandre, G., Lockhart, A., and Duroux, P. 1981. Inhibition of exercise-induced asthma by a calcium antagonist, nifedipine. *Am. Rev. Respir. Dis.* **123**, 156–160.

Chahine, R. A., Raizner, A. E., Ishimori, T., Luchi, R. J., and MacIntosh, H. 1975. The incidence and clinical implications of coronary artery spasm. *Circulation* **52**, 972–978.

Chance, B. 1965. The energy-linked reaction of calcium with mitochondria. *J. Biol. Chem.* **240**, 2729–2748.

Charalampous, F. C., and Hegsted, D. M. 1950. Effect of age and diet on development of cataracts in the diabetic rat. *Am. J. Physiol.* **161**, 540–544.

Cherchi, A., Bina, M., Fonzo, R., and Raffo, M. 1973. Influence of perhexiline on the effort tolerance test in angina pectoris. *Postgrad. Med. J.* **49** (April Suppl.), 67–73.

Cherchi, A., Fonzo, R., and Bina, M. 1975. Influence of nifedipine on the effort tolerance test in angina patients, in *1st International Nifedipine (Adalat) Symposium*, Tokyo, November, 1973, Edited by K. Hashimoto, E. Kimura, and T. Kobayashi, pp. 85–96, University of Tokyo Press, 1975.

Cheung, W. Y. 1980. Calmodulin plays a privotal role in cellular regulation. *Science* **207**, 19–27.

Cho, Y. W., Belej, M., and Aviado, D. M. 1970. Pharmacology of a new antianginal drug: Perhexiline. I. Coronary circulation and myocardial metabolism. *Chest* **58**, 577–581.

Ciplea, A. G., and Bock, P. R. 1976. Kardioprotektion durch perorale Anwendung des Calcium-Antagonisten Sensit® (fendiline). *Arzneimittelforschung (Drug Res.)* **26**, 1819–1826.

Clark, R. E., Christlieb, I. Y., Ferguson, T. B., Weldon, C. S., Marbarger, J. P., Sobel, B. E., Roberts, R., Henry, P. D., Ludbrook, P. A., Biello, D., and Clark, B. K. 1981. Laboratory and initial clinical studies of nifedipine, a calcium antagonist for improved myocardial preservation. *Ann. Surg.* **193**, 719–732.

Clark, R. E., Christlieb, I. Y., Henry, P. D., Fischer, A. E., Nora, J. D., Williamson, J. R., and Sobel, B. E. 1979. Nifedipine: A myocardial protective agent. *Am. J. Cardiol.* **44**, 825–831.

Clark, J. I., Mengel, L., Bagg, A., and Benedek, G. B. 1980. Cortical opacity, calcium concentration and fibre membrane structure in the calf lens. *Exp. Eye Res.* **31**, 399–410.

Clark, A. J., and White, A. C. 1929. The oxygen consumption of the auricles of the frog and of the tortoise. *J. Physiol.* (Lond.), **68**, 406–432.

Coffman, J. D., and Gregg, D. E. 1960. Ventricular fibrillation during uniform myocardial anoxia due to asphyxia. *Am. J. Physiol.* **198**, 955–958.

Cohen. L. S., and Braunwald, E. 1967. Amelioration of angina pectoris in idiopathic hypertrophic subaortic stenosis with beta-adrenergic blockade. *Circulation* **35**, 847–851.

Cohn, A. E., and Levine, S. A. 1925. Beneficial effects of barium chloride on Adams-Stokes disease. *Arch. Intern. Med.* **36,** 1–12.

Coleman, H. N. 1967. Role of acetylstrophanthidin in augmenting myocardial oxygen consumption. *Circ. Res.* **21,** 487–495.

Conn, H. L. 1956. Effects of digitalis and hypoxia on potassium transfer and distribution in the dog heart. *Am. J. Physiol.* **184,** 548–552.

Coumel, P., Attuel, P., and Leclercq, J. F. 1981. The role of calcium antagonists in ventricular arrhythmias, in *Calcium Antagonism in Cardiovascular Therapy,* International Symposium, Florence, October, 1980, Edited by A. Zanchetti and D. M. Krikler, pp. 373–387, Excerpta Medica, Amsterdam-Oxford-Princeton, 1981.

Cranefield, P. F. 1975. *The Conduction of the Cardiac Impulse—The Slow Response and Cardiac Arrhythmias.* Futura, New York.

Cranefield, P. F., Aronson, R. S., and Wit, A. L. 1974. Effect of verapamil on the normal action potential and on a calcium-dependent slow response of canine cardiac Purkinje fibers. *Circ. Res.* **34,** 204–213.

Criley, J. M., Lewis, K. B., White, R. I., and Ross, R. S. 1965. Pressure gradients without obstruction: a new concept of "hypertrophic subaortic stenosis." *Circulation* **32,** 881–887.

Crocker, A. D., Mayeka, I. M., and Wilson, K. A. 1979. The role of calcium and cyclic AMP in the contractile action of angiotensin II upon rat descending colon. *Eur. J. Pharmacol.* **60,** 121–129.

Crompton, M., Cepano, M., and Carafoli, E. 1976. The sodium-induced efflux of calcium from heart mitochondria. A possible mechanism of the regulation of mitochondrial calcium. *Eur. J. Biochem.* **69,** 453–462.

Curry, R. C., Pepine, C. J., Sabom, M. B., and Conti, C. R. 1979. Similarities of ergonovine-induced and spontaneous attacks of variant angina. *Circulation* **59,** 307–312.

Curry, R. C., Pepine, C. J., Sabom, M. B., Feldman, R. L., Christie, L. G., and Conti, C. R. 1977. Effects of ergonovine in patients with and without coronary artery disease. *Circulation* **56,** 803–809.

Curtius, J. M., Goeckenjan, G., Steyer, M., and Hust, M. 1980. Lungenödem als Tokolyse-Komplikation. *Dtsch. Med. Wschr.* **105,** 1320–1324.

Dabrowska, R., Sherry, J. M. F., Aromatorio, D. K., and Hartshorne, D. J. 1978. Modulator protein as a component of the myosin light chain kinase from chicken gizzard. *Biochemistry* **17,** 253–258.

Dargie, H. Rowland, E., and Krikler, D. 1981. Role of calcium antagonists in cardiovascular therapy. *Brit. Heart J.* **46,** 8–16.

Datey, K. K., Bagri, A. K., Kelkar, P. N., Varma, S. R., Bhootra, R. K., and Amin, B. M. 1973. Perhexiline maleate: a new anti-anginal drug. *Postgrad. Med. J.* **49** (April Suppl.), 75–78.

Davignon, J., Lorenz, R. R., and Shepherd, J. T. 1965. Response of human umbilical artery to changes in transmural pressure. *Am. J. Physiol.* **209,** 51–59.

Deth, R., and van Breemen, C. 1974. Relative contributions of Ca^{2+} influx and cellular Ca^{2+} release during drug induced activation of the rabbit aorta. *Pflügers Arch. ges. Physiol.* **348,** 13–22.

Devis, G., Somers, G., van Obberghen, E., and Malaisse, W. J. 1975. Calcium antagonists and islet function. I. Inhibition of insulin release by verapamil. *Diabetes* **24,** 547–551.

Dhalla, N. S., Anand, M. B., and Harrow, J. A. C. 1976. Calcium binding and ATPase activities of heart sarcolemma. *J. Biochem.* (Tokyo) **79,** 1345–1350.

Dhalla, N. S., McNamara, D. B., and Sulakhe, P. V. 1970. Contribution of mitochondria and sarcoplasmic reticulum in the regulation of calcium accumulation in the heart. *Cardiology* **55,** 178–191.

Dhalla, N. S., Sulakhe, P. V., and McNamara, D. B. 1973. Studies on the relationship between adenylate cyclase activity and calcium transport by cardiac sarcotubular membranes. *Biochim. Biophys. Acta* **323,** 276–284.

Dhalla, N. S., Varley, K. G., and Harrow, J. A. C. 1974. Effect of epinephrine and adenosine cyclic

3′,5′-monophosphate on heart mitochondrial and microsomal calcium uptake. *Res. Commun. Chem. Pathol. Pharmacol.* **9**, 489–500.

Dhalla, N. S., Ziegelhoffer, A., and Harrow, J. A. C. 1977. Regulatory role of membrane systems in heart function. *Canad. J. Physiol. Pharmacol.* **55**, 1211–1234.

Dhurandar, R. W., Watt, D. L., Silver, M. D., Trimble, A. S., and Adelman, A. G. 1972. Prinzmetal's variant form of angina with arteriographic evidence of coronary arterial spasm. *Am. J. Cardiol.* **30**, 902–905.

Diekmann, L., and Hösemann, R. 1974. Zur blutdrucksenkenden Wirkung von Verapamil—Untersuchungen und Erfahrungen bei Kindern. *Münch. Med. Wschr.* **116**, 515–520.

Döring, H. J., and Kammermeier, H. 1961. Das Verhalten der energiereichen Phosphor-Verbindungen des Myokards bei unterschiedlichen Belastungsformen sowie bei verschiedenen Arten experimenteller Insuffizienz am Herz-Lungen-Präparat. *Verh. Dtsch. Ges. Kreisl.-Forsch.* **27**, 227–232.

Döring, H. J., and Kammermeier, H. 1963. Änderungen des Herzquerdurchmessers unter dem Einfluss von Sauerstoffmangel, Stoffwechsel-Inhibitoren und erregungshemmenden Substanzen, in *Kreislaufmessungen*, Proceedings of a Symposium, Freiburg (Germany), April 4–6, 1963, Edited by A. Fleckenstein, pp 45–56, Werk Verlag Dr. E. Banaschewski, Munich-Gräfelfing.

Döring, H. J., Kammermeier, H., and Byon, Y. K. 1962. Changes of cardiac tonus and high-energy phosphate concentrations of the heart due to anoxia or metabolic inhibitors. XXII International Congress of Physiological Sciences, Leiden, Sept. 10–17, 1962, Excerpta Med., Internat. Congr. Ser. No. 48, Abstr. No. 39.

Donat, K., and Schlosser, G. A. 1966. Zur Problematik der Angina pectoris-Therapie. *Med. Klin.* **61**, 352–356.

Doyle, A. E., Anavekar, S. N., and Oliver, L. E. 1981. A clinical trial of verapamil in the treatment of hypertension, in *Calcium Antagonism in Cardiovascular Therapy*, International Symposium, Florence, October, 1980, Edited by A. Zanchetti and D. M. Krikler, pp. 252–258, Excerpta Medica, Amsterdam-Oxford-Princeton, 1981.

Drahota, Z., Carafoli, E., Rossi, C. S., Gamble, R. L., and Lehninger, A. L. 1965. The steady state maintenance of accumulated Ca^{++} in rat liver mitochondria. *J. Biol. Chem.* **240**, 2712–2720.

Drake, F. T., Singer, D. H., Haring, O., and Dirnberger, G. 1973. Evaluation of anti-arrhythmic efficacy of perhexiline maleate in ambulatory patients by Holter monitoring. *Postgrad. Med. J.* **49** (April Suppl.), 52–63.

Draper, M. H., and Weidmann, S. 1951. Cardiac resting and action potentials recorded with an intracellular electrode, *J. Physiol.* (Lond.) **115**, 74–94.

Dreifuss, J. J., Grau, J. D., and Nordmann, J. J. 1975. Calcium movements related to neurohypophysical hormone secretion, in *Calcium Transport in Contraction and Secretion*, Edited by E. Carafoli et al., pp. 271–279. North-Holland Publish. Comp., Amsterdam.

Drummond, G. I., and Hemmings, S. J. 1972. Inotropic and chronotropic effects of dibutyryl cyclic AMP, in *Advances in Cyclic Nucleotide Research*, Edited by P. Greengard and G. A. Robison, **1**, 307–316, Raven Press, New York.

Duncan, G., and Bushell, A. R. 1975. Ion analyses of human cataractous lenses. *Exp. Eye Res.* **20**, 223–230.

Duncan, G., and Bushell, A. R. 1976. The bovine lens as an ion exchanger: a comparison with ion levels in human cataractous lenses. *Exp. Eye Res.* **23**, 341–353.

Durbin, R. P., and Jenkinson, D. H. 1961. The calcium dependence of tension development in depolarized smooth muscle. *J. Physiol.* (Lond.) **157**, 90–96.

Eaton, L. W., Weiss, J. L., Bulkley, B. H., Garrison, J. B., and Weisfeldt, M. L. 1979. Regional cardiac dilatation after acute myocardial infarction—Recognition by two dimensional echocardiography. *N. Engl. J. Med.* **300**, 57–62.

Ebashi, S. 1980. Regulation of muscle contraction. The Croonian Lecture 1979: *Proc. Roy. Soc. Lond. Ser. B* **207**, 259–286.

Ebashi, S., and Ebashi, F. 1964. A new protein component participating in the superprecipitation of myosin B. *J. Biochem.* (Tokyo) **55**, 604–613.

Ebashi, S., Ebashi, F., and Kodama, A. 1967. Troponin as the Ca^{2+}-receptive protein in the contractile system. *J. Biochem.* (Tokyo) **62**, 137–138.

Ebashi, S., and Endo, M. 1968. Calcium ions and muscle contraction. *Prog. Biophys. Mol. Biol.* **18**, 123–183.

Ebashi, S., and Kodama, A. 1965. A new protein factor promoting aggregation of tropomyosin. *J. Biochem.* (Tokyo) **58**, 107–108.

Ebashi, S., and Lipmann, F. 1962. Adenosine triphosphate-linked concentration of calcium ions in a particulate fraction of rabbit muscle. *J. Cell. Biol.* **14**, 389–400.

Ebner, F. 1975a. Survey of the results of world-wide clinical trials with nifedipine (Adalat), in *1st International Nifedipine (Adalat) Symposium,* Tokyo, November, 1973, Edited by K. Hashimoto, E. Kimura, and T. Kobayashi, pp. 282–290, University of Tokyo Press, 1975.

Ebner, F. 1975b. Survey and summary of results obtained during the world-wide clinical investigations of Adalat (Nifedipine), in *2nd International Nifedipine (Adalat) Symposium,* Amsterdam, October, 1974, Edited by W. Lochner, W. Braasch, and G. Kroneberg, pp. 348–360, Springer-Verlag, Berlin–Heidelberg–New York, 1975.

Ebner, F., and Dünschede, H. B. 1976. Haemodynamics, therapeutic mechanism of action and clinical findings of Adalat use based on worldwide clinical trials, in *3rd International Nifedipine (Adalat) Symposium,* Rio de Janeiro, October, 1975, Edited by A. D. Jatene and P. R. Lichtlen, pp. 283–300, Excerpta Medica, Amsterdam–Oxford, 1976.

Edman, K. A. P., and Schild, H. O. 1962. The need for calcium in the contractile responses induced by acetylcholine and potassium in the rat uterus. *J. Physiol.* (Lond.) **161**, 424–441.

Edman, K. A. P., and Schild, H. O. 1963. Calcium and the stimulant and inhibitory effects of adrenaline in depolarized smooth muscle. *J. Physiol.* (Lond.) **169**, 404–411.

van Egmond, A. A. J. 1913. Über die Wirkung einiger Arzneimittel beim vollständigen Herzblock. Pflügers *Arch. ges. Physiol.* **154**, 39–65.

Eichelbaum, M., Birkel, P., Grube, E., Gütgemann, U., and Somogyi, A. 1980. Effects of verapamil on P-R-intervals in relation to verapamil plasma levels following single i.v. and oral administration and during chronic treatment. *Klin. Wschr.* **58**, 919–925.

Eichelbaum, M., Dengler, H. J., Somogyi, A., and von Unruh, G. E. 1981. Superiority of stable isotope techniques in the assessment of the bioavailability of drugs undergoing extensive first pass elimination. *Eur. J. Clin. Pharmacol.* **19**, 127–131.

Eichelbaum, M., Ende, M., Remberg, G., Schomerus, M., and Dengler, H.J. 1979. The metabolism of DL-(^{14}C)verapamil in man. *Drug Metabolism and Disposition* **7**, 145–148.

Eichelbaum, M., Somogyi, A., von Unruh, G. E., and Dengler, H. J. 1981. Simultaneous determination of the intravenous and oral pharmacokinetic parameters of D,L-verapamil using stable isotope-labelled verapamil. *Eur. J. Clin. Pharmacol.* **19**, 133–137.

Eisenstein, R., and Zeruolis, L. 1964. Vitamin-D-induced aortic calcification. *Arch. Path.* **77**, 27–35.

van Ekelen, W. A. A. J., and Robles de Medina, E. O. 1978. Variant forms of angina pectoris. *Eur. J. Cardiol.* **8**, 305–317.

Ekelund, L.-G., and Atterhög, J.-H. 1975. Adalat and beta blockers; the mechanism studied with two series of work tests in two groups of patients with angina pectoris, in *2nd International Nifedipine (Adalat) Symposium,* Amsterdam, October, 1974, Edited by W. Lochner, W. Braasch, and G. Kroneberg, pp. 169–173, Springer-Verlag, Berlin–Heidelberg–New York, 1975.

Ekelund, L.-G., Atterhög, J.-H., and Melin, A.-L. 1975. Effect of nifedipine on exercise tolerance in patients with angina pectoris, in *1st International Nifedipine (Adalat) Symposium,* Tokyo, November, 1973, Edited by K. Hashimoto, E. Kimura, and T. Kobayashi, pp. 144–149, University of Tokyo Press, 1975.

Ekelund, L.-G., and Orö, L. 1976. Antianginal efficiency of Adalat with and without a beta-blocker. A subacute study with exercise tests, in *3rd International Adalat® Symposium*, Rio de Janeiro, October 10–11, 1975, Edited by A. D. Jatene and P. R. Lichtlen, pp. 218–225, Excerpta Medica, Amsterdam–Oxford, 1976.

Ellis, E. F., Oelz, O., Roberts, L. J., Payne, N. A., Sweetman, B. J., Nies, A. S., and Oates, J. A. 1976. Coronary arterial smooth muscle contraction by a substance released from platelets: Evidence that it is thromboxane A_2. *Science* **193**, 1135–1137.

Endo, M. 1977. Calcium release from the sarcoplasmic reticulum. *Physiol. Rev.* **57**, 71–108.

Endo, M., Hirosawa, K., Kaneko, N., Hase, K., Inoue, Y., and Konno, S. 1976. Prinzmetal's variant angina. Coronary arteriogram and left ventriculogram during angina attack induced by methacholine. *N. Engl. J. Med.* **294**, 252.

Endo, M., Kanda, I., Hosoda, S., Hayashi, H., Hirosawa, K., and Konno, S. 1975. Prinzmetal's variant form of angina pectoris: re-evaluation of mechanisms. *Circulation* **52**, 33–37.

Endo, M., Tanaka, M., and Ogawa, Y. 1970. Calcium induced release of calcium from the sarcoplasmic reticulum of skinned skeletal muscle fibers. *Nature* **228**, 34–36.

Engstfeld, G., Antoni, H., and Fleckenstein, A. 1961. Die Restitution der Erregungsfortleitung und Kontraktionskraft des K^+-gelähmten Frosch- und Säugetiermyokards durch Adrenalin. *Pflügers Arch. ges. Physiol.* **273**, 145–163.

Enselberg, C. D., Simmons, H. G., and Mintz, A. A. 1950. The effects of potassium upon the heart, with special reference to the possibility of treatment of toxic arrhythmias due to digitalis. *Am. Heart J.* **39**, 713–728.

Entman, M. L. 1974. The role of cyclic AMP in the modulation of cardiac contractility, in *Advances in Cyclic Nucleotide Research*, Edited by P. Greengard and G. A. Robison, **4**, 163–193, Raven Press, New York.

Entman, M. L., Allen, J. C., Bornet, E. P., Gillette, P. C., Wallick, E. T., and Schwartz, A. 1972. Mechanisms of calcium accumulation and transport in cardiac relaxing system (sarcoplasmic reticulum membranes): Effects of verapamil, D 600, X 537 A and A 23187. *J. Mol. Cell. Cardiol.* **4**, 681–687.

Eto, S., Wood, J. M., Hutchins, M., and Fleischer, N. 1974. Pituitary $^{45}Ca^{++}$ uptake and release of ACTH, GH and TSH: effects of verapamil. *Am. J. Physiol.* **226**, 1315–1320.

Evans, D. H. L., Schild, H. O., and Thesleff, S. 1958. Effects of drugs on depolarized plain muscle. *J. Physiol.* (Lond.) **143**, 474–485.

Fabiato, A., and Fabiato, F. 1975. Contractions induced by a calcium-triggered release of calcium from the sarcoplasmic reticulum of single skinned cardiac cells. *J. Physiol.* (Lond.) **249**, 469–495.

Fabiato, A., and Fabiato, F. 1977. Calcium release from the sarcoplasmic reticulum. *Circ. Res.* **40**, 119–129.

Fabiato, A., and Fabiato, F. 1978. Calcium-induced release of calcium from the sarcoplasmic reticulum of skinned cells from adult human, dog, cat, rabbit, rat, and frog hearts and from fetal and newborn rat ventricles. *Ann. N. Y. Acad. Sci.* **307**, 491–522.

Fagerholm, P. P. 1979. The influence of calcium on lens fibers. *Exp. Eye Res.* **28**, 211–222.

Fagher, B., Persson, S., and Svensson, S. E. 1977. Double-blind comparison of verapamil and practolol in the treatment of angina pectoris. *Postgrad. Med. J.* **53**, 61–65.

Fanburg, B., Finkel, R. M., and Martonosi, A. 1964. The role of calcium in the mechanism of relaxation of cardiac muscle. *J. Biol. Chem.* **239**, 2298–2306.

Fawaz, G., and Hawa, E. S. 1953. Phosphocreatine content of mammalian cardiac muscle. *Proc. Soc. Exp. Biol.* (N.Y.) **84**, 277–280.

Fawaz, G., Hawa, E. S., and Tutunji, B. 1957. The effect of dinitrophenol, hypoxaemia and ischaemia on the phosphorus compounds of the dog heart. *Brit. J. Pharmacol.* **12**, 270–272.

Fawcett, D. W., and McNutt, N. S. 1969. The ultra-structure of the cat myocardium. Ventricular papillary muscle. *J. Cell. Biol.* **42**, 1–45.

Fazzini, P. F., Marchi, F., Pucci, P., Ledda, F., and Mugelli, A. 1981. Treatment of "slow response" related premature beats in acute myocardial infarction, in *Calcium Antagonism in Cardiovascular Therapy,* International Symposium, Florence, October, 1980, Edited by A. Zanchetti and D. M. Krikler, pp. 337–341, Excerpta Medica, Amsterdam–Oxford–Princeton, 1981.

Fedelesova, M., and Ziegelhöffer, A. 1975. Enhanced calcium accumulation related to increased protein phosphorylation in cardiac sarcoplasmic reticulum induced by cyclic $3',5'$-AMP or isoproterenol. *Experientia* **31,** 518–520.

Fedelesova, M., Ziegelhöffer, A., Luknarova, O., and Kostolansky, S. 1975. Prevention by K^+, Mg^{2+}-aspartate of isoproterenol-induced metabolic changes in the myocardium, in *Recent Advances in Studies on Cardiac Structure and Metabolism,* Vol. 6, Edited by A. Fleckenstein and G. Rona, pp. 59–73. University Park Press, Baltimore–London–Tokyo.

Feinberg, H., Boyd, E., and Katz, L. N. 1962. Calcium effect on performance of the heart. *Am. J. Physiol.* **202,** 643–648.

Feinsilver, O., Cho, Y. W., and Aviado, D. M. 1970. Pharmacology of a new antianginal drug: Perhexiline. III. Bronchopulmonary system in the dog and humans. *Chest,* **58,** 558–561.

Feinstein, M. 1962. Effects of experimental congestive heart failure, ouabam, and asphyxia on the high-energy phosphate and creatine content of the guinea pig heart. *Circ. Res.* **10,** 333–346.

Ferlemann, H. J., Krehan, L., and Kaltenbach, M. 1979. Wirkung von Perhexilinmaleat auf das Belastungs-EKG von Patienten mit koronarer Herzerkrankung. *Z. Kardiol.* **68,** 826–831.

Ferrer, M. I., Bradley, S. E., Wheeler, H. O., Enson, Y., Preisig, R., and Harvey, R. M. 1965. The effect of digoxin in the splanchnic circulation in ventricular failure. *Circulation* **32,** 524–537.

Ferrier, G. R., and Moe, G. K. 1973. Effect of calcium on acetylstrophanthidin-induced transient depolarizations in canine Purkinje tissue. *Circ. Res.* **33,** 508–515.

Fischer, B. 1911. Über fötale Infektionskrankheiten und fötale Endokarditis, nebst Bemerkungen über Herzmuskelverkalkung. *Frankfurt. Z. Path.* **7,** 83–111.

Fischer, K. 1965. Beitrag zur medikamentösen Behandlung der Koronarinsuffizienz. *Med. Klin.* **60,** 847–851.

Fischer Hansen, J., and Sandøe, E. 1978. Treatment of Prinzmetal's angina due to coronary artery spasm using verapamil: a report of three cases. *Eur. J. Cardiol.* **7,** 327–335.

Fleckenstein, A. 1953. Über Neurosympathomimetica. *Verh. Dtsch. Ges. Inn. Med.* **59,** 17–22.

Fleckenstein, A. 1955. *Der Kalium-Natrium-Austausch als Energieprinzip in Muskel und Nerv.* Springer, Berlin–Göttingen–Heidelberg.

Fleckenstein, A. 1960. Enzymregulation im Herzstoffwechsel, in *Enzymatische Regulationen in der Klinik.* Proceedings 6th International Congress of Internal Medicine, Basel, 1960, Edited by A. Gigon and H. Ludwigs, pp. 37–51, Benno Schwabe, Basel–Stuttgart.

Fleckenstein, A. 1961a. Aktuelle Probleme der Muskelphysiologie und ihre Analyse mit Isotopen, in *Handbuch: Künstliche radioaktive Isotope in Physiologie, Diagnostik und Therapie,* Edited by H. Schwiegk und F. Turba, pp. 179–228. Springer, Berlin–Göttingen–Heidelberg, 1961, 2nd ed.

Fleckenstein, A. 1961b. Die Pathophysiologie des Vorhofs- und Kammerflimmerns, in *Beiträge zur Ersten Hilfe und Behandlung von Unfällen durch elektrischen Strom,* Edited by R. Hauf, pp. 15–37. Verlags- und Wirtschaftsgesellschaft der Elektrizitätswerke, Frankfurt, 1961.

Fleckenstein, A. 1963a. Metabolic aspects of the excitation-contraction coupling, in *The Cellular Functions of Membrane Transport,* Symposium of the Society of General Physiologists in Woods Hole, Mass., September 4–7, 1963. Edited by J. F. Hoffmann, pp. 71–93. Prentice-Hall, Englewood Cliffs, N. J., 1963.

Fleckenstein, A. 1963b. Physiologie und Pathophysiologie des Myokard-Stoffwechsels im Zusammenspiel mit den bioelektrischen und mechanischen Fundamentalprozessen, in *Das Herz des Menschen,* Edited by W. Bargmann und W. Doerr, pp. 355–411. Georg Thieme, Stuttgart, 1963.

Fleckenstein, A. 1964a. Die Bedeutung der energiereichen Phosphate für Kontraktilität und Tonus des Myokards. *Verh. Dtsch. Ges. Inn. Med.*, **70**, 81–99.

Fleckenstein, A. 1964b. Experimentelle Wiederherstellung von Automatie und Erregungsleitung durch Sympathicomimetica. *Verh. Dtsch. Ges. Kreisl. -Forsch.* **30**, 102–113.

Fleckenstein, A. 1967. Stoffwechselprobleme bei der Myokard-Insuffizienz. *Verh. Dtsch. Ges. Path.* **51**, 15–29. Gustav Fischer, Stuttgart.

Fleckenstein, A. 1968a. Myokardstoffwechsel und Nekrose, in *VI Symposium, "Herzinfarkt und Schock"*, *Dtsch. Gesellschaft für Fortschritte auf dem Gebiet der Inneren Medizin*, November 8, 1968, Freiburg, Edited by L. Heilmeyer and H. J. Holtmeier, pp. 94–109, Georg Thieme, Stuttgart.

Fleckenstein, A. 1968b. Experimentelle Pathologie der akuten und chronischen Herzinsuffizienz. *Verh. Dtsch. Ges. Kreisl. -Forsch.* **34**, 15–34.

Fleckenstein, A. 1968c. Experimental heart failure due to disturbances in high-energy phosphate metabolism. Proceedings Vth Eur. Congr. Cardiol. Athens, Sept. 1968, pp. 255–269.

Fleckenstein, A. 1969a. Einfluss antifibrillatorischer Arzneimittel auf die elektrischen Elementarvorgänge. *Verh. Dtsch. Ges. Kreisl. -Forsch.* **35**, 77–87.

Fleckenstein, A. 1969/1971. *Pathophysiologische Kausalfaktoren bei Myocardnekrose und Infarkt.* Research Report at the 14th Cardioangiological Meeting of the Austrian Cardiological Society, Vienna, November 22, 1969, later published in Z. für Inn. Med., **52**, 133–143 (1971).

Fleckenstein, A. 1970/1971a. Specific inhibitors and promoters of calcium action in the excitation-contraction coupling of heart muscle and their role in the production or prevention of myocardial lesions, in *Calcium and the Heart,* Proceedings of the Meeting of the European Section of the International Study Group for Research in Cardiac Metabolism, London, September 6, 1970, Edited by P. Harris and L. Opie, pp. 135–188, Academic Press, London–New York, 1971.

Fleckenstein, A. 1970/1971b. Neuere Ergebnisse zur Physiologie, Pharmakologie und Pathologie der elektromechanischen Koppelungsprozesse im Warmblütermyokard, in *Vorträge der Erlanger Physiologentagung 1970,* Edited by W. D. Keidel and K. H. Plattig, pp. 13–52, Springer-Verlag, Berlin–Heidelberg–New York, 1971.

Fleckenstein, A. 1975. Adalat, a powerful Ca-antagonistic drug, 2nd International Adalat Symposium *New Therapy of Ischemic Heart Disease,* Edited by W. Lochner, W. Braasch, and G. Kroneberg, pp. 56–65, Springer-Verlag, Berlin–Heidelberg–New York.

Fleckenstein, A. 1977. Specific pharmacology of calcium in myocardium, cardiac pacemakers, and vascular smooth muscle. *Ann. Rev. Pharmacol. Toxicol.* **17**, 149–166.

Fleckenstein, A. 1978/1980. Steuerung der myocardialen Kontraktilität, ATP-Spaltung, Atmungsintensität und Schrittmacher-Funktion durch Calcium-Ionen. Wirkungsmechanismus der Calcium-Antagonisten, in *Calcium-Antagonismus,* Proceedings of an International Symposium, 1978, in Frankfort. Edited by A. Fleckenstein and H. Roskamm, pp. 1–28, Springer-Verlag, Berlin–Heidelberg–New York, 1980.

Fleckenstein, A. 1980/1981. Pharmacology and electrophysiology of calcium antagonists, in *Calcium antagonism in cardiovascular therapy: Experience with Verapamil,* International Symposium in Florence, October 2–4, 1980, Edited by A. Zanchetti and D. M. Krikler, pp. 10–29, Excerpta Medica, Amsterdam–Oxford–Princeton, 1981.

Fleckenstein, A. 1981. Fundamental actions of calcium antagonists on myocardial and cardiac pacemaker cell membranes, In *New Perspectives on Calcium Antagonists.* Edited by G. B. Weiss. Clinical Physiology Series, pp. 59–81, *Am. Physiol. Society,* Bethesda.

Fleckenstein, A., and Burn, J. H. 1953. The effect of denervation on the action of sympathomimetic amines on the nictitating membrane. *Brit. J. Pharmacol.* **8**, 69–78.

Fleckenstein, A., and Byon, K. Y. 1974. Prevention by Ca-antagonistic compounds (verapamil, D 600) of coronary smooth muscle contractures due to treatment with cardiac glycosides. *Naunyn-Schmiedebergs Arch. exper. Path. Pharmakol.* Vol. **282** (Suppl.), R 20.

Fleckenstein, A., Döring, H. J., Janke, J., and Byon, Y. K. 1975. Basic actions of ions and drugs on myocardial high-energy phosphate metabolism and contractility, in *Handbook of Experimental Pharmacology. New Series*, Vol. XVI/3, Edited by J. Schmier and O. Eichler, pp. 345–405. Springer-Verlag, Berlin–Heidelberg–New York.

Fleckenstein, A., Döring, H. J., and Kammermeier, H. 1966/1967. Experimental heart failure due to inhibition of utilisation of high-energy phosphates. *Proceedings of an International Symposium on the Coronary Circulation and Energetics of the Myocardium*, Milan, 1966, pp. 220–236. Karger, Basel–New York, 1967.

Fleckenstein, A., Döring, H. J., and Kammermeier, H. 1968. Einfluss von Beta-Receptorenblockern und verwandten Substanzen auf Erregung, Kontraktion und Energiestoffwechsel der Myokardfaser. *Klin. Wschr.* **46**, 343–351.

Fleckenstein, A., Döring, H. J., Kammermeier, H., and Grün, G. 1968. Influence of prenylamine on the utilization of high energy phosphates in cardiac muscle. *Biochim. Applic.* **14** (Suppl. 1), 323–344.

Fleckenstein, A., Döring, H. J., and Leder, O. 1969. The significance of high-energy phosphate exhaustion in the etiology of isoproterenol-induced cardiac necrosis and its prevention by iproveratril, compound D 600 or prenylamine, in *Symposium International on Drugs and Metabolism of Myocardium and Striated Muscle*, Edited by M. Lamarche and R. Royer, pp. 11–22, University of Nancy, France.

Fleckenstein, A., and Fleckenstein-Grün, G. 1975. Further studies on the neutralization of glycoside-induced contractures of coronary smooth muscle by Ca-antagonistic compounds (verapamil, D 600, prenylamine, nifedipine, fendiline or nitrites). *Naunyn-Schmiedebergs Arch. exper. Path. Pharmakol.* **287** (Suppl.), R 38.

Fleckenstein, A., and Fleckenstein-Grün G. 1977. Combined therapy with cardiac glycosides and Ca-antagonistic agents. *Arzneimittelforschung (Drug Res.)* **27**, 736–742.

Fleckenstein, A., and Fleckenstein-Grün, G. 1980. Cardiovascular protection by Ca antagonists. *Europ. Heart Journal* **1**, (Suppl. B), 15–21.

Fleckenstein, A., Fleckenstein-Grün, G., and Byon, Y. K. 1977. Fundamentale Herz- und Gefässwirkungen des Ca^{++}-antagonistischen Koronartherapeutikums Fendilin (Sensit®). *Arzneimittelforschung (Drug Res.)* **27**, 562–571.

Fleckenstein, A., Fleckenstein-Grün, G., Byon, Y. K., Haastert, H. P., and Späh, F. 1979. Vergleichende Untersuchungen über die Ca^{++}-antagonistischen Grundwirkungen von Niludipin (Bay a 7168) und Nifedipin (Bay a 1040) auf Myokard, Myometrium und glatte Gefässmuskulatur. *Arzneimittelforschung (Drug Res.)* **29**, 230–246.

Fleckenstein, A., Fleckenstein-Grün, G., Janke, J., and Frey, M. 1977. Fundamental cardiovascular effects of Ca-antagonists and their therapeutic significance when combined with cardiac glycosides. *Z. Praeklin. Klin. Geriatr.* **7**, 269–284.

Fleckenstein, A., Frey, M., and Keidel, J. 1980/1982. Prevention by verapamil of isoproterenol-induced hypertrophic cardiomyopathy in rats, in *Hypertrophic Myopathy*, Proceedings Symposium in Wertheim, Germany, May 13–14, 1980, Edited by M. Kaltenbach and S. E. Epstein, pp. 115–120, Springer-Verlag, Berlin–Heidelberg–New York, 1982.

Fleckenstein, A., Gerlach, E., Janke, J., and Marmier, P. 1959. Die Bestimmung des Turnovers von ATP, Kreatinphosphat und Orthophosphat in lebenden Muskeln mittels H_2O^{18} und anschliessender Aktivierung durch Protonen-Beschuss. *Naturwissenschaften* **46**, 365–367.

Fleckenstein, A., Gerlach, E., Janke, J., and Marmier, P. 1960. Die Inkorporation von markiertem Sauerstoff aus Wasser in die ATP-, Kreatinphosphat- und Orthophosphat-Fraktion intakter Muskeln bei Ruhe, tetanischer Reizung und Erholung. Neue Wege der intracellulären Turnover-Messung mit Hilfe von H_2O^{18} und anschliessender Aktivierung der O^{18}-haltigen Phosphat-Fraktionen durch Protonen-Beschuss. *Pflügers Arch. ges. Physiol.* **271**, 75–104.

Fleckenstein, A., and Grün, G. 1969. Reversible blockade of excitation-contraction coupling in rat's uterine smooth muscle by means of organic calcium antagonists (iproveratril, D 600, prenylamine). *Pflügers Arch. ges. Physiol.* **307**, 26.

Fleckenstein, A., and Grün, G. 1971/1972. Prinzipielles zur Wirkung von Ca^{++}-Antagonisten auf die bioelektrische und mechanische Funktion glatter Muskelzellen, in *Vascular Smooth Muscle*, Proceedings of a Satellite Symposium of the 25th International Congress of Physiological Sciences, July 20–24, 1971, Tübingen, Edited by E. Betz, pp. 62–65, Springer-Verlag, Berlin–Heidelberg–New York, 1972.

Fleckenstein, A., Grün, G., Byon, Y. K., Döring, H. J., and Tritthart, H. 1975. The basic Ca-antagonistic actions of nifedipine on cardiac energy metabolism and vascular smooth muscle tone, in *New Therapy of Ischemic Heart Disease*, 1st International Nifedipine (Adalat) Symposium, Tokyo, 1973, Edited by K. Hashimoto, E. Kimura and T. Kobayashi, pp. 31–44, University of Tokyo Press, 1975.

Fleckenstein, A., Grün, G., Tritthart, H., and Byon, Y. K. 1971. Uterus-Relaxation durch hochaktive Ca-antagonistische Hemmstoffe der elektromechanischen Koppelung wie Isoptin (Verapamil, Iproveratril), Substanz D 600 und Segontin (Prenylamin). *Klin. Wschr.* **49**, 32–41.

Fleckenstein, A., and Hardt, A. 1949. Der Wirkungsmechanismus der Lokalanästhetica und Antihistaminkörper—ein Permeabilitätsproblem. *Klin. Wschr.* **27**, 360–363.

Fleckenstein, A., and Janke, J. 1958. The turnover rates of labile phosphate compounds in skeletal and heart muscle during activity and rest. An investigation with the use of radiophosphorus and paper chromatography, in *Radioisotopes in Scientific Research*, Proceedings 1st UNESCO International Conference, Paris, 1957, **4**, 60–73, Pergamon Press, London–New York–Paris, 1958.

Fleckenstein, A., and Janke, J. 1959. The metabolism of organophosphates in cardiac tissue as studied with radiophosphorus and paper chromatography, in *Proceedings 2nd International United Nations Conference on Peaceful Uses of Atomic Energy*, Geneva, September, 1958, Session D-14, P/976, Germany (Fed. Rep.), pp. 39–44. Pergamon Press, London–New York–Paris–Los Angeles, 1959.

Fleckenstein, A., and Janke, J. 1964. L'application biologique de l'analyse d'activation de l'oxygène 18, in *L'analyse par radioactivation et ses applications aux sciences biologiques*, 3e Colloque International de Biologie de Saclay en Septembre, 1963, pp. 267–285. Imprimerie des Presses Universitaires de France, Vendôme, 1964.

Fleckenstein, A., Janke, J., Döring, H. J., and Leder, O. 1971. Die intracelluläre Überladung mit Kalzium als entscheidender Kausalfaktor bei der Entstehung nicht-coronarogener Myokard-Nekrosen. *Verh. Dtsch. Ges. Kreisl.-Forsch.* **37**, 345–353.

Fleckenstein, A., Janke, J., Döring, H. J., and Leder, O. 1974. Myocardial fiber necrosis due to intracellular Ca overload—a new principle in cardiac pathophysiology, in *Myocardial Biology, Recent Advances in Studies on Cardiac Structure and Metabolism*, Edited by N. S. Dhalla, Vol.4,pp. 563–580. University Park Press, Baltimore–London–Tokyo.

Fleckenstein, A., Janke, J., Döring, H. J., and Leder, O. 1975. Key role of Ca in the production of noncoronarogenic myocardial necroses, in *Pathophysiology and Morphology of Myocardial Cell Alterations, Recent Advances in Studies on Cardiac Structure and Metabolism*, Edited by A. Fleckenstein, and G. Rona, Vol. **6**, pp. 21–32. University Park Press, Baltimore–London–Tokyo.

Fleckenstein, A., Janke, J., Döring, H. J., and Pachinger, O. 1973. Ca overload as the determinant factor in the production of catecholamine-induced myocardial lesions, in *Cardiomyopathies, Recent Advances in Studies on Cardiac Structure and Metabolism*. Edited by E. Bajusz, and G. Rona, Vol 2, pp. 455–466. University Park Press, Baltimore–London–Tokyo.

Fleckenstein, A., Janke, J., and Fleckenstein-Grün, G. 1978. Kardiotoxische Wirkungen β-adrenerger Tokolytika—Kardioprotektion durch Ca^{++}-Antagonisten, in *Kardiale Probleme bei der Tokolyse*, Proceedings of a Symposium in Freiburg, February, 1976, Edited by H.-G. Hillemanns and R. Trolp, pp. 54–67, Ferdinand Enke Verlag, Stuttgart.

Fleckenstein, A., Janke, J., and Gerlach, E. 1959. Konzentration und Turnover der energiereichen Phosphate des Herzens nach Studien mit Papierchromatographie und Radiophosphor. *Klin. Wschr.* **37**, 451–459.

Fleckenstein, A., Janke, J., and Marmier, P. 1965. Biological application of the activation analysis of O^{18}, in *Isotopes in Experimental Pharmacology*, Edited by L. J. Roth, pp. 33–45. The University of Chicago Press.

Fleckenstein, A., Kammermeier, H., Döring, H. J., and Freund, H. J. 1967. Zum Wirkungsmechanismus neuartiger Koronardilatatoren mit gleichzeitig Sauerstoff-einsparenden Myokard-Effekten, Prenylamin und Iproveratril. *Z. Kreisl.-Forsch.* **56**, 716–744, 839–853.

Fleckenstein, A., Nakayama, K., Fleckenstein-Grün, G., and Byon, Y. K. 1975. Interactions of vasoactive ions and drugs with Ca-dependent excitation-contraction coupling of vascular smooth muscle, in *Calcium Transport in Contraction and Secretion*, Edited by E. Carafoli et al., pp. 555–566, North-Holland, Amsterdam.

Fleckenstein, A., Nakayama, K., Fleckenstein-Grün, G., and Byon, Y. K. 1976a. Mechanism and sites of action of calcium antagonistic coronary therapeutics, in *Coronary Angiography and Angina Pectoris*, Symposium of the European Society of Cardiology, Hanover, March, 1975, Edited by P. R. Lichtlen, pp. 297–316, Georg Thieme, Stuttgart, 1976.

Fleckenstein, A., Nakayama, K., Fleckenstein-Grün, G., and Byon, Y. K. 1976b. Interactions of H ions, Ca-antagonistic drugs and cardiac glycosides with excitation-contraction coupling of vascular smooth muscle, in *Ionic Actions on Vascular Smooth Muscle*, Edited by E. Betz, pp. 117–123, Springer-Verlag, Berlin–Heidelberg–New York, 1976.

Fleckenstein, A., Pachinger, O., Leder, O., Hein, B., and Janke, J. 1972. Verhütung Isoproterenol-induzierter Myocardnekrosen durch Senkung des Plasmacalcium-Spiegels mittels Calcitonin. *Pflügers Arch. ges. Physiol.* Vol. **332** (Suppl.), R40.

Fleckenstein, A., and Schwoerer, W. 1961. Die Bedeutung der Ca-Ionen für die Spaltung von energiereichem Phosphat während verschiedener reversibler Kontrakturen und irreversibler Starre-Verkürzungen des Frosch-Rectus. *Pflügers Arch. ges. Physiol.* **274**, 8–9.

Fleckenstein, A., Schwoerer, W., and Janke, J. 1961. Parallele Beeinflussung der mechanischen Spannungsentwicklung und der Spaltung von energiereichem Phosphat bei der Kalium-Kontraktur des Froschrectus in Lösungen mit variiertem K^+- und Ca^{++}-Gehalt. *Pflügers Arch. ges. Physiol.* **273**, 483–498.

Fleckenstein, A., and Späh, F. 1981/1982. Excitation-contraction uncoupling in cardiac muscle, in *Advances in Pharmacology and Therapeutics II*, Vol. 3: Cardio-Renal and Cell Pharmacology, Proceedings 8th International Pharmacological Congress, Tokyo, July, 1981, Edited by H. Yoshida, Y. Hagihara, and S. Ebashi, pp. 97–110, Pergamon Press, Oxford–New York, (1982).

Fleckenstein, A., and Stöckle, D. 1955. Zum Mechanismus der Wirkungs-Verstärkung und Wirkungs-Abschwächung sympathomimetischer Amine durch Cocain und andere Pharmaca. II. Mitteilung. Die Hemmung der Neurosympathomimetica durch Cocain. *Naunyn-Schmiedebergs Arch. exper. Path. Pharmakol.* **224**, 401–415.

Fleckenstein, A., Tritthart, H., Döring, H. J., and Byon, Y. K. 1972. Bay a 1040 ein hochaktiver Ca^{++}-antagonistischer Inhibitor der elektro-mechanischen Koppelungsprozesse im Warmblüter-Myokard. *Arzneimittelforschung (Drug Res.)* **22**, 22–33.

Fleckenstein, A., Tritthart, H., Fleckenstein, B., Herbst, A., and Grün, G. 1969. A new group of competitive Ca-antagonists (Iproveratril, D 600, Prenylamine) with highly potent inhibitory effects on excitation-contraction coupling in mammalian myocardium. *Pflügers Arch. ges. Physiol.* **307**, R25.

Fleckenstein, A., v. Witzleben, H., Frey, M., and Milner, T. G. 1981. Prevention of cataracts of alloxan-diabetic rats by long-term treatment with verapamil. *Pflügers Arch. ges Physiol.* Vol. **391** (Suppl.), R12.

Fleckenstein-Grün, G., and Fleckenstein, A. 1975. Ca-dependent changes in coronary smooth muscle tone and the action of Ca-antagonistic compounds with special reference to Adalat, in *New Therapy of Ischemic Heart Disease,* 2nd International Adalat Symposium, Amsterdam, 1974, Edited by W. Lochner, W. Braasch, and G. Kroneberg, pp. 66–75, Springer-Verlag, Berlin–Heidelberg–New York, 1975.

Fleckenstein-Grün, G., and Fleckenstein, A. 1978/1980. Calcium-Antagonismus, ein Grundprinzip der Vasodilatation, in *Calcium-Antagonismus,* Proceedings of an International Symposium 1978 in Frankfort, Edited by A. Fleckenstein and H. Roskamm, pp. 191–207, Springer-Verlag, Berlin–Heidelberg–New York, 1980.

Fleckenstein-Grün, G., and Fleckenstein, A. 1980/1981. Calcium antagonism, a basic principle in vasodilation, in *Calcium Antagonism in Cardiovascular Therapy—Experience with Verapamil,* Proceedings of an International Symposium in Florence, October 2–4, 1980, Edited by A. Zanchetti and D. M. Krikler, pp. 30–48, Excerpta Medica, Amsterdam–Oxford–Princeton, 1981.

Fleckenstein-Grün, G., Fleckenstein, A., Byon, Y. K., and Kim, K. W. 1976/1978. Mechanism of action of Ca^{2+}-antagonists in the treatment of coronary disease with special reference to perhexiline maleate. *Proceedings of the Symposium on Perhexiline Maleate,* September 18, 1976, in Strasbourg, pp. 1–22, Excerpta Medica, Amsterdam 1978.

Fleckenstein-Grün, G., Fleckenstein, A., Späh, F., and Assmann, R. 1978/1979. Beeinflussung der elektromechanischen Koppelungsprozesse in der isolierten Herz- und Gefässmuskulatur durch Molsidomin und den Metaboliten SIN-1, in *Proceedings of the Symposium on Molsidomin,* Munich, 1978, Edited by W. Lochner and F. Bender, pp. 56–68, Urban and Schwarzenberg, Munich–Vienna–Baltimore, 1979.

Folkow, B. 1964. Description of the myogenic hypothesis. *Circ. Res.,* Suppl. I to Vols. **14** and **15**, pp. 279–287.

Follis, R. H., Orent-Keiles, E., and McCollum, E. V. 1942. The production of cardiac and renal lesions in rats by a diet extremely deficient in potassium. *Am. J. Path.* **18**, 29–39.

Fondacaro, J. D., Han, J., and Yoon, M. S. 1978. Effects of verapamil on ventricular rhythm during acute coronary occlusion. *Am. Heart J.* **96**, 81–86.

Ford, L. E., and Podolsky, R. J. 1970. Regenerative calcium release within muscle cells. *Science* **67**, 58–59.

Foster, P. R., King, R. M., Nicoll, A. De B., and Zipes, D. P. 1976. Suppression of ouabain-induced ventricular rhythms with aprindine-HCl. *Circulation* **53**, 315–321.

Franklin, D., Millard, R. W., and Nagao, T. 1980. Responses of coronary collateral flow and dependent myocardial mechanical function to the calcium antagonist diltiazem. *Chest* **78** (July Suppl.), 200–204.

Fratz, R., Greeff, K., and Wagner, J. 1967. Über den Einfluss der β-Rezeptorenblocker, des Iproveratrils, Chinidins und Reserpins auf die Wirkung des k-Strophanthins am Meerschweinchenherzen. *Naunyn-Schmiedebergs Arch. exper. Path. Pharmakol.* **256**, 196–206.

Freedman, B., Dunn, R. F., Richmond, D. R., and Kelly, D. T. 1979. Coronary artery spasm—Treatment with verapamil. *Circulation* **60** (Suppl. II), 249.

Frey, M., and Janke, J. 1975. The effect of organic Ca-antagonists (verapamil, prenylamine) on the calcium transport system in isolated mitochondria of rat cardiac muscle. *Pflügers Arch. ges. Physiol.* **359** (Suppl.), R26.

Frey, M., Keidel, J., and Fleckenstein, A. 1978/1980. Verhütung experimenteller Gefäss-Verkalkungen (Mönckeberg's Typ der Arteriosklerose) durch Calcium-Antagonisten, in *Calcium-Antagonismus,* Proceedings International Symposium on Calcium-Antagonism, December, 1978, in Frankfort, Edited by A. Fleckenstein and H. Roskamm, pp. 258–264, Springer-Verlag, Berlin–Heidelberg–New York, 1980.

Froment, R., Normand, J., and Amiel, L. 1973. Angine de potrine du type Prinzmetal: coronaries perméables, mais spasme de l'interventriculaire antérieure en cours de crise. *Arch. Mal. Coeur* **66**, 755–761.

Fühner, H., and Starling, E. H. 1913. Experiments on the pulmonary circulation. *J. Physiol.* (Lond.) **47**, 286–304.

REFERENCES

Fukuzaki, H., Okamoto, R., Yokoyama, M., and Tomomatsu, T. 1975. Clinical study on nifedipine, in *1st International Nifedipine (Adalat) Symposium*, Tokyo, November, 1973, Edited by K. Hashimoto, E. Kimura, and T. Kobayashi, pp. 205–213, University of Tokyo Press, 1975.

Garson, W. P., Gülin, R. C., and Phear, D. N. 1973. Clinical experience with perhexiline maleate in forty-six patients with angina. *Postgrad. Med. J.* **49** (April Suppl.), 90–92.

Garthoff, B. and Kazda, S. 1981. Calcium antagonist nifedipine normalizes high blood pressure and prevents mortality in salt-loaded DS substrain of Dahl rats. *Eur. J. Pharmacol.* **74**, 111–112.

Garvey, H. L. 1969. The mechanism of action of verapamil on the sinus and AV nodes. *Eur. J. Pharmacol.* **8**, 159–166.

Gazes, P. C., Holmes, C. R., Moseley, V., and Pratt-Thomas, H. R. 1961. Acute hemorrhage and necrosis of the intestines associated with digitalization. *Circulation* **23**, 358–364.

Gerlach, E., Deuticke, B., and Dreisbach, R. H. 1963. Der Nucleotid-Abbau im Herzmuskel bei Sauerstoffmangel und seine mögliche Bedeutung für die Coronardurchblutung. *Naturwissenschaften* **50**, 228–229.

Gerry, J. L., Achuff, S. C., Becker, L. C., Pond, M. S., and Greene, H. L. 1979. Predictability of the response to the ergonovine test. Value in the diagnosis of coronary spasm. *JAMA*, **242**, 2858–2861.

Gianelly, R., van der Groeben, J. O., Spivack, A., and Harrison, D. C. 1967. Effect of lidocaine on ventricular arrhythmias in patients with coronary heart disease. *N. Engl. J. Med.* **277**, 1215–1219.

Gitlin, N. 1973. A long-term assessment of perhexiline maleate in the management of patients with angina pectoris. *Postgrad. Med. J.* **49** (April Suppl.), 119–120.

Gitlin, N., and Nellen, M. 1973. Perhexiline maleate in the treatment of angina pectoris: a double-blind trial. *Postgrad. Med. J.* **49** (April Suppl.), 100–104.

Gleichmann, U., Seipel, L., and Loogen, F. 1973. Der Einfluβ von Antiarrhythmika auf die intrakardiale Erregungsleitung (His-Bündel Elektrographie) und Sinusknotenautomatie beim Menschen. *Dtsch. Med. Wschr.* **98**, 1487–1494.

Godfraind, T. 1976. Calcium exchange in vascular smooth muscle, action of noradrenaline and lanthanum. *J. Physiol.* (Lond.) **260**, 21–35.

Godfraind, T., and Kaba, A. 1969a. Actions phasique et tonique de l'adrénaline sur un muscle lisse vasculaire et leur inhibition par des agents pharmacologiques. *Arch. Int. Pharmacodyn.* **178**, 488–491.

Godfraind, T., and Kaba, A. 1969b. Blockade or reversal of the contraction induced by calcium and adrenaline in depolarized arterial smooth muscle. *Brit. J. Pharmacol.* **36**, 549–560.

Godfraind, T., and Sturbois, X. 1975. Inhibition by cinnarizine of heart ionic changes induced by isoprenaline, in *Recent Advances in Studies on Cardiac Structure and Metabolism*, **6**, 127–134, Edited by A. Fleckenstein and G. Rona, University Park Press, Baltimore–London–Tokyo.

Goldberg, S., Reichek, N., Wilson, J., Hirshfeld, J. W., Muller, J., and Kastor, J. A. 1979. Nifedipine in the treatment of Prinzmetal's (variant) angina. *Am. J. Cardiol.* **44**, 804–810.

Golenhofen, K. 1976. Theory of P and T systems for calcium activation in smooth muscle, in *Physiology of Smooth Muscle*, Edited by E. Bülbring and M. F. Shuba, pp. 197–202, Raven Press, New York.

Golenhofen, K., and Hannappel, J. 1978. A tonic component in the motility of the upper urinary tract (renal pelvis-ureter). *Experientia* **34**, 64.

Golenhofen, K., and Lammel, E. 1972. Selective suppression of some components of spontaneous activity in various types of smooth muscle by iproveratril (verapamil). *Pflügers Arch. ges. Physiol.* **331**, 233–243.

Golenhofen, K., and Wegner, H. 1975. Spike-free activation mechanism in smooth muscle of guinea-pig stomach. *Pflügers Arch. ges. Physiol.* **354**, 29–37.

Gollwitzer-Meier, K., and Krüger, E. 1935. Der Einfluss des Sympathikus auf die Coronargefässe. *Pflügers Arch. ges. Physiol.* **236**, 594–605.

Goodman, D., van der Steen, A. B. M., and van Dam, R. T. 1971. Endocardial and epicardial activation pathways of the canine right atrium. *Am. J. Physiol.* **220**, 1–11.

Goodwin, J. F., and Krikler, D. M. 1976. Arrhythmia as a cause of sudden death in hypertrophic cardiomyopathy. *Lancet,* **1976,** 937–940.

Gore, I., and Arons, W. 1949. Calcification of the myocardium. *Arch. Path.* **48,** 1–12.

Gorlin, R., and Lewis, B. M. 1954. Circulatory adjustments to hypoxia in dogs. *J. Appl. Physiol.* **7,** 180–185.

Gould, B. A., Stewart Mann, Kieso, H., Bala Subramanian, V., and Raftery, E. B. 1981. The 24-hour intra-arterial ambulatory profile of blood pressure reduction with verapamil, in *Calcium-Antagonism in Cardiovascular Therapy,* International Symposium, Florence, October, 1980, Edited by A. Zanchetti and D. M. Krikler, pp. 280–289, Excerpta Medica, Amsterdam–Oxford–Princeton, 1981.

Gracey, D. R., and Brandfonbrener, M. 1962. The effect of lanatoside C on coronary vascular resistance. *Clin. Res.* **10,** 172.

Grandjean, T., and Valenti, P. 1979. Effects of nifedipine on effort tolerance and left ventricular function during exercise in patients suffering from severe angina pectoris, in *International Nifedipine (Adalat) Panel Discussion,* Tokyo, September, 1978, Edited by P. Lichtlen, E. Kimura and N. Taira, pp. 118–126, Excerpta Medica, Amsterdam–Oxford–Princeton, 1979.

Greaser, M. L., and Gergely, J. 1971. Reconstitution of troponin activity from three protein components. *J. Biol. Chem.* **246,** 4226–4233.

Greenawalt, J. W., Rossi, C. S., and Lehninger, A. L. 1964. Effect of active accumulation of calcium and phosphate ions on the structure of rat liver mitochondria. *J. Cell. Biol.* **23,** 21–38.

Greene, H. L., and Weisfeldt, M. L. 1977. Determinants of hypoxic and posthypoxic contracture. *Am. J. Physiol.* **232,** H526–533.

Greenspan, A. M., and Morad, M. 1975. Electromechanical studies on the inotropic effects of acetylstrophanthidin in ventricular muscle. *J. Physiol.* (Lond.) **253,** 357–384.

Gremels, H., and Starling, E. H. 1926. On the influence of hydrogen ion concentration and of anoxaemia upon the heart volume. *J. Physiol.* (Lond.) **61,** 297–304.

Grossmann, A., and Furchgott, R. F. 1964. The effects of various drugs on calcium exchange in the isolated guinea-pig left auricle. *J. Pharmacol. Exp. Ther.* **145,** 162–172.

Grün, G., Bayer, M., and Fleckenstein, A. 1972. Der Einfluß des pH auf den Ca^{++}-abhängigen Tonus der Coronargefäss-Muskulatur. *Naunyn-Schmiedebergs Arch. exper. Path. Pharmakol.* **274** (Suppl.), R43.

Grün, G., Byon, Y. K., Kaufmann, R., and Fleckenstein, A. 1972. Differenzierung zwischen den β-adrenolytischen und Ca^{++}-antagonistischen Wirkungskomponenten von β-Rezeptoren-Blockern am Myokard und an glatter Muskulatur unter besonderer Berücksichtigung von Trasicor. *Ärztl. Forsch.* **26,** 369–378.

Grün, G., Byon, Y. K., Tritthart, H., and Fleckenstein, A. 1970. Inhibition of automaticity and contractility of isolated human uterine muscle by Ca-antagonistic compounds. *Pflügers Arch. ges. Physiol.* **319,** (Suppl.) R118.

Grün, G., and Fleckenstein, A. 1971. Ca-antagonism, a new principle of vasodilation. *Naunyn-Schiedebergs Arch. exper. Path. Pharmakol.* **270** (Suppl.), R48.

Grün, G., and Fleckenstein, A. 1972. Die elektromechanische Entkoppelung der glatten Gefässmuskulatur als Grundprinzip der Coronardilatation durch 4-(2′-Nitrophenyl)-2,6-dimethyl-1,4,dihydropyridin-3,5-dicarbonsäure-dimethylester (Bay a 1040, Nifedipin). *Arzneimittelforschung (Drug Res.)* **22,** 334–344.

Grün, G., Fleckenstein, A., and Byon, Y. K. 1971a. Hemmung der Motilität isolierter Uterus-Streifen aus gravidem und nicht-gravidem menschlichen Myometrium durch Ca^{++}-Antagonisten und Sympathomimetica. *Arzneimittelforschung (Drug Res.)* **21,** 1585–1590.

Grün, G., Fleckenstein, A., and Byon, Y. K. 1971b. Ca-antagonism, a new principle of vasodilation, in Proceedings 25th Congress Internat. Union Physiological Sciences, Munich 1971, Vol. 9, p. 221.

Grün, G., Fleckenstein, A., and Byon, Y. K. 1971/1972. Blockierung der Ca^{++}-Effekte auf Tonus und Autoregulation der glatten Gefässmuskulatur durch Ca^{++}-Antagonisten (Verapamil, D 600, Prenylamin, Bay a 1040 u.a.), in *Vascular Smooth Muscle*, Proceedings of a Satellite Symposium 25th Congress Internat. Union Physiological Sciences, Tübingen (Germany), July 20–24, Edited by E. Betz, pp. 69–70, Springer-Verlag, Berlin–Heidelberg–New York, 1972.

Grün, G., Fleckenstein, A., and Tritthart, H. 1969. Excitation-contraction uncoupling on the rat's uterus by some "musculotropic" smooth muscle relaxants. *Pflügers Arch. ges. Physiol.* **264**, 239.

Grün, G., Fleckenstein, A., and Weder, U. 1974. Changes in coronary smooth muscle tone produced by Ca, cardiac glycosides and Ca-antagonistic compounds (verapamil, D 600, prenylamine, etc.). *Pflügers Arch. ges. Physiol.* **347** (Suppl.), R1.

Grün, G., Weder, U., and Fleckenstein, A. 1972. The mutual antagonism between H^+ and Ca^{++} ions in the control of vascular tone and autoregulation. *Pflügers Arch. ges. Physiol.* **335** (Suppl.), R10.

Grundner-Culemann, A. 1952. Experimentelle und morphologische Untersuchungen über Veränderungen des Herzmuskels von Ratten bei Kaliummangelernährung. *Arch. Kreisl.-Forsch.* **18**, 185–210.

Grupp, I. L., Bunde, C. A., and Grupp, G. 1970. Effects of perhexiline maleate on exercise-induced tachycardia. *J. Clin. Pharmacol.* **10**, 312–315.

Guazzi, M., Magrini, F., Fiorentini, C., and Polese. A. 1971. Clinical electrocardiographic, and hemodynamic effects of long-term use of propranolol in Prinzmetal's variant angina pectoris. *Brit. Heart J.* **33**, 889–894.

Guideri, G., Barletta, M., and Lehr, D. 1975. Extraordinary potentiation of isoproterenol cardiotoxicity by corticoid pretreatment (See Lehr, D., Chau, R., Irene, S., 1975, in *Pathophysiology and Morphology of Myocardial Cell Alterations, Recent Advances in Studies on Cardiac Structure and Metabolism*, Edited by A. Fleckenstein, and G. Rona, Vol. **6**, pp. 95–109, University Park Press, Baltimore–London–Tokyo.).

Gunther, S., Green, L., Muller, J. E., Mudge, G. H., and Grossman, W. 1981. Prevention by nifedipine of abnormal coronary vasoconstriction in patients with coronary artery disease. *Circulation* **63**, 849–855.

Haas, H., and Busch, E. 1967. Vergleichende Untersuchungen der Wirkung von α-Isopropyl-α-(N-methyl-N-homoveratryl)-γ-aminopropyl-3,4-dimethoxy-phenyl-acetonitril, seiner Derivate sowie einiger anderer Coronardilatatoren und β-Receptor-affiner Substanzen. *Arzneimittelforschung (Drug Res.)* **17**, 257–271.

Haas, H., and Busch, E. 1968. Antiarrhythmische Wirkungen von Verapamil und seinen Derivaten im Vergleich zu Propranolol, Pronethalol, Chinidin, Procainamid und Ajmalin. *Arzneimittelforschung (Drug Res.)* **18**, 401–407.

Haas, H., and Härtfelder, G. 1962. α-Isopropyl-α-(N-methyl-homoveratryl)-γ-aminopropyl-3,4-dimethoxy-phenylacetonitril, eine Substanz mit coronargefässerweiternden Eigenschaften. *Arzneimittelforschung (Drug Res.)* **12**, 549–558.

Haas, H. G., Kern, R., and Einwächter, H. M. 1970. Electrical activity and metabolism in cardiac tissues. An experimental and theoretical study. *J. Memb. Biol.* **3**, 180–209.

Haastert, H. P. 1973. Besonderheiten der chronotropen, dromotropen und inotropen Wirkung von Ca^{++}-Antagonisten (Verapamil, D 600, Nifedipine) am Herzen in situ und an isolierten Vorhöfen sowie deren Beeinflussung durch Extra-Calcium und Isoproterenol. *Naunyn-Schmiedebergs Arch. exper. Path. Pharmakol.* **227** (Suppl.), R26.

Haastert, H. P., and Fleckenstein, A. 1975. Ca-dependence of supraventricular pacemaker activity and its responsiveness to Ca-antagonistic compounds (verapamil, D 600, nifedipine). *Naunyn-Schmiedebergs Arch. exper. Path. Pharmakol.* **287** (Suppl.), R39.

Haeusler, G. 1972. Differential effect of verapamil on excitation-contraction coupling in smooth muscle and on excitation-secretion coupling in adrenergic nerve terminals. *J. Pharmacol. Exp. Ther.* **180**, 672–682.

Haeusler, G., and Thorens, S. 1976. The pharmacology of vasoactive antihypertensives, in *Vascular Neuroeffector Mechanism*, Edited by J. A. Bevan, G. Burnstock, B. Johansson, R. A. Maxwell, and O.A. Nedergard, pp. 232–241 Karger, Basel.

Hagen, P. S. 1939. The effects of digilanid C in varying dosage upon the potassium and water content of rabbit heart muscle. *J. Pharmacol. Exp. Ther.* **67**, 50–55.

Hanforth, C. P. 1962. Isoproterenol-induced myocardial infarction in animals. *Arch. Pathol.* **73**, 161–165.

Hanna, C., and Schmid, J. R. 1970. Antiarrhythmic actions of coronary vasodilator agents papaverine, dioxyline, and verapamil. *Arch. Int. Pharmacol.* **185**, 228–233.

Harmjanz, D., Böttcher, D., and Schertlein, G. 1971. Correlations of electrocardiographic pattern, shape of ventricular septum, and isovolumetric relaxation time in irregular hypertrophic cardiomyopathy (obstructive cardiomyopathy). *Brit. Heart J.* **33**, 928–937.

Harmjanz, D., and Reale, E. 1981. Overcontraction and excess actin filaments—Basic elements of hypertrophic cardiomyopathy. *Brit. Heart J.*, **45**, 494–499.

Harrison, L. A., Blaschke, J., Phillips, R. S., Price, W. E., de Cotten, M. V., and Jacobson, E. D. 1969. Effects of ouabain on the splanchnic circulation. *J. Pharmacol. Exp. Ther.* **169**, 321–327.

Harrison, D. C., Braunwald, E., Glick, G., Mason, D. T., Chidsey, C. A., and Ross, J. 1964. Effects of beta adrenergic blockade on the circulation, with particular reference to observations in patients with hypertrophic subaortic stenosis. *Circulation* **29**, 84–98.

Hart, C. 1909. Die Herzmuskelverkalkung. *Frankfurt. Z. Path.* **3**, 706–715.

Hart, N. J., Silverman, M. E., and King, S. B. 1974. Variant angina pectoris caused by coronary artery spasm. *Am. J. Med.* **56**, 269–274.

Hartshorne, D. J. 1980. Biochemical basis for contraction of vascular smooth muscle. *Chest* **78** (Suppl. 1), 140–149.

Hartshorne, D. J., and Gorecka, A. 1980. Biochemistry of the contractile proteins of smooth muscle, in *Handbook of Physiology. The Cardiovascular System*. Edited by D. F. Bohr, A. P. Somlyo, and H. V. Sparks, Section 2, Vol. II, chapt. 4, pp. 93–120, American Physiological Society.

Hashimoto, Y., Holman, M. E., and Tille, J. 1966. Electrical properties of the smooth muscle membrane of the guinea-pig vas deferens. *J. Physiol.* (Lond.) **186**, 27–41.

Hashimoto, K., Iijima, T., Hashimoto, K., and Taira, N. 1972. The isolated and cross-circulated AV node preparation of the dog. *Tohoku J. Exp. Med.* **107**, 263–275.

Hashimoto, K., Ono, H., and O'Hara, N. 1978/1980. Blockade of renal autoregulatory vasoconstriction by Ca-antagonists, in *Calcium-Antagonismus*, Proceedings of an International Symposium 1978 in Frankfort. Edited by A. Fleckenstein and H. Roskamm, pp. 221–229, Springer-Verlag, Berlin–Heidelberg–New York, 1980.

Hashimoto, K., Taira, N., Chiba, S., Hashimoto, Jr., K., Endoh, M., Kokubun, M., Kokubun, H., Iijima, T., Kimura, T., Kubota, K., and Oguro, R. 1972. Cardiohemodynamic effects of Bay a 1040 in the dog. *Arzneimittelforschung (Drug Res.)* **22**, 15–21.

Hashimoto, K., Taira, N., Ono, H., Chiba, S., Hashimoto, Jr., K., Endoh, M., Kokubun, M., Kokubun, H., Iijima, T., Kimura, T., Kubota, K., and Oguro, K. 1975. Nifedipine, basis of its pharmacological effect, in *1st International Nifedipine (Adalat) Symposium*, Tokyo, November, 1973, edited by K. Hashimoto, E. Kimura, and T. Kobayashi, pp. 11–22, University of Tokyo Press, 1975.

Hashimoto, K., Takeda, K., Katano, Y., Nakagawa, Y., Tsukada, T., Hashimoto, T., Shimamoto, N., Sakai, K., Otorii, T., and Imai, S. 1979. Effects of niludipine (Bay a 7168) on the cardiovascular system. With a note on its calcium-antagonistic effects. *Arzneimittelforschung (Drug Res.)* **29**, 1368–1373.

Hass, G. M., Trucheart, R. E., Taylor, C. B., and Stumpe, M. 1958. An experimental histologic study of hypervitaminosis D. *Am. J. Path.* **34**, 395–431.

Hasselbach, W., and Makinose, F. 1961. Die Ca^{++}-Pumpe der Erschlaffungsgrana des Muskels und ihre Abhängigkeit von der ATP-Spaltung. *Biochem. Z.* **333**, 518–528.

Hasselbach, W., and Weber, H.H. 1965. Die intrazelluläre Regulation der Muskelaktivität. *Naturwissenschaften* **52**, 121–128.

Hauswirth, O., and Singh, B.N. 1979. Ionic mechanisms in heart muscle in relation to the genesis and the pharmacological control of cardiac arrhythmias. *Pharmacol. Rev.* **30**, 5–63.

Hayase, S., Hirakawa, S., Hosokawa, S., Mori, N., Kanyama, S., and Iwasa, M. 1972. Hemodynamic and therapeutic effect of Bay a 1040 on the patients with ischemic heart disease. *Arzneimittelforschung (Drug Res.)* **22**, 370–373.

Heggtveit, H. A., Herman, L., and Mishra, R. K. 1964. Cardiac necrosis and calcification in experimental magnesium deficiency. A light and electron microscopic study. *Am. J. Path.* **45**, 757–782.

Heilbrunn, L. V., and Wiercinski, F. J. 1947. The action of various cations on muscle protoplasm. *J. Cell. Comp. Physiol.* **29**, 15–32.

Heine, H. W., and Lossnitzer, K. 1976. Verhütung von Myocardnekrosen durch Propranolol beim Krankheitsmodell einer erblichen Kardiomyopathie. *Therapiewoche* **26**, 1744–1767.

Heistracher, P., and Pillat, B. 1962. Elektrophysiologische Untersuchungen über die Wirkung von Chinidin auf die Aconitinvergiftung von Herzmuskelfasern. *Naunyn-Schmiedebergs Arch. exper. Path. Pharmakol.* **244**, 48–62.

Hendrickx, H., and Casteels, R., 1974. Electrogenic sodium pump in arterial smooth muscle cells. *Pflügers Arch. ges. Physiol.* **346**, 299–306.

Heng, M. K., Singh, B. N., Roche, A. H. G., Norris, R. M., and Mercer, C. J. 1975. Effects of intravenous verapamil on cardiac arrhythmias and on the electrocardiogram. *Am. Heart J.* **90**, 487–498.

Henry, P. D. 1976. Protection of ischemic myocardium by nifedipine, in *3rd International Adalat Symposium: New Therapy of Ischemic Heart Disease,* Proceedings of a symposium held at Rio de Janeiro, October, 1975, Edited by A. D. Jatene and P. R. Lichtlen, pp. 55–65, Excerpta Medica, Amsterdam–Oxford, 1976.

Henry, P. D. 1980. Comparative pharmacology of calcium antagonists nifedipine, verapamil and diltiazem. *Am. J. Cardiol.* **46**, 1047–1058.

Henry, P. D., Clark, R. E., and Williamson, J. R. 1978/1980. Protection of the globally ischemic heart with calcium-antagonists: Improved recovery after cardiopulmonary bypass, in *Calcium-Antagonismus,* Proceedings of a Symposium held in Frankfurt, Germany, December, 1978, Edited by A. Fleckenstein and H. Roskamm, pp. 181–190, Springer-Verlag, Berlin–Heidelberg–New York, 1980.

Henry, P. D., Shuchleib, R., Borda, L. J., Roberts, R., Williamson, J. R., and Sobel, B. E. 1978. Effects of nifedipine on myocardial perfusion and ischemic injury in dogs. *Circ. Res.* **43**, 372–380.

Henry, P. D., Shuchleib, R., Clark, R. E., and Perez, J. E. 1979. Effect of nifedipine on myocardial ischemia: Analysis of collateral flow, pulsatile heat and regional muscle shortening. *Am. J. Cardiol.* **44**, 817–824.

Henry, P. D., Shuchleib, R., Davis, J., Weiss, E. S., and Sobel, B.E. 1977. Myocardial contracture and accumulation of mitochondrial calcium in ischemic rabbit heart. *Am. J. Physiol.* **233**, H677–H684.

Hering, H. E. 1904. Über die Wirksamkeit des Accelerans auf die von den Vorhöfen abgetrennten Kammern isolierter Säugetierherzen. *Centralbl. Physiol.* **17**, 1–3.

Hermsmeyer, K., and Sperelakis, N. 1970. Decrease in K^+ conductance and depolarization of frog cardiac muscle produced by Ba^{2+}. *Am. J. Physiol.* **219**, 1108–1114.

den Hertog, A., and van den Akker, 1979. The action of Prostaglandin E_2 on the smooth muscle cell of the guinea-pig taenia coli. *Eur. J. Pharmacol.* **58**, 225–234.

Herzenberg, H. 1929. Studien über die Wirkungsweise des bestrahlten Ergosterins (Vigantol) und die Beziehungen der von ihm gesetzten Veränderungen zur Arteriosklerose. *Beitr. Path. Anat.* **82**, 27–56.

Hess, T., and Stucki, P. 1975. Mesenterialinfarkt bei Digitalis-Intoxikation. *Schweiz. Med. Wschr.* **105**, 1237–1240.

Hester, R. K., Weiss, G. B., and Fry, W. J. 1979. Differing actions of nitroprusside and D 600 on tension and ^{45}Ca fluxes in canine renal arteries. *J. Pharmacol. Exper. Ther.* **208**, 155–160.

Heupler, F. A., and Proudfit, W. L. 1979. Nifedipine therapy for refractory coronary arterial spasm. *Am. J. Cardiol.* **44**, 798–803.

Heupler, F., Proudfit, W., Siegel, W., Shirey, E., Razavi, M., and Sones, F. M. 1975. The ergonovine maleate test for the diagnosis of coronary artery spasm. *Circulation* **52** (Suppl. II), II–11.

Hillemanns, H.-G., and Trolp, R. 1977. Tokolyse-Symposion. 7. Februar 1976 in Freiburg i. Br. *Geburtsh. Frauenheilk.* **37**, 191–193.

Hillis, L. D., and Braunwald, E. 1978. Coronary artery spasm. *N. Engl. J. Med.* **299**, 695–702.

Hinke, J. A. M. 1965. Calcium requirements for noradrenaline and high potassium ion contraction in arterial smooth muscle, in *Muscle*, Edited by W. M. Paul, E. E. Daniel, C. M. Kay, and G. Monckton, pp. 269–284, Pergamon Press, New York.

Hinke, J. A. M., Wilson, M. L., and Burnham, S. C. 1964. Calcium and the contractility of arterial smooth muscle. *Am. J. Physiol.* **206**, 211–217.

Hiraoka, M., Ikeda, K., and Sano, T. 1980. The mechanism of barium-induced automaticity in ventricular muscle fibers. *Adv. Myocardiol.*, Edited by M. Tajuddin, P.K. Das, M. Tarig, and N.S. Dhalla, **1**, 255–266, University Park Press, Baltimore.

Hiraoka, M., Yamagishi, S., and Sano, T. 1968. Role of calcium ions in the contraction of vascular smooth muscle. *Am. J. Physiol.* **214**, 1084–1089.

Hirshleifer, I. 1969. Perhexiline maleate in the treatment of angina pectoris. *Curr. Ther. Res.* **11**, 99–105.

Hiwatari, M. and Taira, N. 1979. Antihypertensive effect of niludipine (Bay a 7168) on conscious renal-hypertensive dogs. *Arzneimittelforschung (Drug Res.)* **29**, 1373–1376.

Hodgkin, A. L., and Huxley, A. F. 1947. Potassium leakage from an active nerve fibre. *J. Physiol.* (Lond.) **106**, 341–367.

Hodgkin, A. L., and Huxley, A. F. 1952a. Currents carried by sodium and potassium ions through the membrane of the giant axon of *Loligo*. *J. Physiol.* (Lond.) **116**, 449–472.

Hodgkin, A. L., and Huxley, A. F. 1952b. The component of membrane conductance in the giant axon of Loligo. *J. Physiol.* (Lond.) **116**, 473–496.

Hodgkin, A. L., and Huxley, A. F. 1952c. The dual effect of membrane potential on sodium conductance in the giant axon of Loligo. *J. Physiol.* (Lond.) **116**, 497–506.

Hodgkin, A. L., and Huxley, A. F. 1953. Movement of radioactive potassium and membrane current in a giant axon. *J. Physiol.* (Lond.) **121**, 403–414.

Hodgkin, A. L., Huxley, A. F. and Katz, B. 1952. Measurements of current-voltage relations in the membrane of the giant axon of Loligo. *J. Physiol.* (Lond.) **116**, 424–448.

Hoekenga, M. T., Bunde, C. A., Cawein, M. J., Kuzma, R. J., and Griffin, C. L. 1973. Clinical results with a new antianginal drug (perhexiline maleate). *Postgrad. Med. J.* **49** (April Suppl.), 95–99.

Hoeschen, R. J. 1977. Effects of verapamil on ($Na^+ + K^+$)- ATPase, Ca^{++}-ATPase, and adenylate cyclase activity in a membrane fraction from rat and guinea pig ventricular muscle. *Can. J. Physiol. Pharmacol.* **55**, 1098–1101.

Hoffman, B. F., and Cranefield, P. F. 1960. *Electrophysiology of the Heart,* McGraw-Hill, New York–Toronto–London.

Hoffman, B. F., and Suckling, E. E. 1952. Cellular potentials of intact mammalian hearts. *Am. J. Physiol.* **170**, 357–362.

Hofmann, H. 1968. Klinische Untersuchungen zur Wirkung von Iproveratril bei Koronarinsuffizienz und zur sympathikolytischen Beeinflussung der Myocardfunktion. *Z. inn. Med.,* **23**, 357–364.

Hofmann, W., Schleich, A., Schroeter, D., Weidinger, H., and Wiest, W. 1977. Der Einfluss von β-Sympathomimetika und sog. Ca^{++}-antagonistischer Hemmstoffe auf den menschlichen Herzmuskel in vitro. *Virchow's Arch. A. Path. Anat.* **373**, 85–95.

Hogan, P.M., and Davis, L.D. 1971. Electrophysiological characteristics of canine atrial plateau fibers. *Circ. Res.* **28**, 62–73.

Holland, W. C., and Briggs, A. H. 1959. Fibrillation and potassium influx. *Science* **129**, 212.

Holtz, P., Kroneberg, G., and Schümann, H. J. 1951. Über die sympathicomimetische Wirksamkeit von Herzmuskelextrakten. *Naunyn-Schmiedebergs Arch. exper. Path. Pharmakol.* **212**, 551–567.

Hopf, R., Kaltenbach, M., and Kober, G. 1981. Verapamil in the treatment of hypertrophic obstructive cardiomyopathy, in *Calcium Antagonism in Cardiovascular Therapy,* International Symposium, Florence, October, 1980, edited by A. Zanchetti and D.M. Krikler, pp. 353–362, Excerpta Medica, Amsterdam–Oxford–Princeton, 1981.

Horn, S., Fyhn, A., Haugaard, N. 1971. Mitochondrial calcium uptake in the perfused contracting rat heart and the influence of epinephrine on calcium exchange. *Biochim. Biophys. Acta.* **226**, 459–466.

Hornykiewicz, O., Hitzenberger, G., and Zellner, H. 1963. Experimentell-pharmakologische Untersuchungen über ein neues Spasmolytikum P 201-1. *Wien. klin. Wschr.* **75**, 189–197.

Horster, F. A. 1975a. Pharmacokinetics of nifedipine-^{14}C in man, in *1st International Nifedipine (Adalat) Symposium,* Tokyo, November, 1973, Edited by K. Hashimoto, E. Kimura, and T. Kobayashi, pp. 67–70, University of Tokyo Press, 1975.

Horster, F. A. 1975b. Pharmacokinetics of nifedipine-^{14}C in man, in *2nd International Nifedipine (Adalat) Symposium,* Amsterdam, October, 1974, Edited by W. Lochner, W. Braasch, and G. Kroneberg, pp. 124–127, Springer Verlag, Berlin–Heidelberg–New York, 1975.

Hosoda, S., Kasanuki, H., Miyata, K., Endoh, M., and Hirosawa, K. 1975. Results of a clinical investigation of nifedipine in angina pectoris with special reference to its therapeutic efficacy in attacks at rest, in *1st International Nifedipine (Adalat) Symposium,* Tokyo, November, 1973, Edited by K. Hashimoto, E. Kimura, and T. Kobayashi, pp. 185–189, University of Tokyo Press, 1975.

Hosoda, S., and Kimura, E. 1976. Efficacy of nifedipine in the variant form of angina pectoris, in *3rd International Nifedipine (Adalat) Symposium,* Rio de Janeiro, October, 1975, Edited by A. D. Jatene and P. Lichtlen, pp. 195–199, Excerpta Medica, Amsterdam–Oxford, 1976.

Hossack, K. F., and Bruce, R. A. 1981. Improved exercise performance in persons with stable angina pectoris receiving diltiazem. *Am. J. Cardiol.* **47**, 95–101.

Houki, S. 1973. Restoration effects of histamine on action potential in potassium-depolarized guinea-pig papillary muscle. *Arch. Int. Pharmacodyn.* **206**, 113–120.

Howse, H. D., Ferrans, V. J., and Hibbs, R. G. 1970. A comparative histochemical and electron microscopic study of the surface coatings of cardiac cells. *J. Mol. Cell. Cardiol.* **1**, 157–168.

Hudak, W. J., Lewis, R. E., and Kuhn, W. L. 1970. Cardiovascular pharmacology of perhexiline. *J. Pharmacol. Exp. Ther.* **173**, 371–382.

Hudak, W. J., Lewis, R. E., Lucas, R. W., and Kuhn, W. L. 1973. Review of the cardiovascular pharmacology of perhexiline. *Postgrad. Med. J.* **49** (April Suppl.), 16–25.

Hudgins, P. M., and Weiss, G. B. 1968. Differential effects of calcium removal upon vascular smooth muscle contraction induced by norepinephrine, histamine and potassium. *J. Pharmacol. Exp. Ther.* **159**, 91–97.

Hudgins, P. M., and Weiss, G. B. 1969. Characteristics of ^{45}Ca binding in vascular smooth muscle. *Am. J. Physiol.* **217**, 1310–1315.

Hüter, J., and Lammers, G. 1973. Beta-Adrenergika bei der Wehenhemmung. *Dtsch. Med. Wschr.* **98**, 2482–2483.

Husaini, M. H., Kvasnicka, J., Ryden, L., and Holmberg, S. 1973. Action of verapamil on sinus node, atrioventricular and intraventricular conduction. *Brit. Heart J.* **35**, 734–737.

Huxley, H. E. 1969. The mechanism of muscular contraction. *Science* **164**, 1356–1366.

Huxley, H. E., and Hanson, J. 1954. Changes in the cross striations of muscle during contraction and stretch and their structural interpretation. *Nature (Lond.)* **173**, 973–976.

Huxley, A. F., and Niedergerke, R. 1954. Structural changes in muscle during contraction. Interference microscopy in living muscle fibres. *Nature (Lond.)* **173**, 971–972.

Iijima, T., Motomura, S., Taira, N., and Hashimoto, K. 1974. Selective suppression of neural excitation by tetrodotoxin injected into the canine atrioventricular node artery. *J. Pharmacol. Exp. Ther.* **189**, 638–645.

Iijima, T., and Taira, N. 1976. Modification by manganese ions and verapamil of the responses of the atrioventricular node to norepinephrine. *Eur. J. Pharmacol.* **37**, 55–62.

Ikeda, M. 1979. Double-blind studies on diltiazem in essential hypertensive patients receiving thiazide therapy, in *New Drug Therapy with a Calcium Antagonist, Diltiazem*, Hakone Symposium 1978, Edited by R.J. Bing, pp. 243–253, Excerpta Medica, Amsterdam–Princeton, 1979.

Imai, S. 1975. Effects of nifedipine on heart and coronary circulation. In: 1st Internat. Nifedipine (Adalat) Symposium, Tokyo, Nov. 1973, Edited by K. Hashimoto, E. Kimura and T. Kobayashi, pp. 23–30, University of Tokyo Press.

Imanishi, S. 1971. Calcium-sensitive discharges in canine Purkinje fibers. *Jpn. J. Physiol.* **21**, 443–463.

Inesi, G., Ebashi, S., and Watanabe, S. 1964. Preparation of vesicular relaxing factor from bovine heart tissue. *Am. J. Physiol.* **207**, 1339–1344.

Inui, J., and Imamura, H. 1976. Restoration by histamine of the calcium-dependent electrical and mechanical response in the guinea-pig papillary muscle partially depolarized by potassium. *Naunyn-Schmiedebergs Arch. exper. Path. Pharmakol.* **294**, 261–269.

Ishizawa, M., and Miyazaki, E. 1977. Calcium and the contractile response to prostaglandin in the smooth muscle of guinea-pig stomach. *Experientia* **33**, 376–377.

Isselhard, W. 1960. Das Verhalten des Energiestoffwechsels im Warmblüterherz bei künstlichem Herzstillstand. *Pflügers Arch. ges. Physiol.* **271**, 347–360.

Itoh, Y., Tawara, I., and Itoh, T. 1975. Clinical experience with nifedipine, in *1st International Nifedipine (Adalat) Symposium*, Tokyo, November, 1973, Edited by K. Hashimoto, E. Kimura, and T. Kobayashi, pp. 251–259, University of Tokyo Press, 1975.

Iversen, L. L. 1965. The uptake of catecholamines at high perfusion concentrations in the rat isolated heart: A novel catecholamine uptake process. *Brit. J. Pharmacol.* **25**, 18–33.

Iwai, M. 1924. Untersuchungen über den Einfluss der Wasserstoffionen-Konzentration auf die Coronargefässe und die Herztätigkeit. *Pflügers Arch. ges. Physiol.* **202**, 356–364.

Iwata, A. 1974. Process of lens opacification and membrane function: A review. *Ophthalmol. Res.* **6**, 138–154.

Janke, J., Döring, H.J., Hein, B., and Fleckenstein, A. 1972. pH-Dependency of catecholamine-induced radiocalcium uptake into the ventricular myocardium of rats in situ. *Pflügers Arch. ges. Physiol.* **335** (Suppl.), R18.

Janke, J., and Fleckenstein, A. 1978. Kardiotoxische Nebenwirkungen der Tokolyse mit β-adrenergen Sympathomimetika und deren Verhütung mit Hilfe des Ca^{++}-Antagonisten Verapamil, in *Fenoterol (Partusisten®) bei der Behandlung in der Geburtshilfe und Perinatologie*, Proceedings of a Symposium, Wiesbaden, October, 1977, Edited by H. Jung and E. Friedrich, pp. 98–107, Georg Thieme, Stuttgart, 1978.

Janke, J., Fleckenstein, A., and Frey, M. 1978. Schutzeffekt von Ca^{++}-Antagonisten bei der Isoproterenol-induzierten hypertrophischen Cardiomyopathie der Ratte. *Verh. Dtsch. Ges. Kreisl.-Forsch.* **44,** 206–207.

Janke, J., Fleckenstein, A., Hein, B., Leder, O., and Sigel, H. 1975. Prevention of myocardial Ca overload and necrotization by Mg and K salts or acidosis, in *Recent Advances in Studies on Cardiac Structure and Metabolism,* Vol. 6, Edited by A. Fleckenstein and G. Rona, pp. 33–42. University Park Press, Baltimore–London–Tokyo.

Janke, J., Fleckenstein, A., and Jaedicke, W. 1970. Hemmung der Isoproterenol-induzierten $^{45}Ca^{++}$-Netto-Aufnahme in das Ventrikelmyokard durch Ca^{++}-antagonistische Hemmstoffe der elektromechanischen Koppelung (Isoptin = Verapamil, Iproveratril und Substanz D 600). *Pflügers Arch. ges. Physiol.* **316,** R10.

Janke, J., Fleckenstein, A., Marmier, P., and Koenig, L. 1966. Steigerung der absoluten ATP-Umsetzungsrate in der isolierten Skelettmuskulatur unter dem Einfluss von 2,4-Dinitrophenol. Turnover-Studien mit P^{32}-markiertem Orthophosphat und H_2O^{18}. *Pflügers Arch. ges. Physiol.* **287,** 9–28.

Janke, J., Hein, B., Pachinger, O., Leder, O., and Fleckenstein, A. 1971/1972. Hemmung arteriosklerotischer Gefässprozesse durch prophylaktische Behandlung mit $MgCl_2$, KCl und organischen Ca^{++}-Antagonisten (quantitative Studien mit Ca^{45} bei Ratten), in *Vascular Smooth Muscle,* Proceedings of a Satellite Symposium 25th Congress International Union Physiological Sciences, Tübingen (Germany), July 20–24, Edited by E. Betz, pp. 71–72, Springer-Verlag, Berlin–Heidelberg–New York, 1972.

Janke, J., Marmier, P., and Fleckenstein, A. 1965. Die Bestimmung der absoluten Umsetzungsraten von ATP, Kreatinphosphat und Orthophosphat in der ruhenden Skelettmuskulatur mit Hilfe von H_2O^{18} als Tracer. *Pflügers Arch. ges. Physiol.* **282,** 119–134.

Jarisch, A., and Wastl, H. 1926. Observations on the effect of anoxaemia upon heart and circulation. *J. Physiol.* (Lond.) **61,** 583–592.

Jasmin, G., and Bajusz, E. 1975. Prevention of myocardial degeneration in hamsters with hereditary cardiomyopathy. *Recent Advances in Studies on Cardiac Structure and Metabolism,* Vol. 6, Edited by A. Fleckenstein and G. Rona, pp. 219–229, University Park Press, Baltimore–London–Tokyo.

Jasmin, G., and Proschek, L. 1978/1980. Prevention of myocardial degeneration in hamsters with hereditary cardiomyopathy, in *Calcium-Antagonismus,* Proceedings of an International Symposium 1978 in Frankfort. Edited by A. Fleckenstein and H. Roskamm, pp. 144–150, Springer-Verlag, Berlin–Heidelberg–New York, 1980.

Jasmin, G., and Solymoss, B. 1975. Prevention of hereditary cardiomyopathy in the hamster by verapamil and other agents (38771). *Proc. Soc. Exp. Biol. Med.* **149,** 193–198.

Jedziniak, J. A., Kinoshita, J. H., Yates, E., Hocker, L., and Benedek, G. B. 1972. Calcium-induced aggregation of bovine lens alpha-crystallin. *Invest. Ophthalmol.* **11,** 905–915.

Jedziniak, J. A., Nicoli, D. F., Yates, E. M., and Benedek, G. B. 1976. On the calcium concentration of cataractous and normal human lenses and protein fractions of cataractous lenses. *Exp. Eye Res.* **23,** 325–332.

Jetley, M., and Weston, A. H. 1980. Some effects of sodium nitroprusside, methoxyverapamil (D 600) and nifedipine on rat portal vein. *Brit. J. Pharmacol.* **68,** 311–319.

Johnson, P. C. 1964. Review of previous studies and current theories of autoregulation. *Circ. Res.* **14** and **15** (Suppl. I), pp. 2–9.

Johnson, A. D., and Detwiler, J. H. 1977. Coronary spasm, variant angina, and recurrent myocardial infarctions. *Circulation* **55,** 947–950.

Johnson, S. M., Mauritson, D. R., Willerson, J. T., Cary, J. R., and Hillis, D. 1981. Verapamil administration in variant angina pectoris—Efficacy shown by ECG monitoring. *JAMA* **245,** 1849–1851.

Josephson, I., Renaud, J., Vogel, S., McLean, M., and Sperelakis, N. 1976. Mechanism of the histamine-induced positive inotropic action in cardiac muscle. *Eur. J. Pharmacol.* **35,** 393–398.

Jouve, A., Guiran, J. B., Viallet, H., Gras, A., Blanc, M., Arnoux, M., Rouvier, M., and Brunel, J. C. 1969. Les modifications électrocardiographiques au cours des crises d'angor spontané. *Arch. Mal. Coeur* **62**, 331–351.

Just, H., v. Mengden, H. J., Kersting, F., and Krebs, R. 1979. Influence of nifedipine on left ventricular dimensions and contractility in patients with coronary artery disease. Comparison with nitrates, in *International Nifedipine (Adalat) Panel Discussion,* Tokyo, September, 1978, Edited by P. Lichtlen, E. Kimura, and N. Taira, pp. 47–56, Excerpta Medica, Amsterdam–Oxford–Princeton, 1979.

Kaltenbach, M. 1970. Medikamentöse Therapie der Angina pectoris. Prüfung verschiedener Medikamente mit Hilfe von Arbeitsversuchen. *Arzneimittelforschung (Drug Res.),* **20**, 1304–1310.

Kaltenbach, M. 1975. Assessment of antianginal substances by means of ST depression in the exercise EKG, in *1st International Nifedipine (Adalat) Symposium,* Tokyo, November, 1973, Edited by K. Hashimoto, E. Kimura, and T. Kobayashi, pp. 126–135, University of Tokyo Press, 1975.

Kaltenbach, M., Becker, H.J., Loos, A., and Kober, G. 1972. Veränderungen der Hämodynamik des linken Herzens unter der Wirkung von Nifedipine (BAY a 1040) im Vergleich mit Nitroglycerin. *Arzneimittelforschung. (Drug Res.)* **22**, 362–365.

Kaltenbach, M., Hopf, R., and Keller, M. 1976. Calciumantagonistische Therapie bei hypertrophobstruktiver Kardiomyopathie. *Dtsch. Med. Wschr.* **101**, 1284–1287.

Kaltenbach, M., Hopf, R., Kober, G., Bussmann, W.-D., Keller, M., and Petersen, Y. 1979. Treatment of hypertrophic obstructive cardiomyopathy with verapamil. *Brit. Heart J.* **42**, 35–42.

Kaltenbach, M., Schulz, W., and Kober, G. 1979. Effects of nifedipine after intravenous and intracoronary administration. *Am. J. Cardiol.* **44**, 832–838.

Kaltenbach, M., and Zimmermann, D. 1968. Zur Wirkung von Iproveratril auf die Angina pectoris und die adrenergischen β-Rezeptoren des Menschen. *Dtsch. Med. Wschr.* **93**, 25–28.

Kambara, H., Fujimoto, K., Wakabayashi, A., and Kawai, C. 1981. Primary pulmonary hypertension: Beneficial therapy with diltiazem. *Am. Heart J.* **101**, 230–231.

Kammermeier, H. 1964. Verhalten von Adenin-Nukleotiden und Kreatinphosphat im Herzmuskel bei funktioneller Erholung nach länger dauernder Asphyxie. *Verh. Dtsch. Ges. Kreisl.-Forsch.* **30**, 206–211.

Kanazawa, T. 1975. The effect of nitrophenyl-dimethyl-dihydro-pyridine-derivative (Bay a 1040) on intercoronary collateral circulation, in *1st International Nifedipine (Adalat) Symposium,* Tokyo, November, 1973, Edited by K. Hashimoto, E. Kimura, and T. Kobayashi, pp. 53–62, University of Tokyo Press, 1975.

Karaki, H., Hester, R. K., and Weiss, G. B. 1980. Cellular basis of nitroprusside-induced relaxation of graded responses to norepinephrine and potassium in canine renal arteries. *Arch. Int. Pharmacodyn. Thér.* **245**, 198–210.

Karaki, H., and Weiss, G. B. 1979. Alterations in high and low affinity binding of ^{45}Ca in rabbit aortic smooth muscle by norepinephrine and potassium after exposure to lanthanum and low temperature. *J. Pharmacol. Exp. Ther.* **211**, 86–92.

Karaki, H., and Weiss, G. B. 1980. Effects of stimulatory agents on mobilization of high and low affinity site ^{45}Ca in rabbit aortic smooth muscle. *J. Pharmacol. Exp. Ther.* **213**, 450–455.

Kass, R. S., and Tsien, R. W. 1975. Multiple effects of calcium antagonists on plateau currents in cardiac Purkinje fibers. *J. Gen. Physiol.* **66**, 169–192.

Katase, A. 1913. Experimentelle Verkalkung am gesunden Tiere. *Beitr. path. Anat.* **57**, 516–550.

Katsuki, S., Arnold, W. P., and Murad, F. 1977. Effects of sodium nitroprusside, nitroglycerin and sodium azide on levels of cyclic nucleotides and mechanical activity of various tissues. *J. Cycl. Nucl. Res.* **3**, 239–247.

Katz, A. M. 1970. Contractile proteins of the heart. *Physiol. Rev.* **50**, 63–158.

Katz, A. M., and Repke, D. I. 1967. Quantitative aspects of dog cardiac microsomal calcium binding and calcium uptake. *Circ. Res.* **21**, 153–162.

Katz, A. M., Repke, D. I., Tada, M., and Corkedale, S. 1974. Propranolol-induced inhibition of cardiac microsomal calcium uptake, calcium-binding, and epinephrine-stimulated adenylate cyclase. *Cardiovasc. Res.* **8**, 541–549.

Kaufmann, R., and Fleckenstein, A. 1965. Ca⁺⁺-kompetitive elektro-mechanische Entkoppelung durch Ni⁺⁺- und Co⁺⁺-Ionen am Warmblütermyokard. *Pflügers Arch. ges. Physiol.* **282**, 290–297.

Kaufmann, R., Fleckenstein, A., and Antoni, H. 1963. Ursachen und Auslösungsbedingungen von Myocard-Kontraktionen ohne reguläres Aktionspotential. *Pflügers Arch. ges. Physiol.* **278**, 435–446.

Kaufmann, R., and Theophile, U. 1967. Automatie-fördernde Dehnungseffekte an Purkinje-Fäden, Papillarmuskeln und Vorhofstrabekeln von Rhesus-Affen. *Pflügers Arch. ges. Physiol.* **297**, 174–189.

Kaumann, A. J., and Aramendia, P. 1968. Prevention of ventricular fibrillation induced by coronary ligation. *J. Pharmacol. Exp. Ther.* **164**, 326–340.

Kavaler, F., and Morad, M. 1966. Paradoxial effects of epinephrine on excitation-contraction coupling in cardiac muscle. *Circ. Res.* **18**, 492–501.

Kazda, S., and Hoffmeister, F., 1979. Effect of some cerebral vasodilators on the postischemic impaired cerebral reperfusion in cats. *Naunyn-Schmiedebergs Arch. exper. Path. Pharmakol.* **307** (Suppl.), R43.

Kazda, S., Hoffmeister, F., Garthoff, B., and Towart, R. 1979. Prevention of the postischaemic impaired reperfusion of the brain by nimodipine (Bay e 9736). *Acta Neurol. Scand.* **60**, (Suppl. 72) 302–303.

Keatinge, W. R. 1968a. Ionic requirements for arterial action potential. *J. Physiol. (Lond.)* **194**, 169–182.

Keatinge, W. R. 1968b. Reversal of electrical response of arterial smooth muscle to noradrenaline in calcium-deficient solution. *J. Physiol. (Lond.)* **198**, 20–22P.

Kehar, N. D., Hooker, D. R. 1935. Evidences of an altered tissue state in ventricular fibrillation. *Am. J. Physiol.* **112**, 301–306.

Kerber, E. R., and Abboud, F. M. 1975. Effect of alterations of arterial blood pressure and heart rate on segmental dyskinesis during acute myocardial ischemia and following coronary reperfusion. *Circ. Res.* **36**, 145–155.

Kerin, N., and MacLeod, C. A. 1974. Coronary artery spasm associated with variant angina pectoris. *Brit. Heart J.* **36**, 224–227.

Kerridge, D. F., Mazurkie, S. J., and Verel, D. 1961. A clinical trial of prenylamine lactate. A long-lasting coronary dilator drug. *Canad. Med. Assoc. J.* **85**, 1352–1353.

Kimura, E., and Kishida, H. 1981. Treatment of variant angina with drugs: A survey of 11 cardiology institutes in Japan. *Circulation* **63**, 844–848.

King, M. J., Zir, L. M., Kaltman, A. J., and Fox, A. C. 1973. Variant angina associated with angiographically demonstrated coronary artery spasm and REM sleep. *Am. J. Med. Sci.* **265**, 419–422.

Kinney, E. L., Moskowitz, R. M., and Zelis, R. 1981. The pharmacokinetics and pharmacology of oral diltiazem in normal volunteers. *J. Clin. Pharmacol.* **21**, 337–342.

Kirchberger, M. A., Tada, M., and Katz, A. M. 1974. Adenosine 3′,5′-monophosphate-dependent protein kinase-catalyzed phosphorylation reaction and its relationship to calcium transport in cardiac sarcoplasmic reticulum. *J. Biol. Chem.* **249**, 6166–6173.

Kirchberger, M. A., Tada, M., Repke, D. I., and Katz, A. M. 1972. Cyclic adenosine 3′,5′-monophosphate-dependent protein kinase stimulation of calcium uptake by canine cardiac microsomes. *J. Mol. Cell. Cardiol.* **4**, 673–680.

Kirk, D., and Duthie, H. L. 1977. Electrical activity of human taenia coli in vitro. *Gastroenterology* **72**, 1080.

Kitamura, K., Kuriyama, H., and Suzuki, H. 1976. Effect of noradrenaline on the membrane properties and on the contraction of the rabbit main pulmonary artery. *J. Physiol. (Lond.)* **263**, 164–165 P.

Kitazawa, T. 1976. Physiological significance of Ca uptake by mitochondria in the heart in comparison with that by cardiac sarcoplasmic reticulum. *J. Biochem. (Tokyo)* **80**, 1129–1147.

Kiyomoto, A. 1978/1979. Antihypertensive effects of diltiazem in rats, in *New Drug Therapy with a Calcium Antagonist, Diltiazem*, Hakone Symposium, 1978, Edited by R. J. Bing, pp. 112–125, Excerpta Medica, Amsterdam–Princeton, 1979.

Klein, W. 1982. Ergebnisse einer Vergleichsuntersuchung zwischen Nifedipin und Diltiazem bei essentieller arterieller Hypertonie, in: *Calciumantagonisten zur Behandlung der Angina pectoris, Hypertonie und Arrhythmie, International Symposium on Diltiazem*, Copenhagen, June 25–27, 1981, Edited by F. Bender and K. Greeff, pp. 210–218, Excerpta Medica, Amsterdam–Oxford–Princeton, 1982.

Klein, I., and Levey, G. S. 1971. Activation of myocardial adenyl cyclase by histamine in guinea-pig, cat and human heart. *J. Clin. Invest.* **50**, 1012–1015.

Kobayashi, M. 1965. Effects of Na and Ca on the generation and conduction of excitation in the ureter. *Am. J. Physiol.* **208**, 715–719.

Kobayashi, T., Ito, Y., and Tawara, I. 1972. Clinical experience with a new coronary-active substance (Bay a 1040). *Arzneimittelforschung (Drug Res.)* **22**, 380–389.

Kober, G., Berlad, T., Hopf, R., and Kaltenbach, M. 1981. Die Wirkung von Diltiazem und Nifedipin auf die ST-Senkung und Herzfrequenz im Belastungs-EKG bei Patienten mit koronarer Herzerkrankung. *Z. Kardiol.* **70**, 59–65.

Kochsiek, K., Bretschneider, H. J., and Scheler, F. 1960. Vergleichende experimentelle Untersuchungen über die Coronargefäss-erweiternde Wirkung von Phenyl-propyl-diphenyl-propyl-amin. *Arzneimittelforschung (Drug Res.)* **10**, 576–583.

Kochsiek, K., and Neubaur, J. 1972. Die Wirkung von 4-(2'-Nitrophenyl)-2,6-dimethyl-1,4-dihydropyridin-3,5-dicarbonsäuredimethylester auf den Myokardstoffwechsel, die Hämodynamic, die Blutgase und den allgemeinen Stoffwechsel des Menschen. *Arzneimittelforschung (Drug Res.)* **22**, 353–358.

Kodama, I., Hirata, Y., Toyama, J., and Yamada, K. 1980. Effects of niludipine (Bay-a-7168) on transmembrane action potentials of rabbit sinus node cells and atrial muscle fibers. *J. Cardiovasc. Pharmacol.* **2**, 145–153.

Kölle, E. U., Ochs, H. R., Thomann, P., and Neurath, G. 1982. Pharmacokinetics of diltiazem in man. *Naunyn-Schmiedeberg's Arch. exper. Path. Pharmacol.*, Suppl. to Vol **319**, R 83.

Koepcke, E., and Seidenschnur, G. 1973. Zur klinischen Anwendung von wehenhemmenden Substanzen. *Z. ärztl. Fortbild.* **67**, 533–539.

Kohlhardt, M., Bauer, B., Krause, H., and Fleckenstein, A. 1971. Selective inhibition of Ca conductivity of mammalian cardiac fibre membranes by Ca-antagonistic compounds (verapamil, D 600), in Proceedings 25th Congress Internat. Union Physiological Sciences, Munich 1971, Vol. 9, p. 313.

Kohlhardt, M., Bauer, B., Krause, H., and Fleckenstein, A. 1972. Differentiation of the transmembrane Na and Ca channel in mammalian cardiac fibres by the use of specific inhibitors. *Pflügers Arch. ges. Physiol.* **335**, 309–322.

Kohlhardt, M., Bauer, B., Krause, H., and Fleckenstein, A. 1973. Selective inhibition of the transmembrane Ca conductivity of mammalian myocardial fibres by Ni, Co and Mn ions. *Pflügers Arch. ges. Physiol.* **338**, 115–123.

Kohlhardt, M., Figulla, H. R., and Tripathi, O. 1976. The slow membrane channel as the predominant mediator of the excitation process of the sinoatrial pacemaker cell. *Basic Res. Cardiol.* **71**, 17–26.

Kohlhardt, M., and Fleckenstein, A. 1977. Inhibition of the slow inward current by nifedipine in mammalian ventricular myocardium. *Naunyn-Schmiedebergs Arch. exper. Path. Pharmakol.* **298**, 267–272.

Kohlhardt, M., Haap, K., and Figulla, H. R. 1976. Influence of low extracellular pH upon the Ca inward current and isometric contractile force in mammalian ventricular myocardium. *Pflügers Arch. ges. Physiol.* **366**, 31–38.

Kohlhardt, M., Haastert, H. P., and Krause, H. 1973. Evidence of non-specificity of the Ca channel in mammalian myocardial fibre membranes. Substitution of Ca by Sr, Ba or Mg as charge carriers. *Pflügers Arch. ges. Physiol.* **342**, 125–136.

Kohlhardt, M., and Kaufmann, R. 1970. Differential influence of Ca^{++}-ions on the automaticity of the sinus node and of Ba^{++}-induced ventricular pacemakers. *Pflügers Arch. ges. Physiol.* **316**, R9.

Koidl, B., and Tritthart, H. A. 1980. Excitation and contraction is not uncoupled in single cultured pacemaker fibres by D 600. *Naunyn-Schmiedebergs Arch. exper. Path. Pharmakol.* **311** (Suppl.), R35.

Koidl, B., and Tritthart, H. A. 1982. D-600 blocks spontaneous discharge, excitability and contraction of cultured embryonic chick heart cells. *J. Mol. Cell. Cardiol.* **14**, 251–257.

Kolm, R., and Pick, E. 1920. Über die Bedeutung des Kaliums für die Selbststeuerung des Herzens. *Pflügers Arch. ges. Physiol.* **185**, 235–247.

van der Kooi, M. W., Durrer, D., van Dam, R. T., and van der Tweel, L. H. 1956. Electrical activity in sinus node and atrioventricular node. *Am. Heart J.* **51**, 684–700.

Kornberg, A., and Endicott, K. M. 1946. Potassium deficiency in the rat. *Am. J. Physiol.* **145**, 291–298.

von Kossa, J. 1901. Über die im Organismus künstlich erzeugbaren Verkalkungen. *Beitr. path. Anat.* **29**, 163–202.

Kotowski, H., Antoni, H., Vahlenkamp, H., and Fleckenstein, A. 1961. Effekte von ATP und Kalium auf die Schrittmacher-Automatie bei Frosch- und Warmblüterherzen. *Pflügers Arch. ges. Physiol.* **273**, 45–61.

Krayer, O. 1931. Versuche am insuffizienten Herzen. *Naunyn-Schmiedebergs Arch. exper. Path. Pharmakol.* **162**, 1–28.

Krayer, O., and Schütz, E. 1932. Mechanische Leistung und einphasisches Elektrogramm am Herz-Lungen-Präparat des Hundes. *Z. Biol.* **92**, 453–461.

Kreitner, D. 1975. Evidence for the existence of a rapid sodium channel in the membrane of rabbit sinoatrial cells. *J. Mol. Cell. Cardiol.* **7**, 655–662.

Krikler, D. 1974a. A fresh look at cardiac arrhythmias. *Lancet 1974*, pp. 851, 913, 974, and 1034.

Krikler, D. 1974b. Verapamil in cardiology. *Eur. J. Cardiol.* **2**, 3–10.

Krikler, D., Spurrell, R. A. J. 1972. Asystole after verapamil. *Brit. Med. J.* **2**, 405.

Krikler, D., and Spurrell, R. A. J. 1974. Verapamil in the treatment of paroxysmal supraventricular tachycardia. *Postgrad. Med. J.* **50**, 447–453.

Kroeger, E. A., Marshall, J. M., and Bianchi, C. P. 1975. Effect of isoproterenol and D 600 on calcium movements in rat myometrium. *J. Pharmacol. Exp. Ther.* **193**, 309–316.

Kroeger, E. A., and Stephens, N. L. 1975. Effect of tetraethylammonium on tonic airway smooth muscle: initiation of phasic electrical activity. *Am. J. Physiol.* **228**, 633–636.

Kroneberg, G. 1975. Pharmacology of nifedipine (Adalat[R]), in *1st International Nifedipine (Adalat) Symposium,* Tokyo, November, 1973, Edited by K. Hashimoto, E. Kimura, and T. Kobayashi, pp. 3–10, University of Tokyo Press, 1975.

Kruta, V. 1934. Sur l'activité automatique de l'oreillette gauche isolée du coeur de mammifère. *Arch. Int. Physiol.* **40**, 140–157.

Kübler, W., and Shinebourne, E. A. 1970/1971. Calcium and the mitochondria, in *Calcium and the Heart,* Edited by P. Harris and L. Opie, pp. 93–123. Academic Press, London–New York, 1971.

Kukovetz, W. R., Holzmann, S., Wurm, A., and Pöch, G. 1979. Evidence of cyclic GMP-mediated relaxant effects of nitro-compounds in coronary smooth muscle. *Naunyn-Schmiedebergs Arch. exper. Path. Pharmakol.* **310**, 129–138.

Kukovetz, W. R., and Pöch, G. 1970. Cardiostimulatory effects of cyclic 3′,5′-adenosine monophosphate and its acylated derivatives. *Naunyn-Schmiedebergs Arch. exper. Path. Pharmakol.* **266**, 236–254.

Kukovetz, W. R., and Pöch, G. 1972. The positive inotropic effect of cyclic AMP, in *Advances in Cyclic Nucleotide Research,* Edited by P. Greengard and G. A. Robison, **1,** 261–290, Raven Press, New York.

Kukovetz, W. R., Pöch, G., and Wurm, A. 1973. Effect of catecholamines, histamine and oxyfedrine on isotonic contraction and cyclic AMP in the guinea-pig heart. *Naunyn-Schmiedebergs Arch. exper. Path. Pharmakol.* **278,** 403–424.

Kumagai, H., Ebashi, S., and Takeda, F. 1955. Essential relaxing factor in muscle other than myokinase and phosphokinase. *Nature* (Lond.) **176,** 166.

Kurita, A. 1975. Effect of nifedipine on the left ventricular haemodynamics in angina pectoris, in *1st International Nifedipine (Adalat) Symposium,* Tokyo, November, 1973, Edited by K. Hashimoto, E. Kimura and T. Kobayashi, pp. 121–125, University of Tokyo Press, 1975.

Kuriyama, H., Ohshima, K., and Sakamoto, Y. 1971. The membrane properties of the smooth muscle of the guinea-pig portal vein in isotonic and hypertonic solutions. *J. Physiol.* (Lond.) **217,** 179–199.

Kuriyama, H., Osa, T., and Toida, N. 1967a. Electrophysiological study of the intestinal smooth muscle of the guinea-pig. *J. Physiol.* (Lond.) **191,** 239–255.

Kuriyama, H., Osa, T., and Toida, N. 1967b. Membrane properties of the smooth muscle of guinea-pig ureter. *J. Physiol.* (Lond.) **191,** 225–238.

Kurland, G., Williams, J., and Lewiston, N.J. 1979. Fatal myocardial toxicity during continuous infusion intravenous isoproterenol therapy of asthma. *J. Allerg. Clinic. Immun.* **63,** 407–411.

Lakatta, E. G., Nayler, W. G., and Poole-Wilson, P. A. 1979. Calcium overload and mechanical function in post-hypoxic myocardium. Biphasic effect of pH during hypoxia. *Eur. J. Cardiol.* **10,** 77–87.

Lamprecht, W., Michal, G., and Nägle, S. 1961. Der Stoffwechsel des hypoxischen und anoxischen Herzmuskels. *Klin. Wschr.* **39,** 358–364.

Landmark, K., and Amlie, J. P. 1976. A study of the verapamil-induced changes in conductivity and refractoriness and monophasic action potentials of the dog heart in situ. *Eur. J. Cardiol.* **4,** 419–427.

Langer, G. A. 1964. Kinetic studies of calcium distribution in ventricular muscle of the dog. *Circ. Res.* **15,** 393–405.

Langer, G. A. 1973. Excitation-contraction coupling. *Ann. Rev. Physiol.* **35,** 55–86.

Langer, G. A., and Brady, A. J. 1963. Calcium influx in the mammalian ventricular myocardium. *J. Gen. Physiol.* **46,** 703–719.

Langer, G. A., Frank, J. S., Nudd, L. M., and Seraydarian, K. 1976. Sialic acid: Effect of removal on calcium exchangeability of cultured heart cells. *Science,* **193,** 1013–1015.

Langer, G. A., Serena, S. D., and Nudd, L. M. 1975. Localization of contractile dependent Ca: comparison of Mn and verapamil in cardiac and skeletal muscle. *Am. J. Physiol.* **229,** 1003–1007.

Laplane, D., Bousser, M. G., Bouche, P., and Touboul, P. J. 1976/1978. Peripheral neuropathies caused by perhexiline maleate, in *Perhexiline Maleate,* Proceedings of a Symposium, Strasbourg, September 18, 1976, pp. 89–96, Excerpta Medica, Amsterdam–Princeton, 1978.

Ledda, F., Fantozzi, R., Mugelli, A., Moroni, F., and Mannaioni, P. F. 1974. The antagonism of the positive inotropic effects of histamine and noradrenaline by H_1 and H_2-receptor blocking agents. *Agents Actions* **4,** 193–194.

Leder, O., and Fleckenstein, A. 1963/1965 Verteilung und Stapelung von C^{14}-Noradrenalin im Körper der Ratte, in *Radioisopes in Endocrinology,* 1st Ann. Meeting Dtsch. Ges. Nuclearmedizin, Freiburg 17.–19. Oct. 1963, Edited by G. Hoffmann and W. Keiderling, pp. 423–429. F. K. Schattauer-Verlag Stuttgart, 1965.

Lederballe Pedersen, O. 1978. Does verapamil have a clinically significant antihypertensive effect? *Eur. J. Clin. Pharmacol.* **13,** 21–24.

Lederballe Pedersen, O., Christensen, N. J., and Rämsch, K. D. 1980. Comparison of acute effects of nifedipine in normotensive and hypertensive men. *J. Cardiovasc. Pharmacol.* **2,** 357–366.

Lederballe Pedersen, O., and Mikkelsen, E. 1978. Acute and chronic effects of nifedipine in arterial hypertension. *Eur. J. Clin. Pharmacol.* **14**, 375–381.

Lee, K. S., and Klaus, W. 1971. The subcellular basis for the mechanism of inotropic action of cardiac glycosides. *Pharmacol. Rev.* **23**, 193–261.

Lee, K. S., Ladinsky, H., Choi, S. J., and Kasuya, Y. 1966. Studies on the in vitro interaction of electrical stimulation and Ca^{++} movement in sarcoplasmic reticulum. *J. Gen. Physiol.* **49**, 689–715.

de Leeuw, P. W., Smout, A. J. P. M., Willemse, P. J., and Birkenhäger, W. H. 1981. Effects of verapamil in hypertensive patients, in *Calcium Antagonism in Cardiovascular Therapy*, International Symposium, Florence, October, 1980, Edited by A. Zanchetti and D. M. Krikler, pp. 233–237, Excerpta Medica, Amsterdam, 1981.

Legato, M. J., Spiro, D., and Langer, G. A. 1968. Ultrastructural alterations produced in mammalian myocardium by variation in perfusate ionic composition. *J. Cell Biol.* **37**, 1–12.

Lehninger, A. L. 1970. Mitochondria and calcium ion transport. *Biochem. J.* **119**, 129–138.

Lehr, D., Chau, R., and Irene, S. 1975. Possible role of magnesium loss in the pathogenesis of myocardial fiber necrosis. In *Recent Advances in Studies on Cardiac Structure and Metabolism*, Vol. 6, Edited by A. Fleckenstein, and G. Rona, pp. 95–109, University Park Press, Baltimore–London–Tokyo, 1975.

Lehr, D., Chau, R., and Kaplan, J. 1972. Prevention of experimental myocardial necrosis by electrolyte solutions, in *Recent Advances in Studies on Cardiac Structure and Metabolism*, Vol. 1, Edited by E. Bajusz and G. Rona, pp. 684–698, University Park Press, Baltimore–London–Tokyo.

Lenfant, J., Mironneau, J., Gargouil, Y. M., and Galand, G. 1968. Analyse de l'activité électrique spontanée du centre de l'automatisme cardiaque de lapin par les inhibiteurs de perméabilités membranaires. *C. R. Acad. Sci. Ser. D.* **266**, 901–904.

Leonetti, G., Pasotti, C., Ferrari, G. P., and Zanchetti, A. 1981. Double-blind comparison of the antihypertensive effects of verapamil and propranolol, in *Calcium Antagonism in Cardiovascular Therapy*, International Symposium, Florence, October, 1980, Edited by A. Zanchetti and D. M. Krikler, pp. 260–267, Excerpta Medica, Amsterdam–Oxford–Princeton, 1981.

Lewis, G. R. J., Morley, K. D., Lewis, B. M., and Bones, P. J. 1978. The treatment of hypertension with verapamil. *N. Zeal. Med. J.* **87**, 351–354.

Lewis, G. R. J., Stewart, D. J., Lewis, B. M., Bones, P. J., Morley, K. D., and Janus, E. D. 1981. The antihypertensive effect of oral verapamil—acute and long-term administrations and its effects on the high-density lipoprotein values in plasma, in *Calcium Antagonism in Cardiovascular Therapy*, International Symposium, Florence, October, 1980, Edited by A. Zanchetti and D. M. Krikler, pp. 270–277, Excerpta Medica, Amsterdam–Oxford–Princeton, 1981.

Lichstein, E., Chudda, K. D., and Gupta, P. K. 1973. Atrioventricular block with lidocaine therapy. *Am. J. Cardiol.* **31**, 277–281.

Lichtlen, P. R. 1975. The influence of nifedipine on left ventricular and coronary dynamics at rest and during exercise in patients with coronary artery disease, in *1st International Nifedipine (Adalat) Symposium*, Tokyo, November, 1973, Edited by K. Hashimoto, E. Kimura, and T. Kobayashi, pp. 114–120, University of Tokyo Press, 1975.

Lichtlen, P. R., Engel, H. -J., Wolf, R., and Hundeshagen, H. 1979. Effect of nifedipine on regional myocardial blood flow at rest and in pacing-induced ischemia. *Circulation* **60** (Suppl. II), 249.

Lichtlen, P. R., Engel, H. -J., Wolf, R., and Pretschner, P. 1979. Regional myocardial blood flow in patients with coronary artery disease after nifedipine, in *International Nifedipine (Adalat) Panel Discussion*, Tokyo, September, 1978, Edited by P. R. Lichtlen, E. Kimura and N. Taira, pp. 69–85, Excerpta Medica, Amsterdam–Oxford–Princeton, 1979.

Lindner, E. 1960. Phenyl-propyl-diphenyl-propyl-amin, eine neue Substanz mit coronargefäss-erweiternder Wirkung. *Arzneimittelforschung (Drug Res)* **10**, 569–573.

Lindner, E. 1971. The pharmacology of prenylamine (Synadrin; Segontin). *Clin. Trials J.* **8** (Suppl. 1), 6–17.

Lindner, E., and Kaiser, J. 1975. Die antiarrhythmische Wirkung des Segontin (N-(3'-phenyl-propyl-(2'))-1,1-diphenyl-propyl-(3)amin = prenylamin). Herz/Kreislauf 7, 88–94.

Livesley, B., Catley, P. F., Campbell, R. C., and Oram, S. 1973. Double-blind evaluation of verapamil, propranolol, and isosorbide dinitrate against a placebo in the treatment of angina pectoris. Brit. Med. J. 1973/I, 375–378.

Locke, T. S., and Rosenheim, O. 1907. Contributions to the physiology of the isolated heart. The consumption of dextrose by mammalian cardiac muscle. J. Physiol. (Lond.) 36, 205–220.

Loewi, O. 1917. Über den Zusammenhang zwischen Digitalis-und Calciumwirkung. Naunyn-Schmiedebergs Arch. exper. Path. Pharmakol. 82, 131–158.

Loewy, A., and Mayer, E. 1926. Über experimentell erzeugte akute Herzerweiterungen beim Menschen. Klin. Wschr. 5, 1213–1216.

Loos, A., and Kaltenbach, M. 1972. Die Wirkung von Nifedipine (Bay a 1040) auf das Belastungs-Elektrokardiogramm von Angina-pectoris-Kranken. Arzneimittelforschung (Drug Res.) 22, 358–362.

Lossnitzer, K. 1975. Genetic induction of a cardiomyopathy, in Handbook of Experimental Pharmacology. New Series, Vol. XVI/3. Edited by J. Schmier and O. Eichler, pp. 309–344, Springer-Verlag, Berlin–Heidelberg–New York.

Lossnitzer, K., Janke, J., Hein, B., Stauch, M., and Fleckenstein, A. 1975. Disturbed myocardial calcium metabolism: A possible pathogenetic factor in the hereditary cardiomyopathy of the Syrian hamster, in Recent Advances in Studies on Cardiac Structure and Metabolism Vol. 6, Edited by A. Fleckenstein and G. Rona, pp. 207–217, University Park Press, Baltimore–London–Tokyo.

Lossnitzer, K., Konrad, A., and Jakob, M. 1978/1980. Kardioprotektion durch Kalzium-Antagonisten bei erblich kardiomyopathischen Hamstern, in Calcium-Antagonismus, Proceedings of an International Symposium, 1978, in Frankfort. Edited by A. Fleckenstein and H. Roskamm, pp. 151–171 Springer-Verlag, Berlin–Heidelberg–New York, 1980.

Lossnitzer, K., and Mohr, W. 1973. Prevention of myocardial necroses in myopathic hamsters. Int. Res. Commun. Syst. (73–10) 1–5–9.

Lossnitzer, K., Mohr, W., Konrad, A., and Guggenmoos, R. 1978. Hereditary cardiomyopathy in the Syrian golden hamster: Influence of verapamil as calcium antagonist, in Cardiomyopathy and Myocardial Biopsy, Edited by M. Kaltenbach, F. Loogen, and E. G. J. Olsen, pp. 27–37, Springer-Verlag, Berlin–Heidelberg–New York.

Lossnitzer, K., Mohr, W., and Stauch, M. 1975. Die Verhütung von Myokardnekrosen bei der erblichen Kardiomyopathie des syrischen Goldhamsters. Verh. Dtsch. Ges. Inn. Med. 81, 335–338.

Lossnitzer, K., Steinhardt, B., Grewe, N., and Stauch, M. 1975. Characteristic electrolyte changes in the hereditary myopathy and cardiomyopathy of the Syrian golden hamster (strain BIO 8262). Basic Res. Cardiol. 70, 508–520.

Lowenhaupt, E., Schulman, M. P., and Greenberg, D. M. 1950. Basic histologic lesions of magnesium deficiency in the rat, Arch. Path., 49, 427–433.

Lown, B., Salzberg, H., Enselberg, C. D., and Weston, R. E. 1951. Interrelation between potassium metabolism and digitalis toxicity in heart failure, Proc. Soc. Exp. Biol. (N.Y.) 76, 797–801.

Lu, H. H., and Brooks, C.Mc C. 1969. Role of calcium in cardiac pacemaker cell action. Bull. N. Y. Acad. Med. 45, 100.

Luebs, E. D., Cohen, A., Zaleski, E., and Bing, R. J. 1966. Effect of nitroglycerin, intensain, isoptin and papaverine on coronary blood flow in man. Am. J. Cardiol. 17, 535–541.

Lüthy, E. 1978. Feldstudie über Fendilin (Sensit[R]). Schweiz. Rundsch. Med. (Praxis) 67, 71–77.

Luisada, A. A., and Neumann, M. 1963. Double-blind study with "coronary drugs" in old patients. Acta. Sec. Convent. Med. Internat. Hung., Cardiologia, Budapest, 1963, 94–98.

Lupi, G. A., Urthaler, F., and James, T. N. 1979. Effects of verapamil on automaticity and conduction with particular reference to tachyphylaxis. Eur. J. Cardiol. 9, 345–368.

Lydtin, H., Lohmöller, G., Lohmöller, R., and Walter, I. 1975. Hemodynamic studies on nifedipine in man, in *1st International Nifedipine (Adalat) Symposium*, Tokyo, November, 1973, Edited by K. Hashimoto, E. Kimura, and T. Kobayashi, pp. 97–106, University of Tokyo Press, 1975.

Lynch, P., Dargie, H., Krikler, S., and Krikler, D. 1980. Objective assessment of antianginal treatment: a double-blind evaluation of propranolol, nifedipine, and their combination. *Brit. Med. J.* **281**, 184–187.

Mabuchi, G., Kishida, H., and Suzuki, K. 1975. Clinical effect of nifedipine on variant form of angina pectoris, in *1st International Nifedipine (Adalat) Symposium*, Tokyo, November, 1973, Edited by K. Hashimoto, E. Kimura, and T. Kobayashi, pp. 177–184, University of Tokyo Press, 1975.

MacGregor, G. A., Markandu, N. D., Bayliss, J., Brown, M., and Roulston, J. E. 1981. Circumstantial evidence that an abnormality of calcium transport may be important in essential hypertension. *Clin. Sci.* **60**, 6P–7P.

McAllister, R. E., Noble, D., and Tsien, R. W. 1975. Reconstruction of the electrical activity of cardiac Purkinje fibres. *J. Physiol. (Lond.)* **251**, 1–59.

McDonald, T. F., Nawrath, H., and Trautwein, W. 1975. Membrane currents and tension in cat ventricular muscle treated with cardiac glycosides. *Circ. Res.* **37**, 674–682.

McDonald, T. F., Pelzer, D., and Trautwein, W. 1980. On the mechanism of slow calcium channel block in heart. *Pflügers Arch. ges. Physiol.* **385**, 175–179.

McDonald, T. F., and Trautwein, W. 1978a. The potassium current underlying delayed rectification in cat ventricular muscle. *J. Physiol. (Lond.)* **274**, 217–246.

McDonald, T. F., and Trautwein, W. 1978b. Membrane currents in cat myocardium: Separation of inward and outward components. *J. Physiol. (Lond.)* **274**, 193–216.

McElroy, W. T., Gerdes, A. J., and Brown, E. B. 1958. Effects of CO_2, bicarbonate and pH on the performance of isolated perfused guinea pig hearts. *Am. J. Physiol.* **195**, 412–416.

McMurtry, I. F., Davidson, A. B., Reeves, J. T., and Grover, R. F. 1976. Inhibition of hypoxic pulmonary vasoconstriction by calcium antagonists in isolated rat lungs. *Circ. Res.* **38**, 99–104.

McNeill, J. H., and Muschek, L. D. 1972. Histamine effects on cardiac contractibility, phosphorylase and adenyl cyclase. *J. Mol. Cell. Cardiol.* **4**, 611–624.

McNeill, J. H., and Verma, S. C. 1974. Blockade by burimamide of the effects of histamine and histamine analogs on cardiac contractibility, phosphorylase activation and cyclic adenosine monophosphate. *J. Pharmacol. Exp. Ther.* **188**, 180–188.

Maeda, K., Takasugi, T., Tsukano, Y., Tanaka, Y., and Shiota, K. 1981. Clinical study on the hypotensive effect of diltiazem hydrochloride. *Internat. J. Clin. Pharmacol. Ther. Toxicol.* **19**, 47–55.

Maggi, G. C. 1975. Clinical observations on the efficacy of nifedipine versus timed disintegration capsules of pentaerythrityl tetranitrate, in *1st International Nifedipine (Adalat) Symposium*, Tokyo, November, 1973, Edited by K. Hashimoto, E. Kimura, and T. Kobayashi, pp. 160–162, University of Tokyo Press, 1975.

Maggi, G. C., and Piscitello, F. 1975. Clinical observations on the efficacy of Adalat compared with a pentaerythrityl tetranitrate preparation, in *2nd International Nifedipine (Adalat) Symposium*, Amsterdam, October, 1974, Edited by W. Lochner, W. Braasch, and G. Kroneberg, pp. 281–284, Springer-Verlag, Berlin–Heidelberg–New York, 1975.

Magometschnigg, D., and Pichler, M. 1981. Effective and safe treatment of hypertensive crisis with nifedipine. *Am. J. Cardiol.* **47**, 469.

Mandel, W. J., Hayakawa, H., Allen, H., Danzig, R., and Kermaier, A. I. 1972. Assessment of sinus node function in patients with the sick sinus syndrome. *Circulation* **46**, 761–769.

Mandrek, K., and Golenhofen, K. 1977. Activation of gastro-intestinal smooth muscle induced by the calcium ionophore A23187. *Pflügers Arch. ges. Physiol.* **371**, 119–124.

Maroko, P. R. 1971. Factors influencing infarct size following experimental coronary artery occlusions. *Circulation* **43**, 67–86.

Maroko, P. R., Braunwald, E., and Covell, J. W. 1970. The effect of digitalis on the severity of myocardial ischemic injury following experimental coronary occlusion. *Pharmacologist* **12**, 212.

Marsh, B. B. 1951. A factor modifying muscle fibre synaeresis. *Nature* (Lond.) **167**, 1065–1066.

Marshall, J. M. 1962. Regulation of activity in uterine smooth muscle. *Physiol. Rev.* **42** (Suppl. No 5), 213–227.

Mascher, D. 1970. Electrical and mechanical responses from ventricular muscle fibres after inactivation of the sodium carrying system. *Pflügers Arch. ges. Physiol.* **317**, 359–372.

Mascher, D., and Peper, K. 1969. Two components of inward current in myocardial muscle fibres. *Pflügers Arch. ges. Physiol.* **307**, 190–203.

Maseri, A., L'Abbate, A., Baroldi, G., Chierchia, S., Marzilli, M., Ballestra, A. M., Severi, S., Parodi, O., Biagini, A., Distante, A., and Pesola, A. 1978. Coronary vasospasm as a possible cause of myocardial infarction. *N. Engl. J. Med.* **299**, 1271–1277.

Maseri, A., L'Abbate, A., Chierchia, S., Parodi, O., Severi, S., Biagini, A., Distante, A., Marzilli, M., and Ballestra, A. M. 1979. Significance of spasm in the pathogenesis of ischemic heart disease. *Am. J. Cardiol.* **44**, 788–792.

Maseri, A., Parodi, O., Severi, S., and Pesola, A. 1976. Transient transmural reduction of myocardial blood flow, demonstrated by thallium-201 scintigraphy, as a cause of variant angina. *Circulation* **54**, 280–288.

Maseri, A., Severi, S., De Nes, M., L'Abbate, A., Chierchia, S., Marzilli, M., Ballestra, A. M., Parodi, O., Biagini, A., and Distante, A. 1978. "Variant" angina: One aspect of a continuous spectrum of vasospastic myocardial ischemia. Pathogenetic mechanisms, estimated incidence and clinical and coronary arteriographic findings in 138 patients. *Am. J. Cardiol.* **42**, 1019–1035.

Massingham, R. 1973. A study of compounds which inhibit vascular smooth muscle contraction. *Eur. J. Pharmacol.* **22**, 75–82.

Mathey, D., Montz, R., Hanrath, P., Kuck, K. H., and Bleifeld, W. 1980. Nicht-invasive Methode zur Erkennung des Koronar-Arterien-Spasmus. [201]Thallium Szintigraphie des Myocards nach Ergotamin. *Dtsch. Med. Wschr.* **105**, 509–515.

Mathison, G. C. 1910. The action of asphyxia upon the spinal animal. *J. Physiol. (Lond.)* **41**, 416–449.

Matsuda, K. 1973. see Watanabe, Y. 1980.

Matsuda, K., Hoshi, T., and Kameyama, S. 1959. Effects of aconitine on the cardiac membrane potential of the dog. *Jpn. J. Physiol.* **9**, 419–429.

Matsuo, S., Cho, Y. W., and Aviado, D. M. 1970. Pharmacology of a new antianginal drug: Perhexiline. II. Heart rate and transmembrane potential of cardiac tissue. *Chest* **58**, 581–585.

Matthews, E. K., and Sakamoto, Y. 1975. Electrical characteristics of pancreatic islet cells. *J. Physiol. (Lond.)* **246**, 421–437.

Mayer, C. J., van Breemen, C., and Casteels, R. 1972. The action of lanthanum and D 600 on the calcium exchange in the smooth muscle cells of the guinea-pig taenia coli. *Pflügers Arch. ges. Physiol.* **337**, 333–350.

Mayer, C. J., Ruppin, H., Riemer, J., Kölling, K., Domschke, W., Wünsch, E., and Demling, L. 1977. "Minute-rhythm"-type contractions induced by motilin and acetylcholine in the circular muscle layer of rabbit duodenum. *Pflügers Arch. ges. Physiol.* **368**, R24.

Meinertz, T., Nawrath, H., and Scholz, H. 1973a. Dibutyryl cyclic AMP and adrenaline increase contractile force and [45]Ca uptake in mammalian cardiac muscle. *Naunyn-Schmiedebergs Arch. exper. Path. Pharmakol.* **277**, 107–112.

Meinertz, T., Nawrath, H., and Scholz, H. 1973b. Stimulatory effects of DB-c-AMP and adrenaline on myocardial contraction and [45]Ca exchange. Experiments at reduced calcium concentration and low frequencies of stimulation. *Naunyn-Schmiedebergs Arch. exper. Path. Pharmakol.* **279**, 327–338.

Meller, J., Pichard, A., and Dack, S. 1976. Coronary arterial spasm in Prinzmetal's angina: a proved hypothesis. *Am. J. Cardiol.* **37**, 938–940.

Melville, K. I., Shister, H. E., and Huq, S. 1964. Iproveratril: Experimental data on coronary dilatation and antiarrhythmic action. *Canad. Med. Assoc. J.* **90**, 761–770.

Menges, H., Brandenburg, R. O., and Brown, A. L. 1961. The clinical, hemodynamic, and pathologic diagnosis of muscular subvalvular aortic stenosis. *Circulation* **24**, 1126–1136.

Mercker, H. 1943. Zur Frage der Herzinsuffizienz im Sauerstoffmangel. *Luftfahrtmedizin* **8**, 217–223.

Merker, H. -J., and Guenther, T. 1970. Das elektronenmikroskopische Bild der Rattenaorta bei Mg-Mangel. *Z. klin. Chem. klin. Biochem.*, **8**, 374–378.

Midtbø, K., and Hals, O. 1980. Verapamil in the treatment of hypertension. *Curr. Ther. Res.* **27**, 830–838.

Millard, R. W. 1980. Changes in cardiac mechanics and coronary blood flow of regionally ischemic porcine myocardium induced by diltiazem. *Chest* **78** (July Suppl.), 193–199.

Mines, G. R. 1913. On functional analysis by the action of electrolytes. *J. Physiol. (Lond.)* **46**, 188–235.

Mizuno, K., Tanaka, K., Honda, Y., and Kimura, E. 1979. Suppression of repeatedly occurring ventricular fibrillation with nifedipine in variant form of angina pectoris, in *International Nifedipine (Adalat) Panel Discussion,* Tokyo, September 20, 1978, Edited by P. R. Lichtlen, E. Kimura, and N. Taira, pp. 61–67, Excerpta Medica, Amsterdam–Oxford–Princeton, 1979.

Mohr, W., Hersener, J., and Lossnitzer, K. 1973. Der Nachweis von Calcium-Phosphat in der Herzmuskulatur mittels Röntgenmikroanalyse. *Virchow's Arch. A. Path. Anat.* **358**, 259–264.

Mommaerts, W. F. H. M. 1969. Energetics of muscular contraction. *Physiol. Rev.* **49**, 427–508.

Moore, L. A., Hallman, E. T., and Sholl, L. B. 1938. Cardiovascular and other lesions in calves fed diets low in magnesium. *Arch. Path.* **26**, 820–838.

Morad, M. 1969. Contracture and catecholamines in mammalian myocardium. *Science* **166**, 505–506.

Morad, M., and Rolett, E. 1972. Relaxing effects of catecholamines on mammalian heart. *J. Physiol. (Lond.)* **224**, 537–558.

Morgenstern, M., Noack, E., and Köhler, E. 1972. The effects of isoprenaline and tyramine on the [45]calcium uptake, the total calcium content and the contraction force of isolated guinea-pig atria in dependence on different extracellular hydrogen ion concentrations. *Naunyn-Schmiedebergs Arch. exper. Path. Pharmakol.* **274**, 125–137.

Morledge, J. 1973. Effects of perhexiline maleate in angina pectoris: a double-blind clinical evaluation with ECG-treadmill exercise testing. *Postgrad. Med. J.* **49** (April Suppl.), 64–67.

Morledge, J., Adams, D., Hudak, W. J., Powell, R. L., and Kuzma, R. J. 1976/1978. Effects of perhexiline maleate versus placebo in angina pectoris. Symptomatic and treadmill exercise double-blind evaluation. in *Perhexiline Maleate,* Proceedings of a Symposium, Strasbourg, September 18, 1976, pp. 178–190, Excerpta Medica, Amsterdam–Princeton, 1978.

Mosler, K. H. 1972. Potenzierung der Uterushemmung beta-adrenerger Sympathomimetika durch neue kardioprotektive Substanzen, in *Methoden der pharmakologischen Geburtserleichterung und Uterus-Relaxation,* Bad Aachen, June 1970, Edited by H. Jung, pp. 170–177, Georg Thieme, Stuttgart, 1972.

Muggia, F. M. 1967. Hemorrhagic necrosis of the intestine: its occurrence with digitalis intoxication. *Am. J. Med. Sci.* **253**, 263.

Muiesan, G., Agabiti-Rosei, E., Alicandri, C., Beschi, M., Castellano, M., Corea, L., Fariello, R., Romanelli, G., Pasini, C., and Platto, L. 1981. Influence of verapamil in catecholamines, renin and aldosterone in essential hypertensive patients, in *Calcium Antagonism in Cardiovascular Therapy,* International Symposium, Florence, October 1980, Edited by A. Zanchetti and D. M. Krikler, pp. 238–249, Excerpta Medica, Amsterdam–Oxford–Princeton, 1981.

Muller, J. E., and Gunther, S. 1978. Nifedipine therapy for Prinzmetal's angina. *Circulation* **57**, 137–139.

Muscholl, E. 1959. Die Konzentration von Noradrenalin und Adrenalin in den einzelnen Abschnitten des Herzens. *Naunyn-Schmiedebergs Arch. exper. Path. Pharmakol.* **237**, 350–364.

Muscholl, E. 1966. Indirectly acting sympathomimetic amines. *Pharmacol. Rev.* **18,** 551–559.

Nägle, S., Hockerts, Th., and Bögelmann, G. 1964. Die Beeinflussung des Kreatin-phosphokinase-Gleichgewichts durch pH-Abfall im Herzmuskel unter ischämischen Bedingungen. *Klin. Wschr.* **42,** 780–784.

Nagao, T., Matlib, M. A., Franklin, D., Millard, R. W., and Schwartz, A. 1980. Effects of diltiazem, a calcium antagonist, on regional myocardial function and mitochondria after brief coronary occlusion. *J. Mol. Cell. Cardiol.* **12,** 29–43.

Nahas, G. G. 1957. Effect of hydrocortisone on acidotic failure of the isolated heart. *Circ. Res.* **5,** 489–492.

Nakajima, H., Hoshiyama, M., Yamashita, K., and Kiyomoto, A. 1975. Effect of diltiazem on electrical and mechanical activity of isolated cardiac ventricular muscle of guinea pig. *Jpn. J. Pharmacol.* **25,** 383–392.

Nakamura, M., Etoh, Y., Hamanaka, N., Kuroiwa, A., Tomoike, H., and Ishihara, Y. 1975. Effects of selective coronary hypotension and nitroglycerin or Bay a 1040 on the distribution of ^{86}Rb clearance in the canine heart, in *1st International Nifedipine (Adalat) Symposium,* Tokyo, November, 1973, Edited by K. Hashimoto, E. Kimura, and T. Kobayashi, pp. 63–66, University of Tokyo Press, 1975.

Nakamura, M., Kikuchi, Y., Senda, Y., Yamada, A., and Koiwaya, Y. 1980. Myocardial blood flow following experimental coronary occlusion. Effects of diltiazem. *Chest* **78** (July Suppl.), 205–209.

Nakao, K., Oka, M., Chen, C., Bajusz, E., and Angrist, A. 1970. Studies of the spontaneous myocardiopathy in the BIO 14.6 strain of hamster. *Path. Microbiol. (Basel)* **35,** 118–124.

Nakayama, K., Byon, Y. K., and Fleckenstein-Grün, G. 1976. Identical responses of isolated smooth muscle preparations from brain (A. basilaris) and coronary arteries upon electric field stimulation. *Pflügers Arch. ges. Physiol.* **362** (Suppl.), R2.

Nakayama, K., Fleckenstein, A., Byon, Y. K., and Fleckenstein-Grün, G. 1978. Fundamental physiology of coronary smooth musculature from extramural stem arteries of pigs and rabbits (electric excitability, tension development, influence of Ca, Mg, H and K ions). *Eur. J. Cardiol.* **8,** 319–335.

Narimatsu, A., and Taira, N. 1976. Effects on atrio-ventricular conduction of calcium-antagonistic coronary vasodilators, local anaesthetics and quinidine injected into the posterior and the anterior septal artery of the atrio-ventricular node preparation of the dog. *Naunyn-Schmiedebergs Arch. exper. Path. Pharmakol.* **294,** 169–177.

Nauth, H. F., Hort, W., and Hubinger, R. 1979. Localization of sclerotic lesions in the coronary arteries and their epicardial branches. *Z. Kardiol.* **68,** 832–838.

Nawrath, H., Ten Eick, R. E., McDonald, T. F., and Trautwein, W. 1977. On the mechanism underlying the action of D 600 on slow inward current and tension in mammalian myocardium. *Circ. Res.* **40,** 408–414.

Nayler, W. G. 1967. Some factors involved in the maintenance and regulation of cardiac contractility. *Circ. Res.* **21** (Suppl. III), 213–221.

Nayler, W. G., and Berry, D. 1975. Effect of drugs on the cyclic 3′,5′-monophosphate-dependent protein kinase-induced stimulation of calcium uptake by cardiac microsomal fractions. *J. Mol. Cell. Cardiol.* **7,** 387–395.

Nayler, W. G., Fassold, E., and Yepez, C. 1978. The pharmacological protection of mitochondrial function in hypoxic heart muscle: effect of verapamil, propranolol and methylprednisolone. *Cardiovasc. Res.* **12,** 151–161.

Nayler, W. G., Ferrari, R., Poole-Wilson, P. A., and Yepez, C. E. 1979. A protective effect of a mild acidosis on hypoxic heart muscle. *J. Mol. Cell. Cardiol.* **11,** 1053–1071.

Nayler, W. G., Ferrari, F., and Slade, A., 1978/1980. Cardioprotective actions of calcium-antagonists in myocardial anoxia and ischemia, in *Calcium-Antagonism,* Proceedings of an Internat. Symposium, 1978, in Frankfort, Edited by A. Fleckenstein and H. Roskamm, pp. 119–137, Springer-Verlag, Berlin–Heidelberg–New York, 1980.

Nayler, W. G., Grau, A., and Slade, A. 1976. A protective effect of verapamil on hypoxic heart muscle. *Cardiovasc. Res.* **10**, 650–662.

Nayler, W. G., and Merrillees, N. C. R. 1970/1971. Cellular exchange of calcium, in *Calcium and the Heart,* Proceedings of the Meeting of the European Section of the International Study Group for Research in Cardiac Metabolism, London, September 6, 1970, Edited by P. Harris and L. Opie, p. 24–65 Academic, London–New York, 1971.

Nayler, W. G., and Szeto, J. 1972. Effect of verapamil on contractility, oxygen utilization and calcium exchangeability in mammalian heart muscle. *Cardiovasc. Res.* **6**, 120–128.

Neubüser, D. 1974. Über die Wirkung der Kalziuminhibitoren Verapamil (Isoptin) und D 600 auf die Nebenwirkungen der klinischen Tokolyse mit dem Beta-Stimulator Th 1165a (Partusisten). *Geburtsh. Frauenheilk.* **34**, 782–787.

Neumann, M., and Luisada, A. A. 1966. Double blind evaluation of orally administered iproveratril in patients with angina pectoris. *Am. J. Med. Sci.* **251**, 552–556.

Neuss, H., and Schlepper, M. 1971. Der Einfluss von Verapamil auf die atrio-ventrikuläre Überleitung. Lokalisation des Wirkungsortes mit His-Bündel Elektrogrammen. *Verh. Dtsch. Ges. Kreisl.-Forsch.* **37**, 433–438.

Newman, R. K., Leroux, E. J., Peterson, D. F., Bishop, V. S., and Horwitz, L. D. 1976. Effects of verapamil on cardiac performance in conscious dogs. *Clin. Res.* **24**(1), 5A.

Nickerson, M., Karr, G. W., and Dresel, P. E. 1961. Pathogenesis of "electrolyte-steroid-cardiopathy." *Circ. Res.* **9**, 209–217.

Niedergerke, R. 1955. Local muscular shortening by intracellularly applied calcium. *J. Physiol.* (Lond.), **128**, 12–13P.

Niedergerke, R. 1957. The rate of action of calcium ions on the contraction of the heart. *J. Physiol.* (Lond.) **138**, 506–515.

Niitani, H., and Fujimaki, T. 1975. Clinical experience with nifedipine for ischemic heart disease, in *1st International Nifedipine (Adalat) Symposium,* Tokyo, November, 1973, Edited by K. Hashimoto, E. Kimura, and T. Kobayashi, pp. 268–278, University of Tokyo Press, 1975.

Noble, D., and Tsien, R. W. 1969. Reconstruction of the repolarization process in cardiac Purkinje fibres based on voltage clamp measurements of the membrane current. *J. Physiol.* (Lond.) **200**, 234–254.

Nonomura, Y., Hotta, Y., and Ohashi, H. 1966. Tetrodotoxin and manganese ions: Effects on electrical activity and tension in taenia coli of guinea pig. *Science* **152**, 97–99.

van Noorden, S., Olsen, E. G. J., and Pearse, A. G. E. 1971. Hypertrophic obstructive cardiomyopathy, a histological, histochemical, and ultrastructural study of biopsy material. *Cardiovasc. Res.* **5**, 118–131.

Ochi, R. 1970. The slow inward current and the action of manganese ions in guinea-pig's myocardium. *Pflügers Arch. ges. Physiol.* **316**, 81–94.

Ochi, R., and Trautwein, W. 1971. The dependence of cardiac contraction on depolarization and slow inward current. *Pflügers Arch. ges. Physiol.* **323**, 187–203.

Ohnishi, T., and Ebashi, S. 1963. Spectrophotometric measurements of instantaneous calcium binding of the relaxing factor of muscle. *J. Biochem.* (Tokyo) **54**, 506–511.

Oliva, P. B., and Breckinridge, J. C. 1977. Arteriographic evidence of coronary arterial spasm in acute myocardial infarction. *Circulation* **56**, 366–374.

Oliva, P. B., Potts, D. E., and Pluss, R. G. 1973. Coronary arterial spasm in Prinzmetal angina: documentation by coronary arteriography. *N. Engl. J. Med.* **288**, 745–751.

Olivari, M. T., Bartorelli, C., Polese, A., Fiorentini, C., Moruzzi, P., and Guazzi, M. 1979. Treatment of hypertension with nifedipine, a calcium-antagonistic agent. *Circulation* **59**, 1056–1062.

deOliveira, J. M., Loyola, S. F., and Da Cunha Chaves, J. L. 1973. Perhexiline maleate: eighteen months of continuous administration in patients with angina pectoris. *Postgrad. Med. J.* **49** (April Suppl.), 78–84.

Onishi, S., Bajusz, E., Büchner, F., and Rickers, K. 1970. Herzmuskelhypertrophie bei erbbedingter Myopathie des syrischen Hamsters nach elektronenmikroskopischen Untersuchungen. *Beitr. path. Anat.* **140**, 119–141.

Ono, H., Kokubun, H., and Hashimoto, K. 1974. Abolition by calcium-antagonists of the autoregulation of renal blood flow. *Naunyn-Schmiedebergs Arch. exper. Path. Pharmakol.* **285**, 201–207.

Opitz, E., and Schneider, M. 1950. Über die Sauerstoffversorgung des Gehirns und den Mechanismus von Mangelwirkungen. *Ergebn. Physiol.* **46**, 126–260.

Orent-Keiles, E., and McCollum, E. V. 1941. Potassium in animal nutrition. *J. Biol. Chem.* **140**, 337–352.

Orentlicher, M., Reuben, J. P., Grundfest, H., and Brandt, P. W. 1974. Calcium binding and tension development in detergent-treated muscle fibres. *J. Gen. Physiol.* **63**, 168–186.

Osakada, G., Kumada, T., Gallagher, K. P., Kemper, W. S., and Ross, J. 1981. Effect of verapamil on exercise-induced regional myocardial dysfunction in conscious dogs. *Am. J. Cardiol.* **47**, 416.

Overkamp, H. 1960. Doppelblindversuche mit dem Coronartherapeuticum Segontin. *Med. Klin.* **55**, 1423–1426.

Owen, N. E., Feinberg, H., and Le Breton, G. C. 1980. Epinephrine induces Ca^{2+} uptake in human blood platelets. *Am. J. Physiol.* **239**, H 483–H 488.

Paes de Carvalho, A. 1961. Cellular electrophysiology of the atrial specialized tissues, in *The Specialized Tissues of the Heart,* Edited by A. Paes de Carvalho, W. C. de Mello, and B. F. Hoffman, pp. 115–133, Elsevier, Amsterdam.

Paes de Carvalho, A., Hoffman, B. F., and de Paula Carvalho, M. 1969. Two components of the cardiac action potential. I. Voltage time course and the effect of acetylcholine on atrial and nodal cells of the rabbit heart. *J. Gen. Physiol.* **54**, 607–635.

Paes de Carvalho, A., de Mello, W. C., and Hoffman, B. F. 1959. Electrophysiological evidence for specialized fiber types in rabbit atrium. *Am. J. Physiol.* **196**, 483–488.

Pappano, A. J. 1970. Calcium-dependent action potentials produced by catecholamines in guinea pig atrial muscle fibers depolarized by potassium. *Circ. Res.* **27**, 379–390.

Paradise, R. R. 1963. Influence of potassium and calcium on behavior of isolated rat atria. *Proc. Soc. Exp. Biol. Med.* **112**, 483–486.

Parodi, O., Maseri, A., and Simonetti, I. 1979. Management of unstable angina at rest by verapamil. A double-blind cross-over study in coronary care unit. *Brit. Heart J.* **41**, 167–174.

Parodi, O., Severi, S., Maseri, A., and Biagini, A. 1978. Reversible reduction of regional myocardial blood flow as cause of "primary" angina at rest: relationship with electrocardiographic S-T changes, in *Primary and Secondary Angina Pectoris,* Edited by A. Maseri, G. A. Klassen, and M. Lesch, pp. 227–237, Grune and Stratton, New York.

Patel, K. R. 1981. Calcium antagonists in exercise-induced asthma. *Brit. Med. J.* **282**, 932–933.

Patriarca, P., and Carafoli, E. 1968. A study of the intracellular transport of calcium in rat heart. *J. Cell. Comp. Physiol.* **72**, 29–37.

Patterson, J. W. 1953. Effect of lowered blood sugar on development of diabetic cataracts. *Am. J. Physiol.* **172**, 77–82.

Patzschke, K., Duhm, B., Maul, W., Medenwald, H., and Wegner, L. A. 1975. Pharmacokinetics of Adalat in animal experiments, in *2nd International Nifedipine (Adalat) Symposium,* Amsterdam, October, 1974, Edited by W. Lochner, W. Braasch, and G. Kroneberg, pp. 27–32, Springer-Verlag, Berlin-Heidelberg-New York, 1975.

Peiper, U., Griebel, L., and Wende, W. 1971. Activation of vascular smooth muscle of rat aorta by noradrenaline and depolarization: Two different mechanisms. *Pflügers Arch. ges. Physiol.* **330**, 74–89.

Peper, K., and Trautwein, W. 1966. Über den Mechanismus der Extrasystolen des Aconitin-vergifteten Herzmuskels. *Pflügers Arch. ges. Physiol.* **291**, R 16.

Pepine, C. J., Schang, S. J., and Bemiller, C. R. 1973. Alteration of left ventricular responses to ischemia with oral perhexiline. *Postgrad. Med. J.* **49** (April Suppl.), 43–46.

Pepine, C. J., Schang, S. J., and Bemiller, C. R. 1974. Effects of perhexiline on symptomatic and hemodynamic responses to exercise in patients with angina pectoris. *Am. J. Cardiol.* **33,** 806–812.

Perry, S. V., and Grey, T. C. 1956. A study of the effects of substrate concentration and certain relaxing factors on the magnesium-activated myofibrillar adenosine triphosphatase. *Biochem. J.* **64,** 184–192.

Pfitzer, P., Knieriem, H. -J., Dietrich, H., and Herbertz, G. 1972. Hypertrophie des Rattenherzens nach Isoproterenol. *Virchow's Arch. Abt. B. Zellpath.* **12,** 22–38.

Philipson, K. D., Bers, D. M., Nishimoto, A. Y., and Langer, G. A. 1980. Binding of Ca^{2+} and Na^+ to sarcolemmal membranes: Relation to control of myocardial contractility. *Am. J. Physiol. 238/2,* H 373–H 378.

Philipson, K. D., and Langer, G. A. 1979. Sarcolemmal-bound calcium and contractility in the mammalian myocardium. *J. Mol. Cell. Cardiology* **11,** 857–875.

Piepho, R. W., Bloedow, D. C., Lacz, J. P., Runser, D. J., Dimmit, D. C., and Browne, R. K. 1982. Pharmacokinetics of diltiazem in selected animal species and human beings. *Am. J. Cardiol.* **49,** 525–528.

Pilcher, J., Chandrasekhar, K. P., Russell Rees, J., Boyce, M. J., Peirce, T. H., and Ikram, H. 1973. Long-term assessment of perhexiline maleate in angina pectoris. *Postgrad. Med. J.* **49** (April Suppl.), 115–118.

Polansky, B. J., Berger, R. L., and Byrne, J. J. 1964. Massive nonocclusive intestinal infarction associated with digitalis toxicity. *Circulation* **29/30** (Suppl. III), 141.

de Ponti, C., Mauri, F., Ciliberto, G. R., and Carù, B. 1979. Comparative effects of nifedipine, verapamil, isosorbide dinitrate and propranolol on exercise-induced angina pectoris. *Eur. J. Cardiol.* **10,** 47–58.

Pool, P. E., Seagren, S. C., Bonanno, J. A., Salel, A. F., and Dennish, G. W. 1980. The treatment of exercise-inducible chronic stable angina with diltiazem. *Chest* **78,** (Suppl. 1), 234–238.

Poole-Wilson, P. A. 1978. Inhibition of calcium uptake by acidosis in the myocardium of the rabbit. *J. Physiol.* (Lond.) **277,** 79P.

Pretorius, P. J., Pohl, W. G., Smithen, C. S., and Inesi, G. 1969. Structural and functional characterization of dog heart microsomes. *Circ. Res.* **25,** 487–499.

Prinzmetal, M., Kennamer, R., Merliss, R., Wada, T., and Bor, N. 1959. Angina pectoris: a variant form of angina pectoris. *Am. J. Med.* **27,** 375–388.

Prosser, C. L. 1962. Conduction in nonstriated muscle. *Physiol. Rev.* **42,** 193–212.

Pruitt, R. D., and Essex, H. E. 1960. Potential changes attending the excitation process in the atrioventricular conduction system of bovine and canine hearts. *Circ. Res.* **8,** 149–174.

Pueschner, H., and Gussmann, S. 1970. Die spontane Arteriosklerose bei Haustieren. *Z. Gerontol.* **3,** 364–372.

Raab, W. 1953. *Hormonal and Neurogenic Cardiovascular Disorders.* Williams and Wilkins, Baltimore.

Raab, W. 1963. Neurogenic multifocal destruction of myocardial tissue. *Rev. Canad. Biol.* **22,** 217–239.

Racz, P., and Kellermayer, M. 1978. Non-dialysable calcium, sodium and potassium in normal and senile cataractous lenses. *Ophthalmol. Res.* **10,** 63–66.

Raemsch, K.-D. 1981. Zur Pharmakokinetik von Nifedipin. Zeitschr. *Schwerpunktmedizin* **4,** 55–61.

Raff, G. L., Brundage, B. H., Ports, T. A., and Chatterjee, K. 1981. Dissociation between acute hemodynamic effects and clinical response to verapamil in hypertrophic cardiomyopathy. *Clin. Res.* **29,** 79A.

Raff, W. K., Kosche, F., and Lochner, W. 1972. Untersuchungen mit Nifedipine, einer coronargefässerweiternden Substanz mit schneller sublingualer Wirkung. *Arzneimittelforschung (Drug Res.)* **22,** 33–39.

Rakusan, K., Tietzova, H., Turek, Z., and Poupa, O. 1965. Cardiomegaly after repeated application of isoprenaline in the rat. *Physiol. Bohemoslov.* **14,** 456.

Rapela, C. E., and Green, H. D. 1964. Autoregulation of canine cerebral blood flow. *Circ. Res.* **14** and **15** (Suppl. I), 206–212.

Raschack, M. 1976a. Differences in the cardiac actions of the calcium antagonists verapamil and nifedipine. *Arzneimittelforschung (Drug Res.)* **26,** 1330–1333.

Raschack, M. 1976b. Relationship of antiarrhythmic to inotropic activity and antiarrhythmic qualities of the optical isomers of verapamil. *Naunyn-Schmiedebergs Arch. exper. Path. Pharmakol.* **294,** 285–291.

Rayner, B., and Weatherall, M. 1957. Digoxin, ouabain and potassium movements in rabbit auricles. *Brit. J. Pharmacol.* **12,** 371–381.

Reddy, K. M., Etlinger, J. D., Fischman, D. A., Rabinowitz, M., and Zak, R. 1975. Removal of Z lines and α-actinin from isolated myofibrils by a calcium-activated neutral protease. *J. Biol. Chem.* **250,** 4278–4289.

Refsum, H. 1975. Calcium-antagonistic and anti-arrhythmic effects of nifedipine on the isolated rat atrium. *Acta Pharmacol. Toxicol.* **37,** 377–386.

Refsum, H., and Landmark, K. 1975. The effect of a calcium-antagonistic drug, nifedipine, on the mechanical and electrical activity of the isolated rat atrium. *Acta Pharmacol. Toxicol.* **37,** 369–376.

Reimer, K. A., Lowe, J. E., and Jennings, R. B. 1977. Effect of the calcium antagonist verapamil on necrosis following temporary coronary artery occlusion in dogs. *Circulation* **55,** 581–587.

Rein, H. 1931. Die Physiologie der Herz-Kranz-Gefässe. *Z. Biol.* **92,** 115–127.

Reiner, O., and Marshall, J. M. 1975. Action of D 600 on spontaneous and electrically stimulated activity of parturient rat uterus. *Naunyn-Schmiedebergs Arch. exper. Path. Pharmakol.* **290,** 21–28.

Reiner, O., and Marshall, J. M. 1976. Action of prostaglandin, PGF 2_α, on the uterus of the pregnant rat. *Naunyn-Schmiedebergs Arch. Exper. Path. Pharmakol.* **292,** 243–250.

Reinhardt, D., Schmidt, U., Brodde, O. E., and Schümann, H. J. 1977. H_1- and H_2-receptor mediated responses to histamine on contractility and cyclic AMP of atrial and papillary muscles from guinea-pig hearts. *Agents and Actions* **7,** 1–12.

Reinhardt, D., Wagner, J., and Schümann, H. J. 1974. Differentiation of H_1- and H_2-receptors mediating positive chrono- and inotropic responses to histamine on atrial preparations of the guinea-pig. *Agents and Actions* **4,** 217–221.

Reiter, M., and Noé, J. 1959. Die Bedeutung von Calcium, Magnesium, Kalium und Natrium für die rhythmische Erregungsbildung in Sinusknoten des Warmblüterherzens. *Plügers Arch. ges. Physiol.* **269,** 366–374.

Remberg, G., Ende, M., Eichelbaum, M., and Schomerus, M. 1980. Mass spectrometric identification of DL-verapamil metabolites. *Arzneimittelforschung. (Drug Res.)* **30,** *398–401.*

Repke, K. R. H. 1964. Über den biochemischen Wirkungsmodus von Digitalis. *Klin. Wschr.* **42,** 157–165.

Reuben, S. R., and Kuan, P. 1980. The acute haemodynamic effects of intravenous verapamil in hypoxic lung disease. *Bull. Eur. Physiopathol. Respir.* **16,** P 111–P 113.

Reuter, H. 1965. Über die Wirkung von Adrenalin auf den cellulären Ca-Umsatz des Meerschwein-chenvorhofs. *Naunyn-Schmiedebergs Arch. exp. Path. Pharmakol.* **251,** 401–412.

Reuter, H. 1973. Divalent cations as charge carriers in excitable membranes. *Prog. Biophys. Mol. Biol.* **26,** 1–43.

Reuter, H. 1974. Localization of beta-adrenergic receptors, and effects of noradrenaline and cyclic nucleotides on action potentials, ionic currents and tension in mammalian cardiac muscle. *J. Physiol. (Lond.)* **242,** 429–451.

Reuter, H., and Beeler, G. W. 1969. Calcium current and activation of contraction in ventricular myocardial fibers. *Science* **162,** 399–401.

Reuter, H., and Seitz, N. 1968. Dependence of calcium efflux from cardiac muscle on temperature and external ion composition. *J. Physiol. (Lond.)* **195**, 451–470.

Riemer, J., Dörfler, F., Mayer, C. -J., and Ulbrecht, G. 1974. Calcium-antagonistic effects on the spontaneous activity of guinea-pig taenia coli. *Pflügers Arch. ges. Physiol.* **351**, 241–258.

Ries, G. H. 1979. Kasuistische Mitteilung über das Auftreten einer Myokardischämie unter medikamentöser Tokolyse mit Ritodrin (Pre-Par®). *Geburtsh. Frauenheilk.* **39**, 33–37.

Ringer, S. 1882. A further contribution regarding the influence of the different constituents of the blood on the contraction of the heart. *J. Physiol. (Lond.)* **4**, 29–42.

Ringqvist, T. 1974. Effect of verapamil in obstructive airways disease. *Eur. J. Clin. Pharmacol.* **7**, 61–64.

Rink, H., Münnighoff, J., and Hockwin, O. 1977. Sodium, potassium and calcium contents of bovine lenses in dependence on age. *Ophthalm. Res.* **9**, 129–135.

Robb-Nicholson, C., Currie, W. D., and Wechsler, A. S. 1978. Effects of verapamil on myocardial tolerance to ischemic arrest: Comparison to potassium arrest. *Circulation* **58** (Suppl. I), 119–124.

Rodrigues-Pereira, E., and Viana, A. P. 1968. Actions of verapamil on experimental arrhythmias. *Arzneimittelforschung (Drug Res.)* **18**, 175–179.

Rona, G., Chappel, C. I., Balazs, T., and Gaudry, R. 1959. An infarct-like myocardial lesion and other toxic manifestations produced by isoproterenol in the rat. *Arch. Pathol.* **67**, 443–455.

Rona, G., Chappel, C. I., and Kahn, D. S. 1963. The significance of factors modifying the development of isoproterenol-induced myocardial necrosis. *Am. Heart J.,* **66**, 389–395.

Rona, G., Kahn, D. S., and Chappel, C. I. 1963. Studies on infarct-like myocardial necrosis produced by isoproterenol: A review. *Rev. Canad. Biol.* **22**, 241–255.

Rona, G., Kahn, D. S., and Chappel, C. I. 1965. The effect of electrolytes on experimental infarct-like myocardial necrosis, in *Electrolytes and Cardiovascular Diseases.* Edited by E. Bajusz, pp. 181–191. Karger, Basel–New York.

Rosenberger, L. B., Ticku, M. K., and Triggle, D. J. 1979. The effects of Ca^{2+} antagonists on mechanical responses and Ca^{2+} movements in guinea pig ileal longitudinal smooth muscle. *Canad. J. Physiol.* **57**, 333–347.

Rosenblum, I., Wohl, A., and Stein, A. 1965. Studies in cardiac necrosis. III. Metabolic effects of sympathomimetic amines producing cardiac lesions. *Toxicol. Appl. Pharmacol.* **7**, 344–351.

Rosenmann, E., Gazenfield, E., Laufer, A., and Davies, A. M. 1964. Isoproterenol-induced myocardial lesions in the immunized and nonimmunized rat. *Path. Microbiol. (Basel),* **27**, 303–309.

Rosing, D. R., Kent, K. M., Borer, J. S., Seides, S. F., Maron, B. J., and Epstein, S. E. 1979. Verapamil therapy: A new approach to the pharmacologic treatment of hypertrophic cardiomyopathy. I. Hemodynamic effects. *Circulation* **60**, 1201–1207.

Rosing, D. R., Kent, K. M., Maron, B. J., and Epstein, S. E. 1979. Verapamil therapy: A new approach to the pharmacologic treatment of hypertrophic cardiomyopathy. II. Effects on exercise capacity and symptomatic status. *Circulation* **60**, 1208–1213.

Roskamm, H., Fröhlich, G. J., and Reindell, H. 1966. Die Wirkung verschiedener Koronardilatatoren auf den Sauerstoffverbrauch, die Herzfrequenz und den Blutdruck bei standardisierter Belastung auf dem Ergometer. *Arzneimittelforschung (Drug Res.)* **16**, 835–841.

Rothberger, C. J., and Winterberg, H. 1911. Über die experimentelle Erzeugung extrasystolischer ventrikulärer Tachykardie durch Acceleransreizung. (Ein Beitrag zur Herzwirkung von Barium und Calcium). *Pflügers Arch. ges. Physiol.* **142**, 461–522.

Rovei, V., Gomeni, R., Mitchard, M., Larribaud, J., Blatrix, C., Thebault, J. J., and Morselli, P. L. 1980. Pharmacokinetics and metabolism of diltiazem in man. *Acta Cardiol.* **35**, 35–45.

Rowe, G. G., Stenlund, R. R., Thomsen, J. H., Corliss, R. J., and Sialer, S. 1971. The systemic and coronary hemodynamic effects of iproveratril. *Arch. Int. Pharmacodyn. Ther.* **193**, 381–390.

Rowland, E., Evans, T., and Krikler, D. 1979. Effect of nifedipine on atrioventricular conduction as compared with verapamil. *Brit. Heart J.* **42**, 124–127.

Roy, P. R., Spurrell, R. A. J., and Sowton, E. 1974. The effect of verapamil on the cardiac conduction system in man. *Postgrad. Med. J.* **50**, 270–275.

Rudolph, W., Kriener, J., and Meister, W. 1971. Die Wirkung von Verapamil auf Coronardurchblutung, Sauerstoffutilisation und Kohlendioxydproduktion des menschlichen Herzens. *Klin. Wschr.* **49**, 982–988.

Rüegg, J. C. 1971. Smooth muscle tone. *Physiol. Rev.* **51**, 201–248.

Ruigrok, T. J. C., Boink, A. B. T. J., Spies, F., Blok, F. J., Maas, A. H. J., and Zimmerman, A. N. E. 1978. Energy dependence of the calcium paradox. *J. Mol. Cell. Cardiol.* **10**, 991–1002.

Ruigrok, T. J. C., Boink, A. B. T. J., Zimmerman, A. N. E., and Meijler, F. L. 1978/1980. Effect of verapamil on energy consumption and development of contracture during the calcium paradox, in *Calcium-Antagonismus*, Proceedings of an International Symposium, 1978, in Frankfort, Edited by A. Fleckenstein and H. Roskamm, pp. 138–142, Springer-Verlag, Berlin–Heidelberg–New York, 1980.

Rushmer, R. F. 1961. *Cardiovascular dynamics*, Saunders, Philadelphia–London.

Russell, J. T., and Thorn, N. A. 1974. Calcium and stimulus-secretion coupling in the neurohypophysis. II. Effects of lanthanum, a verapamil analogue (D 600) and prenylamine on 45-calcium transport and vasopressin release in isolated rat neurohypophyses. *Acta Endocrinol. Copenhagen* **76**, 471–487.

Ryden, L., and Korsgren, M. 1969. The effect of lignocaine on the stimulation threshold and conduction disturbances in patients treated with pacemakers. *Cardiovasc. Res.* **3**, 415–418.

Sacks, H., and Kennelly, B. M. 1972. Verapamil in cardiac arrhythmias. *Brit. Med. J.* **2**, 716.

Salit, P. W. 1933. Calcium content and weight of human cataractous lenses. *Arch. Ophthalmol.* **9**, 571–578.

Sampson, J. J., Alberton, E. C., and Kondo, B. 1943. The effect on man of potassium administration in relation to digitalis glycosides, with special reference to blood serum potassium, the electro-cardiogram, and ectopic beats. *Am. Heart J.* **26**, 164–179.

Sampson, J. J., and Anderson, E. M. 1932. The treatment of certain cardiac arrhythmias with potassium salts. *JAMA* **99**, 2257–2261.

Sanadi, D. R. 1965. Energy-linked reactions in mitochondria. *Ann. Rev. Biochem.* **34**, 21–48.

Sanborn, W. D., and Langer, G. A. 1970. Specific uncoupling of excitation and contraction in mammalian cardiac tissue by lanthanum. *J. Gen. Physiol.* **56**, 191–217.

Sandahl, B., Ulmsten, U., and Andersson, K. E. 1979. Trial of the calcium antagonist nifedipine in the treatment of primary dysmenorrhoea. *Arch. Gynecol.* **227**, 147–151.

Sandler, G., Clayton, G. A., and Thornicroft, S. G. 1968. Clinical evaluation of verapamil in angina pectoris. *Brit. Med. J.* **1968**, 224–227.

Sandow, A. 1952. Excitation-contraction coupling in muscular response. *Yale J. Biol. Med.* **25**, 176–201.

Sano, T. 1976. Conduction in the heart, in *The Theoretical Basis of Electrophysiology*, Edited by C. V. Nelson and D. B. Geselowitz, pp. 70–119, Clarendon Press, Oxford.

Sano, T., and Yamagishi, S. 1965. Spread of excitation from the sinus node. *Circ. Res.* **16**, 423–430.

Sato, M., Nagao, T., Yamaguchi, I., Nakajima, H., and Kiyomoto, A. 1971. Pharmacological studies on a new 1,5-benzothiazepine derivative (CRD-401 = Diltiazem). *Arzneimittelforschung (Drug Res.)* **21**, 1338–1343.

Satoh, K., Yanagisawa, T., and Taira, N. 1979. Effects on atrioventricular conduction and blood flow of enantiomers of verapamil and of tetrodotoxin injected into the posterior and the anterior septal artery of the atrioventricular node preparation of the dog. *Naunyn-Schmiedebergs Arch. exper. Path. Pharmakol.* **308**, 89–98.

Scarpa, A., and Graziotti, P. 1973. Mechanisms for intracellular calcium regulation in heart. I. Stopped-flow measurements of Ca^{++} uptake by cardiac mitochondria. *J. Gen. Physiol.* **62**, 756–772.

Schädler, M. 1967. Proportionale Aktivierung von ATPase-Aktivität und Kontraktionsspannung durch Calciumionen in isolierten kontraktilen Strukturen verschiedener Muskelarten. *Pflügers Arch. ges. Physiol.* **296**, 70–90.

Schaefer, J., Schwarzkopf, H.-J., Schoettler, M., and Wilms, R. 1975a. Action of nifedipine on oxygen extraction and lactate metabolism of the myocardium of patients with bradycardic disturbances of rhythm and angina pectoris during pacing induced tachycardia, in *1st International Nifedipine (Adalat) Symposium,* Tokyo, November, 1973, Edited by K. Hashimoto, E. Kimura, and T. Kobayashi, pp. 107–113, University of Tokyo Press, 1975.

Schaefer, J., Schwarzkopf, H. -J., Schoettler, M., and Wilms, R. 1975b. Effect of nifedipine (Adalat) on myocardial oxygen extraction and lactate metabolism and ST-T segment changes in patients with coronary insufficiency during artificial stimulation of the heart. in *2nd International Nifedipine (Adalat) Symposium,* Amsterdam, October, 1974, Edited by W. Lochner, W. Braasch, and G. Kroneberg, pp. 141–144, Springer-Verlag, Berlin-Heidelberg-New York, 1975.

Schärer, K., Alatas, H., and Bein, G. 1977. Die Behandlung der renalen Hypertension mit Verapamil im Kindesalter. *Mschr. Kinderheilk.* **125**, 706–712.

Schamroth, L. 1971. Immediate effects of intravenous verapamil on atrial fibrillation. *Cardiovasc. Res.* **5**, 419–424.

Schamroth, L., Krikler, D. M., and Garrett, C. 1972. Immediate effects of intravenous verapamil in cardiac arrhythmias. *Brit. Med. J.* **1972**, 660–662.

Schatzmann, H. J. 1964. Erregung und Kontraktion glatter Vertebratenmuskeln. *Ergebn. Physiol.* **55**, 28–130.

Scher, A. M., Rodriguez, M. I., Liikane, J., and Young, A. C. 1959. Mechanism of atrioventricular conduction. *Circ. Res.* **7**, 54–67.

Schildberg, F. W., and Fleckenstein, A. 1965. Die Bedeutung der extracellulären Calciumkonzentration für die Spaltung von energiereichem Phosphat in ruhendem und tätigem Myokardgewebe. *Pflügers Arch. Ges. Physiol.* **283**, 137–150.

Schlepper, M., and Witzleb, E. 1962. Tierexperimentelle Untersuchungen über die Veränderung von Coronardurchblutung und Sauerstoffverbrauch des Herzens nach α-Isopropyl-α - ((N-methyl-N-homoveratryl)-γ-amino-propyl)-3,4-dimethoxyphenylacetonitril. *Arzneimittelforschung (Drug Res.)* **12**, 559–561.

Schlossmann, K., Medenwald, H., and Rosenkranz, H. 1975. Investigations on the metabolism and protein binding of nifedipine, in *2nd International Nifedipine (Adalat) Symposium,* Amsterdam, October, 1974, Edited by W. Lochner, W. Braasch, and G. Kroneberg, pp. 33–39, Springer-Verlag, Berlin–Heidelberg–New York, 1975.

Schmid, J. R., and Hanna, C. 1967. Comparison of the antiarrhythmic action of two new synthetic compounds iproveratril (verapamil) and MJ 1999, with quinidine and pronethalol. *J. Pharmacol. Exp. Ther.* **156**, 331–338.

Schmid, P., Pavek, P., and Klein, W. 1979. Echokardiographische und hämodynamische Untersuchungen zur Beeinflussung der hypertrophischen obstruktiven Kardiomyopathie durch Verapamil. *Z. Kardiol.* **68**, 89–92.

Schmidt, R. F. 1960. Versuche mit Aconitin zum Problem der spontanen Erregungsbildung im Herzen. *Pflügers Arch. ges. Physiol.* **271**, 526–536.

Schneider, J. A., and Sperelakis, N. 1975. Slow Ca^{2+} and Na^+ responses induced by isoproterenol and methylxanthines in isolated perfused guinea pig hearts exposed to elevated K^+. *J. Mol. Cell. Cardiol.* **7**, 249–273.

Schomerus, M., Spiegelhalder, B., Stieren, B., and Eichelbaum, M. 1976. Physiological disposition of verapamil in man. *Cardiovasc. Res.* **10**, 605–612.

Schrader, G. A., Prickett, C. O., and Salmon, W. D. 1937. Symptomatology and pathology of potassium and magnesium deficiencies in the rat. *J. Nutr.* **14**, 85–109.

Schreiber, S. S. 1956. Potassium and sodium exchange in the working frog heart. Effects of overwork, external concentrations of potassium and ouabain. *Am. J. Physiol.* **185,** 337–347.

Schroeder, J. S., Bolen, J. L., Quint, R. A., Clark, D. A., Hayden, W. G., Higgens, C. B., and Wexler, L. 1977. Provocation of coronary spasm with ergonovine maleate. New test with results in 57 patients undergoing coronary arteriography. *Am. J. Cardiol.* **40,** 487–491.

Schroeder, J. S., Rosenthal, S., Ginsburg, R., and Lamb, I. 1980. Medical therapy of Prinzmetal's variant angina. *Chest* **78** (July Suppl.), 231–233.

Schroeder, J., Silverman, J. F., and Harrison, D. C. 1974. Right coronary arterial spasm causing Prinzmetal's variant angina. *Chest* **65,** 573–574.

Schümann, H. J., Görlitz, B. D., and Wagner, J. 1975. Influence of papaverine, D 600 and nifedipine on the effects of noradrenaline and calcium on the isolated aorta and mesenteric artery of the rabbit. *Naunyn-Schmiedebergs Arch. exper. Path. Pharmakol.* **289,** 409–418.

Schultz, K. D., Schultz, K., and Schultz, G. 1977. Sodium nitroprusside and other smooth muscle-relaxants increase cyclic GMP levels in rat ductus deferens. *Nature* (Lond.) **265,** 750–751.

Schwartz, A. 1970/1971. Calcium and the sarcoplasmic reticulum, in *Calcium and the Heart,* Proceedings of the Meeting of the European Section of the International Study Group for Research in Cardiac Metabolism, London, September 6, 1970, Edited by P. Harris and L. Opie, pp. 66–92, Academic Press, London-New York, 1971.

Schwartz, A., Lindenmayer, G. E., and Allen, J. C. 1975. The sodium-potassium adenosine triphosphatase: Pharmalogical, physiological and biochemical aspects. *Pharmacol. Rev.* **27,** 3–134.

Schwartz, A., Nagao, T., and Matlib, M. A. 1978/1979. The reaction of diltiazem on occlusive-induced regional myocardial damage: a beneficial effect on mitochondria in situ, in *New Drug Therapy with a Calcium Antagonist, Diltiazem,* Hakone Symposium, 1978, Edited by R. J. Bing, pp. 48–58, Excerpta Medica, Amsterdam–Princeton, 1979.

Schwiegk, H. 1931. Kreislaufwirkung eines Glykosides aus Digitalis lanata. *Naunyn-Schmiedebergs Arch. exper. Path. Pharmakol.* **162,** 56–69.

Seabra-Gomes, R., Rickards, A., and Sutton, R. 1976. Hemodynamic effects of verapamil and practolol in man. *Eur. J. Cardiol.* **4,** 79–85.

Seidel, J. C., and Gergely, J. 1963. Studies on myofibrillar adenosine triphosphatase with calcium-free adenosine triphosphate. *J. Biol. Chem.* **238,** 3648–3653.

Seifen, E., Flacke, W., and Alper, M. H. 1964. Effects of calcium on isolated mammalian heart. *Am. J. Physiol.* **207,** 716–720.

Seifen, E., Schaer, H., and Marshall, J. M. 1964. Effect of calcium on the membrane potentials of single pacemaker fibres and atrial fibres in isolated rabbit atria. *Nature* (Lond.) **202,** 1223–1224.

Seipel, L., and Breithardt, G. 1978/80. Effects of calcium antagonists on automaticity and conduction in man, in *Calcium Antagonismus,* Proceedings of an International Symposium 1978 in Frankfurt, Edited by A. Fleckenstein and H. Roskamm, pp. 87–96, Springer-Verlag, Berlin-Heidelberg-New York, 1980.

Selye, H. 1958. Prophylactic treatment of an experimental arteriosclerosis with magnesium and potassium salts. *Am. Heart J.* **55,** 805–809.

Selye, H. 1960. *Elektrolyte, Stress und Herznekrose,* Schwabe, Basel.

Selye, H., and Bajusz, E. 1959. Sensitization by potassium deficiency for the production of myocardial necrosis by stress. *Am. J. Path.* **35,** 525–535.

Senges, J., Randolf, U., and Katus, H. 1977. Ventricular arrhythmias in cardiac anaphylaxis. *Naunyn-Schmiedebergs Arch. exper. Path. Pharmakol.* **300,** 115–121.

Sepaha, G. C., Jain, S. R., and Jain, P. 1971. The treatment of angina pectoris. A double-blind study of prenylamine (Synadrin; Segontin). *Clin. Trials J.* **8,** 43–46.

Serruys, P. W., Brower, R. W., Ten Katen, H. J., Bom, A. H., and Hugenholtz, P. G. 1981. Regional wall motion from radiopaque markers after intravenous and intracoronary injections of nifedipine. *Circulation* **63**, 584–591.

Serruys, P. W., Steward, R., Booman, F., Michels, R., Reiber, J. H. C., and Hugenholtz, P. G. 1980. Can unstable angina pectoris be due to increased coronary vasomotor tone? *Eur. Heart J.* **1**, (Suppl. B), 71–85.

Shanbour, L. L., Jacobson, E. D., Brobmann, G. F., and Hinshaw, L. B. 1971. Effects of ouabain on splanchnic hemodynamics in the rhesus monkey. *Am. Heart J.* **81**, 511–515.

Shanes, A. M. 1950. Drug and ion effects in frog muscle. *J. Gen. Physiol.* **33**, 729–744.

Shen, A. C., and Jennings, R. B. 1972a. Myocardial calcium and magnesium in acute ischemic injury. *Am. J. Path.* **67**, 417–440.

Shen, A. C., and Jennings, R. B. 1972b. Kinetics of calcium accumulation in acute myocardial ischemic injury. *Am. J. Path.* **67**, 441–452.

Sherry, J. M. F., Gorecha, A., Aksoy, M. O., Dabrowska, R., and Hartshorne, D. J. 1978. Roles of calcium and phosphorylation in the regulation of the activity of gizzard myosin. *Biochemistry* **17**, 4411–4418.

Shibata, S., and Briggs, A. H. 1966. The relationships between electrical and mechanical events in rabbit aortic strips. *J. Pharmacol. Exp. Ther.* **153**, 466–470.

Shine, K. I., Serena, S. D., and Langer, G. A. 1971. Kinetic localization of contractile calcium in rabbit myocardium. *Am. J. Physiol.* **221**, 1408–1417.

Siegelbaum, S. A., Tsien, R. W., and Kass, R. S. 1977. Role of intracellular calcium in the transient outward current of calf Purkinje fibres. *Nature,* (Lond.) **269**, 611–613.

Simonneau, G., Escourrou, P., Duroux, P., and Lockhart A. 1981. Inhibition of hypoxic pulmonary vasoconstriction by nifedipine. *N. Engl. J. Med.* **304**, 1582–1585.

Singh, B. N., and Vaughan Williams, E. M. 1972. A fourth class of antidysrhythmic action? Effect of verapamil on ouabain toxicity, on atrial and ventricular intracellular potentials and on other features of cardiac function. *Cardiovasc. Res.* **6**, 109–119.

Sitrin, M. D., and Bohr, D. F. 1971. Ca and Na interaction in vascular smooth muscle contraction. *Am. J. Physiol.* **220**, 1124–1128.

Skelton, C. L., Levey, G. S., and Epstein, S. E. 1970. Positive inotropic effects of dibutyryl cyclic adenosine $3',5'$-monophosphate. *Circ. Res.* **26**, 35–43.

Slater, E. C., and Cleland, K. W. 1953. The effect of calcium on the respiratory and phosphorylative activities of heart muscle sarcosomes. *Biochem. J.* **55**, 566–580.

Slezak, J., and Tribulova, N. 1975. Morphological changes after combined administration of isoproterenol and K^+, Mg^{2+}-aspartate as a physiological Ca^{2+} antagonist, in *Recent Advances in Studies on Cardiac Structure and Metabolism,* Vol. 6, Edited by A. Fleckenstein, and G. Rona, pp. 75–84, University Park Press, Baltimore-London-Tokyo, 1975.

Smith, H. J., Singh, B. N., Nisbet, H. D., and Norris, R. M. 1975. Effects of verapamil on infarct size following experimental coronary occlusion. *Cardiovasc. Res.* **9**, 569–578.

Solaro, R. J., Wise, R. M., Shiner, J. S., and Briggs, F. N. 1974. Calcium requirements for cardiac myofibrillar activation. *Circ. Res.* **34**, 525–530.

Solberg, L. E., Nissen, R. G., Vlietstra, R. E., and Callahan, J. A. 1978. Prinzmetal's variant angina—Response to verapamil. *Mayo Clin. Proc.* **53**, 256–259.

Somlyo, A. P., and Somlyo, A. V. 1968. Vascular smooth muscle. I. Normal structure, pathology, biochemistry, and biophysics. *Pharmacol. Rev.* **20**, 197–272.

Somlyo, A. P., and Somlyo, A. V. 1970. Vascular smooth muscle. II. Pharmacology of normal and hypertensive vessels. *Pharmacol. Rev.* **22**, 249–353.

Sordahl, L. A., and Silver, B. B. 1975. Pathological accumulation of calcium by mitochondria: Modulation by magnesium, in *Recent Advances in Studies on Cardiac Structure and Metabolism,* Vol.

6, Edited by A. Fleckenstein and G. Rona, pp. 85–93, University Park Press, Baltimore-London-Tokyo, 1975.

Späh, F., and Fleckenstein, A. 1979. Evidence of a new, preferentially Mg-carrying, transport system besides the fast Na and the slow Ca channels in the excited myocardial sarcolemma membrane. *J. Molec. Cell. Cardiol.* **11**, 1109–1127.

Späh, F. and Fleckenstein, A. 1978/80. Nachweis einer strengen quantitativen Korrelation zwischen Hemmung des transmembranären Calcium-Influx und der mechanischen Spannungsentwicklung des Myocards unter dem Einfluß verschiedener Calcium-Antagonisten, in *Calcium Antagonismus,* Proceedings of an International Symposium 1978 in Frankfort, Edited by A. Fleckenstein and H. Roskamm, pp. 29–41, Springer-Verlag, Berlin-Heidelberg-New York, 1980.

Sparks, Jr., H. V. 1964. Effect of quick stretch on isolated vascular smooth muscle. *Circ. Res.* **14** and **15** (Suppl. I), 254–260.

Sparks, Jr., H. V., and Bohr, D. F. 1962. Effect of stretch on passive tension and contractility of isolated vascular smooth muscle. *Am. J. Physiol.* **202**, 835–840.

Spector, A., Adams, D., and Krul, K. 1974. Calcium and high molecular weight protein aggregates in bovine and human lens. *Invest. Ophthalmol.* **13**, 982–990.

Spector, A., and Rothschild, C. 1973. The effect of calcium upon the reaggregation of alpha crystallin. *Invest. Ophthalmol.* **12**, 225–231.

Spiel, R., and Enenkel, W. 1976. Wirkung von Fendilin auf die Belastungsuntersuchung Koronarkranker. *Wien. Med. Wschr.* **126**, 186–189.

Spies, H. F., Koch, E., Appel, E., Palm, D., and Kaltenbach, M. 1978. Einfluss oraler Langzeittherapie mit Verapamil und Metoprolol auf arteriellen Blutdruck, Herzfrequenz und Plasmakatecholamine bei Hypertonikern. *Verh. Dtsch. Ges. Kreisl.-Forsch.* **44**, 251.

Spurrell, R., Krikler, D., and Sowton, E. 1974a. Concealed bypasses of the atrioventricular node in patients with paroxysmal supraventricular tachycardia revealed by intracardiac electrical stimulation and verapamil. *Am. J. Cardiol.* **33**, 590–595.

Spurrell, R., Krikler, D., and Sowton, E. 1974b. Effects of verapamil on electrophysiological properties of anomalous atrioventricular connexion in Wolff-Parkinson-White syndrome. *Brit. Heart J.* **36**, 256–264.

Stämpfli, R. 1954. A new method for measuring membrane potential with external electrodes. *Experientia* (Basel), **10**, 508–509.

Stanton, H. C., Brenner, G., and Mayfield, E. D. 1969. Studies on isoproterenol-induced cardiomegaly in rats. *Am. Heart J.* **77**, 72–80.

Stanton, H. C., and Schwartz, A. 1967. Effects of a hydrazine monoamine oxidase inhibitor (phenelzine) on isoproterenol-induced myocardiopathies in the rat. *J. Pharmacol. Exp. Ther.* **157**, 649–658.

Stein, I. 1949. Observations on the action of ergonovine on the coronary circulation and its use in the diagnosis of coronary artery insufficiency. *Am. Heart J.* **37**, 36–45.

Stein, G. 1975. Effect and duration of effect of nifedipine in patients in the post-infarction phase under standardized loading (double-blind study) and tolerance test (safety test) in the form of an open clinical study, in *1st International Nifedipine (Adalat) Symposium,* Tokyo, November, 1973, Edited by K. Hashimoto, E. Kimura, and T. Kobayashi, pp. 192–199, University of Tokyo Press, 1975.

Steinberg, M. I., and Holland, D. R. 1975. Separate receptors mediating the positive inotropic and chronotropic effect of histamine in guinea-pig atria. *Eur. J. Pharmacol.* **34**, 95–104.

Steiness, E., Bille-Brahe, N. E., Hansen, J. F., Lomholdt, N., and Ring-Larsen, H. 1978. Reduced myocardial blood flow in acute and chronic digitalization. *Acta Pharmacol. (Kbh.)* **43**, 29–35.

Stephens, N. L., Kroeger, E. A., and Kromer, U. 1975. Induction of a myogenic response in tonic airway smooth muscle by tetraethylammonium. *Am. J. Physiol.* **228**, 628–632.

Stolte, M. 1981. *Anatomie und Pathologie der Koronararterien. Beiträge zur Kardiologie,* Volume 21, Edition Perimed, Erlangen.

Strässle, B., and Burckhardt, D. 1965. Isoptin (D-365), klinische Untersuchungen zur Behandlung coronarer Herzkrankheit. *Schweiz. Med. Wschr.* **95**, 667–672.

Strubelt, O., and Siegers, C. -P. 1975. Role of cardiovascular and ionic changes in pathogenesis and prevention of isoprenaline-induced cardiac necrosis, in *Recent Advances in Studies on Cardiac Structure and Metabolism,* Vol. 6, Edited by A. Fleckenstein and G. Rona, pp. 135–142. University Park Press, Baltimore-London-Tokyo, 1975.

Strughold, H. 1930. A cinematographic study of systolic and diastolic heart size with special reference to the effects of anoxemia. *Am. J. Physiol.* **94**, 641–655.

Strunz, U., Domschke, W., Mitznegg, P., Domschke, S., Schubert, E., Wünsch, E., Jaeger, E., and Demling, L. 1975. Analysis of the motor effects of 13-norleucine motilin on the rabbit, guinea pig, rat, and human alimentary tract in vitro. *Gastroenterology* **68**, 1485–1491.

Stull, J. T., and Sanford, C. F. 1981. Differences in skeletal, cardiac, and smooth muscle contractile element regulation by calcium, in *New Perspectives on Calcium-Antagonists,* Edited by G. B. Weiss, Clinical Physiology Series, pp. 35–46, Am. Physiol. Society, Bethesda.

Sukerman, M. 1973. Clinical evaluation of perhexiline maleate in the treatment of chronic cardiac arrhythmias of patients with coronary heart disease. *Postgrad. Med. J.* **49**, (April Suppl.), 46–52.

Sutherland, E. W., Robison, G. A., and Butcher, R. W. 1968. Some aspects on the biological role of adenosine 3'-5'-monophosphate (cyclic AMP). *Circulation* **37**, 279–306.

Swan, D. A., Bell, B., Oakley, C. M., and Goodwin, J. 1971. Analysis of symptomatic course and prognosis and treatment of hypertrophic obstructive cardiomyopathy. *Brit. Heart J.* **33**, 671–685.

Syllm-Rapoport, I., and Strassburger, I. 1956. Herz-, Gefäss- und Nierenverkalkung bei experimentellem Magnesium-Mangel. *Klin. Wschr.* **34**, 762–763.

Szekeres, L., and Schein, M. 1959. Cell metabolism of overloaded mammalian heart in situ. *Cardiologia* **34**, 19–27.

Szeli, J., Molina, E., Zappia, L., and Bertaccini, G. 1977. Action of some natural polypeptides on the longitudinal muscle of the guinea pig ileum. *Eur. J. Pharmacol.* **43**, 285–287.

Szent-Györgyi, A. 1947. *Chemistry of Muscular Contraction,* Academic Press, New York.

Tada, M., Kirchberger, M. A., and Katz, A. M. 1975. Phosphorylation of a 22,000-dalton component of the cardiac sarcoplasmic reticulum by adenosine 3',5'-monophosphate-dependent protein kinase. *J. Biol. Chem.* **250**, 2640–2647.

Tada, M. Kirchberger, M. A., Repke, D. I., and Katz, A. M. 1974. The stimulation of calcium transport in cardiac sarcoplasmic reticulum by adenosine 3',5'-monophosphate-dependent protein kinase. *J. Biol. Chem.* **249**, 6174–6180.

Tada, M., Yamamoto, T., and Tonomura, Y. 1978. Molecular mechanism of active calcium transport by sarcoplasmic reticulum. *Physiol. Rev.* **58**, 1–79.

Taira, N. 1978/1979. Effects of diltiazem and other calcium-antagonists on cardiac functions and coronary blood flow as assessed in blood perfused dog-heart preparations, in *New Drug Therapy with a Calcium Antagonist, Diltiazem,* Hakone Symposium, 1978, Edited by R. J. Bing, pp. 91–103, Excerpta Medica, Amsterdam–Princeton, 1979.

Taira, N., Motomura, S., Narimatsu, A., and Iijima, T. 1975. Experimental pharmacological investigations of effects of nifedipine on atrioventricular conduction in comparison with those of other coronary vasodilators, in *New Therapy of Ischemic Heart Disease,* 2nd International Adalat Symposium. Edited by W. Lochner, W. Braasch, and G. Kroneberg, pp. 40–48, Springer Verlag, Berlin-Heidelberg-New York, 1975.

Taira, N., Motomura, S., Narimatsu, A., Satoh, K., and Yanagisawa, T. 1978/1980. The effect of calcium-antagonists on atrioventricular conduction, in *Calcium-Antagonismus,* Proceeding of an International Symposium, 1978, in Frankfort. Edited by A. Fleckenstein and H. Roskamm, pp. 42–43, Springer-Verlag, Berlin-Heidelberg-New York, 1980.

Taira, N., and Narimatsu, A. 1975. Effects of nifedipine, a potent calcium-antagonistic coronary vasodilator, on atrioventricular conduction and blood flow in the isolated atrioventricular node preparation of the dog. *Naunyn Schmiedebergs Arch. exper. Path. Pharmacol.* **290**, 107–112.

Takeuchi, K. 1925. The relation between the size of the heart and the oxygen content of the arterial blood. *J. Physiol.* (Lond.) **60**, 208–214.

Teare, D. 1958. Asymmetrical hypertrophy of the heart in young adults. *Brit. Heart J.* **20**, 1–8.

Thorens, S., and Haeusler, G. 1979. Effects of some vasodilators on calcium translocation in intact and fractionated vascular smooth muscle. *Eur. J. Pharmacol.* **54**, 79–91.

Thorn, W., Heimann, J., Müldener, B., Isselhard, W., and Gercken, G. 1959. Herzstoffwechsel in Abhängigkeit von Versuchsanordnung, Gewebsgewinnung und anoxischer Belastung. *Pflügers Arch. ges. Physiol.* **269**, 214–231.

Thurau, K., and Kramer, K. 1959. Weitere Untersuchung zur myogenen Natur der Autoregulation des Nierenkreislaufes. *Pflügers Arch. ges. Physiol.* **269**, 77–93.

Thyrum, P. 1974. Inotropic stimuli and systolic transmembrane calcium flow in depolarized guinea pig atria. *J. Pharmacol. Exp. Ther.* **188**, 166–179.

Titus, E., and Dengler, H. J. 1966. The mechanism of uptake of norepinephrine. *Pharmacol. Rev.* **18**, 525–535.

Toda, N. 1980. Mechanisms of ouabain-induced arterial muscle contraction. *Am. J. Physiol.* **239**, H199–H205.

Toda, N., and West, T. C. 1967. Interaction between Na, Ca, Mg, and vagal stimulation in the S.A. node of the rabbit. *Am. J. Physiol.* **212**, 424–430.

Torok, T. L., Vizi, E. S., and Knoll, J. 1974. Depolarizing effect of PGE on taenia coli. *Naunyn Schmiedebergs Arch. exper. Path. Pharmakol.* **284**, R84.

Trautwein, W. 1973. Membrane currents in cardiac muscle fibers. *Physiol. Rev.* **53**, 793–835.

Trautwein, W., Gottstein, U., and Dudel, J. 1954. Der Aktionsstrom der Myokardfaser im Sauerstoff-Mangel. *Pflügers Arch. ges. Physiol.* **260**, 40–60.

Trautwein, W., and Schmidt, R. F. 1960. Zur Membranwirkung des Adrenalins an der Herzmuskelfaser. *Pflügers Arch. ges. Physiol.* **271**, 715–726.

Trautwein, W., and Zink, K. 1952. Über Membran- und Aktionspotentiale einzelner Myokardfasern des Kalt- und Warmblüterherzens. *Pflügers Arch. ges. Physiol.* **256**, 68–84.

Treat, E., Ulano, H. B., and Jacobson, E. D. 1971. Effects of intraarterial ouabain on mesenteric and carotid hemodynamics. *J. Pharmacol. Exp. Ther.* **179**, 144–148.

Trendelenburg, U. 1960. The action of histamine and 5-hydroxytryptamine on isolated mammalian atria. *J. Pharmacol. Exp. Ther.* **130**, 450–460.

Tritthart, H., Fleckenstein, B., and Fleckenstein, A. 1970/1971. Some fundamental actions of antiarrhythmic drugs on the excitability and the contractility of single myocardial fibres. Proceed. Joint Meeting of the Italian and German Pharmacol. Soc., Heidelberg, 27–30. Sept. 1970, *Naunyn-Schmiedebergs Arch. exper. Path. Pharmakol.* **269**, 212–219 (1971).

Tritthart, H., Fleckenstein, A., Kaufmann, R., and Bayer, R. 1968. Die spezifische Beschleunigung des Erschlaffungsprozesses durch sympathische Überträgerstoffe und die Hemmung dieses Effektes durch β-Rezeptoren-Blockade. Versuche an isolierten Papillarmuskeln von Rhesus-Affen und Meerschweinchen sowie an Ventrikalstreifen vom Frosch. *Pflügers Arch. ges. Physiol.* **303**, 350–365.

Tritthart, H., Grün, G., Byon, Y. K., and Fleckenstein, A. 1970. Influence of Ca-antagonistic inhibitors of excitation-contraction coupling on isolated uterine muscle, studied with the sucrose gap method. *Pflügers Arch. ges. Physiol.* **319**, R117.

Tritthart, H., Grundy, H. F., Haastert, H. -P., and Herbst, A. 1972. Studies on the rising phase of the action potential in mammalian cardiac ventricular fibers. *Pflügers Arch. ges. Physiol.* **332**, 1–9.

Tritthart, H., Volkmann, R., Weiss, R., and Fleckenstein, A. 1973. Calcium-mediated action potentials in mammalian myocardium. Alteration of membrane response as induced by changes of Ca or by promoters and inhibitors of transmembrane Ca inflow. *Naunyn-Schmiedebergs Arch. exper. Path. Pharmakol.* **280**, 239–252.

Tritthart, H., Weiss, R., Volkmann, R., and Späh, F. 1974. The effects of cardiac glycosides on Ca-mediated action potentials in the mammalian myocardium. *Naunyn-Schmiedebergs Arch. exper. Path. Pharmakol.* **282**, R99.

Troesch, M., Hirzel, H. O., Jenni, R., and Krayenbühl, H. P. 1979. Langzeittherapie mit Verapamil bei hypertropher Kardiomyopathie. *Schweiz. Med. Wschr.* **109**, 1683.

Tschirdewahn, B., and Klepzig, H. 1963. Klinische Untersuchung über die Wirkung von Isoptin und Isoptin S bei Patienten mit Koronarinsuffizienz. *Dtsch. Med. Wschr.* **88**, 1702–1707.

Tse, W. W., and Han, J. 1975. Effects of manganese chloride and verapamil on automaticity of digitalized Purkinje fibers. *Am. J. Cardiol.* **36**, 50–55.

Tsien, R. W. 1973. Adrenaline-like effects of intracellular iontophoresis of cyclic AMP in cardiac Purkinje fibers. *Nature New Biol.* **245**, 120–122.

Tsien, R. W., Giles, W., and Greengard, P. 1972. Cyclic AMP mediates the effects of adrenaline on cardiac Purkinje fibers. *Nature New Biol.* **240**, 181–183.

Tucker, H., Carson, P., Bass, N., and Massey, J. 1974. Prenylamine in treatment of angina. *Brit. Heart J.* **36**, 1001–1004.

Tucker, V. L., Hanna, H., Kaiser, C. J., and Darrow, D. C. 1963. Cardiac necrosis accompanying potassium deficiency and administration of corticoids. *Circ. Res.* **13**, 420–431.

Ueda, K., Kuwajima, I., Ito, H., Kuramoto, K., and Murakami, M. 1979. Nifedipine in the management of hypertension, in *International Nifedipine (Adalat) Panel Discussion,* Tokyo, September 20, 1978, Edited by P. R. Lichtlen, E. Kimura, and N. Taira, pp. 105–114, Excerpta Medica, Amsterdam-Oxford-Princeton, 1979.

Ulmsten, U., Andersson, K. E., and Forman, A. 1978. Relaxing effects of nifedipine on the nonpregnant human uterus in vitro and in vivo. *Obstet. Gynecol.* **52**, 436–441.

Ulmsten, U., Andersson, K. E., and Wingerup, L. 1980. Treatment of premature labor with the calcium antagonist nifedipine. *Arch. Gynecol.* **229**, 1–5.

Urbanek, E., Vasku, J., Bednarik, B., Praslicka, M., and Pospisil, M. 1975. Electrolyte changes in myocardial injury, in *Recent Advances in Studies on Cardiac Structure and Metabolism,* Vol. 6, Edited by A. Fleckenstein and G. Rona, pp. 43–58. University Park Press, Baltimore-London-Tokyo.

Urbanek, E., Vasku, J., Bednarik, B., and Urbankova, H. 1969. Influence of Na_2-EDTA upon development of experimental cardiomyopathies, in *Proceedings of the Second Annual Meeting of the International Study Group for Research in Cardiac Metabolism,* Istituto Lombardo, Fondazione Baselli, pp. 242–249.

Urthaler, F., and James, T. N. 1973. Effect of tetrodotoxin on A-V conduction and A-V junctional rhythm. *Am. J. Physiol.* **224**, 1155–1161.

Vassilev, V., Stoyanov, I., Lukanov, Y., and Vassileva, P. 1975. The action of acetylcholine and some blockers on the preparations of complex stomach smooth muscles. *Aggressologie* **16**, 101–105.

Vassort, G., Rougier, O., Garnier, D., Sauviat, M. P., Coraboeuf, E., and Gargouil, Y. M. 1969. Effects of adrenaline on membrane inward current during the cardiac action potential. *Pflügers Arch. ges. Physiol.* **309**, 70–81.

Vater, W., Kroneberg, G., Hoffmeister, F., Kaller, H., Meng, K., Oberdorf, A., Puls, W., Schlossmann, K., and Stoepel, K. 1972. Zur Pharmakologie von 4-(2'Nitrophenyl)-2,6-dimethyl-1,4-dihydropyridin-3,5-dicarbonsäuredimethylester (Nifedipin, Bay a 1040). *Arzneimittelforschung (Drug Res.).* **22**, 1–14.

Vatner, S. F., Higgins, C. B., Franklin, D., and Braunwald, E. 1971. Effects of a digitalis glycoside on coronary and systemic dynamics in conscious dogs. *Circ. Res.* **28**, 470–479.

Vatner, S. F., Higgins, C. B., McKown, D. P., Franklin, D., and Braunwald, E. 1970. Coronary vasoconstriction due to digitalis in the conscious dog. *Clin. Res.* **18**, 526.

Vaughan-Neil, E. F., Snell, N. J. C., and Bevan, G. 1972. Hypotension after verapamil. *Brit. Med. J.* **2**, 529.

Vaughan Williams, E. M. 1965. The mode of action of anti-fibrillatory drugs, in *Proceedings of the 2nd International Pharmacology Meeting*, Vol. 15, p. 119. Pergamon Press.

Vaughan Williams, E. M. 1975. Classification of antiarrhythmic drugs. *J. Pharmacol. Ther.* **1**, 115–138.

Verhaeghe, R. H., and Shepherd, J. T. 1976. Effect of nitroprusside on smooth muscle and adrenergic nerve terminals in isolated blood vessels. *J. Pharmacol. Exp. Ther.* **199**, 269–277.

Vitale, J. J., Hellerstein, E. E., Nakamura, M., and Lown, B. 1961. Effects of magnesium-deficient diets upon puppies. *Circulation Res.* **9**, 387–394.

Vitek, M., and Trautwein, W. 1971. Slow inward current and action potential in cardiac Purkinje fibres. *Pflügers Arch. ges. Physiol.* **323**, 204–218.

Vornovitskii, E. G., Ignat'eva, V. B., and Khodorov, B. I. 1974. Effect of histamine on electrical and mechanical activity of the myocardial fibers of the guinea pig heart after blocking of the fast sodium channels. *Bull. Exp. Biol. Med.* **78**, 1241–1244.

Waldhausen, J. A., Kilman, J. W., Herendeen, T. L., and Abel, F. L. 1965. Effects of acetylstrophanthidin on coronary vascular resistance and myocardial oxygen consumption. *Circ. Res.* **16**, 203–209.

Washizu, Y. 1966. Grouped discharges in ureter muscle. *Comp. Biochem. Physiol.*, **19**, 713–728.

Watanabe, Y. 1978/1980. Effects of altered calcium concentrations on A.V. conduction and interactions of verapamil and sodium or calcium, in *Calcium-Antagonismus*, Proceedings of an International Symposium, 1978, in Frankfort. Edited by A. Fleckenstein and H. Roskamm, pp. 97–107, Springer-Verlag, Berlin-Heidelberg-New York, 1980.

Watanabe, A. M., and Besch, Jr., H. R. 1974a. Cyclic adenosine monophosphate modulation of slow calcium influx channels in guinea-pig hearts. *Circ. Res.* **35**, 316–324.

Watanabe, A. M., and Besch, Jr., H. R. 1974b. Subcellular myocardial effects of verapamil and D 600: comparison with propranolol. *J. Pharmacol. Exp. Ther.* **191**, 241–251.

Watanabe, A. M., and Besch, Jr., H. R. 1975. The relationship between adenosine 3',5'-monophosphate levels and systolic transmembrane calcium flux, in *Basic Functions of Cations in Myocardial Activity. Recent Advances in Studies on Cardiac Structure and Metabolism*. Vol. 5, Edited by A. Fleckenstein and N. S. Dhalla, pp. 95–102, University Park Press, Baltimore-London-Tokyo, 1975.

Waters, D. D., Szlachcic, J., and Theroux, P. 1981. Prognosis of variant angina patients treated with calcium antagonist drugs. *Am. J. Cardiol.* **47**, 463.

Waters, D. D., Theroux, P., Dauwe, F., Crittin, J., Affaki, G., and Mizgala, H. F. 1979. Ergonovine testing to assess the effects of calcium antagonist drugs in variant angina. *Circulation* **60** (Suppl. II), 248.

Watkins, R. W., and Davidson, I. W. F. 1980. Comparative effects of nitroprusside and nitroglycerin; actions on phasic and tonic components of arterial smooth muscle contraction. *Eur. J. Pharmacol.* **62**, 191–200.

Waugh, W. H. 1962. Role of calcium in contractile excitation of vascular smooth muscle by epinephrine and potassium. *Circ. Res.* **11**, 927–940.

Weber, H. H. 1934. Die Muskeleiweisskörper und der Feinbau des Skelettmuskels. *Ergebn. Physiol.* **36**, 109–150.

Weber, A., and Herz, R. 1963. The binding of calcium to actomyosin systems in relation to their biological activity. *J. Biol. Chem.* **238**, 599–605.

Weber, A., Herz, R., and Reiss, I. 1967. The nature of the cardiac relaxing factor. *Biochem. Biophys. Acta* **131**, 188–194.

Weber, A., and Murray, J. M. 1973. Molecular control mechanism in muscle contraction. *Physiol. Rev.* **53**, 612–673.

Weber, A., and Winicur, S. 1961. The role of calcium in the superprecipitation of actomyosin. *J. Biol. Chem.* **236**, 3198–3202.

Weder, U., and Grün, G. 1973. Ca^{++}-antagonistische elektro-mechanische Entkoppelung der glatten Gefässmuskulatur als Wirkungsprinzip vasodilatatorischer Nitroverbindungen. *Naunyn-Schmiedebergs Arch. exper. Path. Pharmakol.* **277** (Suppl.), R88.

Weidinger, H. 1976. Tokolyse. *Schweiz. Rundsch. Med. Praxis* **65**, 175–180.

Weidinger, H., and Wiest, W. 1971. Behandlung der vorzeitigen Wehentätigkeit mit einem neuen Tokolytikum und Isoptin. *Z. Fortschr. Medizin* **89**, 1380–1381.

Weidinger, H., and Wiest, W. 1973a. Die Behandlung des Spätabortes und der drohenden Frühgeburt mit Th 1165a in Kombination mit Isoptin. *Z. Geburtsh. Perinat.* **177**, 233–237.

Weidinger, H., and Wiest, W. 1973b. Die Auswirkungen langdauernder Wehenhemmung mit Th 1165a und Isoptin auf Herz-, Kreislauf-, Organ-, und Stoffwechsel-parameter der Mutter. *Z. Geburtsh. Perinat.* **177**, 238–244.

Weidinger, H., Wiest, W., Dietze, S., and Witzel, K. 1973. Wirkungen der Wehenhemmung mit Th 1165a und Isoptin auf den Fet, das Neugeborene und den Säugling. *Z. Geburtsh. Perinat.* **177**, 366–372.

Weidmann, S. 1955. Effects of calcium ions and local anaesthetics on electrical properties of Purkinje-fibres. *J. Physiol.* (Lond.) **129**, 568–582.

Weidmann, S. 1956. *Elektrophysiologie der Herzmuskelfaser.* Huber, Bern-Stuttgart.

Weishaar, R., Ashikawa, K., and Bing, R. J. 1979. Effect of diltiazem, a calcium antagonist, on myocardial ischemia. *Am. J. Cardiol.* **43**, 1136–1143.

Weiss, G. B. 1977. Calcium and contractility in vascular smooth muscle, in *Advances in General and Cellular Pharmacology*, Vol. 2, Edited by T. Narahashi and C. P. Bianchi, pp. 71–154, Plenum Press.

Welman, E., Carroll, B. J., Scott Lawson, J., Selwyn, A. P., and Fox, K. M. 1978. Effects of nifedipine on creatine kinase release during myocardial ischemia in dogs. *Eur. J. Cardiol.* **7**, 379–389.

Wende, W., Bleifeld, W., Meyer, J., and Stühlen, H. W. 1975. Reduction of the size of acute experimental myocardial infarction by verapamil. *Basic Res. Cardiol.* **70**, 198–208.

Wende, W., and Peiper, U. 1970. Wechselwirkung von Kalium und Noradrenalin auf die Spannungsentwicklung des isolierten Gefäßmuskels. *Pflügers Arch. ges. Physiol.* **320**, 133–141.

West, T. C. 1955. Ultramicroelectrode recording from the cardiac pacemaker. *J. Pharmacol. Exp. Ther.* **115**, 283–290.

Wette, K., Heimsoth, V., and Jansen, F. K. 1966. Einfluß von Isproveratril auf EKG-Veränderungen bei Hochdruckpatienten mit Angina pectoris. *Münch. Med. Wschr.* **108**, 1238–1242.

Wheeler, E. S., and Weiss, G. B. 1979. Correlation between response to norepinephrine and removal of ^{45}Ca from high-affinity binding sites by extracellular EDTA in rabbit aortic smooth muscle. *J. Pharmacol. Exp. Ther.* **211**, 353–359.

Wilbrandt, W. 1955. Zum Wirkungsmechanismus der Herzglykoside. *Schweiz. Med. Wschr.* **85**, 315–320.

Williamson, J. R., Woodrow, M. L., and Scarpa, A. 1975. Calcium binding to cardiac sarcolemma, in *Recent Advances in Studies on Cardiac Structure and Metabolism*, Vol. 5, *Basic Functions of Cations in Myocardial Activity*, Edited by A. Fleckenstein and G. Rona, pp. 61–71, University Park Press, Baltimore-London-Tokyo.

Winegrad, S. 1971. Studies of cardiac muscle with a high permeability to calcium produced by treatment with ethylenediamine-tetraacetic acid. *J. Gen. Physiol.* **58**, 71–93.

Winsor, T. 1970. Clinical evaluation of perhexiline maleate. *Clin. Pharmacol. Ther.* **11**, 85–89.

Winsor, T., Bleifer, K., Cole, S., Goldman, I. R., Karpman, H., Kaye, H., Oblath, R., and Stone, S. H. 1971. Prenylamine (Synadrin) in angina pectoris. A double-blind, double cross-over trial. *Clin. Trials J.* **8** (Suppl. 1), 24–34.

Wit, A. L., and Cranefield, P. F. 1974. Effect of verapamil on the sinoatrial and atrioventricular nodes of the rabbit and the mechanism by which it arrests reentrant atrioventricular nodal tachycardia. *Circ. Res.* **35**, 413–425.

v. Witzleben, H., Frey, M., Keidel, J., and Fleckenstein, A. 1980. Normalization of blood pressure in spontaneously hypertensive rats by long-term oral treatment with verapamil and nifedipine. *Pflügers Arch. ges. Physiol.* **384** (Suppl), R9.

Wolf, R., Habel, F., Witt, E., Nötges, A., Everling, F., and Hochrein, H. 1977. Wirkung von Verapamil auf die Hämodynamik und Grösse des akuten Herzinfarktes. *Herz* **2**, 110–119.

Wollenberger, A. 1947. On the energy-rich phosphate supply of the failing heart. *Am. J. Physiol.* **150**, 733–745.

Wollenberger, A. 1975. The role of cyclic AMP in the adrenergic control of the heart, in *Contraction and Relaxation in the Myocardium*, Edited by W. G. Nayler, pp. 113–190. Academic Press, London-New York-San Francisco.

Wood, E. H., and Moe, S. K. 1938. Studies on the effect of digitalis glycosides on potassium loss from the heart of the heart lung preparation. *Am. J. Physiol.* **123**, 219–220.

Wrogemann, K., Blanchaer, M. C., Thakar, J. H., and Mezon, B. J. 1975. On the role of mitochondria in the hereditary cardiomyopathy of the Syrian hamster, in *Recent Advances in Studies on Cardiac Structure and Metabolism*, Vol. 6, Edited by A. Fleckenstein and G. Rona, pp. 231–241, University Park Press, Baltimore-London-Tokyo.

Wrogemann, K., and Nylen, E. G. 1978. Mitochondrial calcium overloading in cardiomyopathic hamsters. *J. Mol. Cell. Cardiol.* **10**, 185–195.

Yamagishi, S., and Sano, T. 1966. Effect of tetrodotoxin on the pacemaker action potential on the sinus node. *Proc. Jpn. Acad.* **42**, 1194–1196.

Yamashita, K., Takagi, T., and Hotta, K. 1977. Mobilization of cellular calcium and contraction relaxation of vascular smooth muscle. *Jpn. J. Physiol. (Tokyo)* **27**, 551–564.

Yasue, H. 1980. Pathophysiology and treatment of coronary arterial spasm. *Chest* **78** (July suppl.) 216–223.

Yasue, H., Nagao, M., Omote, S., Takizawa, A., Miwa, K., and Tanaka, S. 1978. Coronary arterial spasm and Prinzmetal's variant form of angina induced by hyperventilation and Tris-buffer infusion. *Circulation* **58**, 56–62.

Yasue, H., Omote, S., Takizawa, A., Nagao, M., Miwa, K., and Tanaka, S. 1979. Circadian variation of exercise capacity in patients with Prinzmetal's variant angina: role of exercise-induced coronary arterial spasm. *Circulation* **59**, 938–948.

Yasue, H., Touyama, M., Kato, H., Tanaka, S. and Akiyama, F. 1976. Prinzmetal's variant form of angina as a manifestation of alpha-adrenergic receptor-mediated coronary artery spasm: documentation by coronary arteriography. *Am. Heart J.* **91**, 148–155.

Yasue, H., Touyama, M., Shimamoto, M., Kato, H., Tanaka, S., and Akiyama, F. 1974. Role of autonomic nervous system in the pathogenesis of Prinzmetal's variant form of angina. *Circulation* **50**, 534–539.

Zelis, R. F., and Kinney, E. L. 1982. The pharmacokinetics of diltiazem in healthy American men. *Am. J. Cardiol.* **49**, 529–532.

Zimmer, H. G., and Gerlach, E. 1978. Stimulation of myocardial adenine nucleotide biosynthesis by pentoses and pentitols. *Pflügers Arch. ges. Physiol.* **376**, 223–227.

Zimmer, H. G., Ibel, H., Steinkopff, G., and Korb, G. 1979. Reduction of isoproterenol-induced myocardial cell damage by long-term application of ribose in rats. *J. Mol. Cell. Cardiol.* **11**, Suppl. 2, 69.

Zimmerman, A. N. E., and Hülsmann, W. C. 1966. Paradoxical influence of calcium ions on the permeability of the cell membranes of the isolated rat heart. *Nature* **211**, 646–647.

REFERENCES

Zipes, D. P., and Fischer, J. C. 1974. Effects of agents which inhibit the slow channel on sinus node automaticity and atrioventricular conduction in the dog. *Circ. Res.* **34,** 184–192.

Zipes, D. P., and Mendez, C. 1973. Action of manganese ions and tetrodotoxin on atrioventricular nodal transmembrane potentials in isolated rabbit hearts. *Circ. Res.* **32,** 447–454.

Zondek, H. 1919. Herzbefunde bei Leuchtgasvergifteten. Ein Beitrag zur Lehre von der Organdisposition des Herzens. *Dtsch. Med. Wschr.* **45,** 678–680.

Zsoter, T. T., Henein, N. F., and Wolchinsky, C. 1977. The effect of sodium nitroprusside on the uptake and efflux of ^{45}Ca from rabbit and rat vessels. *Europ. J. Pharmacol.* **45,** 7–12.

Index

Acetylcholine:
abbreviation of action potential in frog
heart and mammalian atria, 43, 44
coronary vasoconstrictor action, 250-254,
272, 298
enhancement of atrial fibrillation by increase in K efflux, 193
generation of Ca-carried spike potentials
in visceral smooth muscle, 213, 215
induction of TTX-insensitive, Ca-dependent contractions on normal and
depolarized visceral smooth muscle,
221, 222, 223
loss of contractile potency on frog skeletal muscle upon Ca withdrawal, 2
Aconitine:
neutralization by reduction of extracellular Na or administration of procaine
amide, quinidine or TTX, 189
production of Na-dependent type of ventricular ectopic automaticity, 189
Action potentials:
adult Na-dependent ventricular action
potentials, see Na⁺-K⁺ exchange
Ca-dependent action potentials of SA and
AV node, ectopic pacemakers, embryonic hearts, and partially depolarized adult myocardium, see Ca⁺⁺-
K⁺ exchange
Mg-induced action potentials of partially
depolarized myocardium, 69-75, 86-92
mixed Mg/Ca-mediated action potentials
of partially depolarized myocardium, 70-75, 87-92
responsiveness of Mg-induced and of
mixed Mg/Ca-mediated action

potentials to adrenergic β-receptor
stimulation, H₂-receptor stimulation, dibutyryl cAMP and Ca antagonists, 69-75, 86-92
shortening of frog ventricular and mammalian atrial action potentials by
acetylcholine, 43, 44
Adenine, and ATP degradation, 10, 11
Adenosine:
and ATP degradation, 10, 11
coronary arteriolar vasodilation, 227,
241, 247
ADP (adenosine diphosphate), 5-12
Adrenaline (epinephrine), direct action on
adrenergic α- and β-receptors, see
Adrenergic α-receptor stimulation,
Adrenergic β-receptor stimulation,
Sympathomimetic amines
Adrenergic β-receptor blocking agents
(heart):
with Ca-antagonistic side effects:
dichloroisoproterenol, 34-35
pronethalol (Alderlin, Nethalide), 34-35
propranolol (Inderal, Dociton), 34-35,
164
without Ca-antagonistic side effects:
atenolol, 164
oxprenolol, 35
pindolol, 35, 86
sotalol, 35
contraindication in spastic coronary disease, 203, 255, 300, 322
inability in neutralizing the promoter
effects of H₂-receptor stimulation or
dibutyryl cAMP on slow inward Ca
current 80, 93